Pregnancy
from preconception to birth

babycentre™

Pregnancy

from preconception to birth

London • New York • Munich • Melbourne • Delhi

For BabyCentre
Project editor Victoria Farrimond
Contributing editor Martine Gallie
Editor Sasha Miller

For DK
Project editor Hilary Mandleberg
Project designers Hannah Moore and Kevin Smith
Senior editor Emma Maule
Senior art editor Isabel de Cordova
Designer Saskia Janssen
Photographer Ruth Jenkinson
Photography art direction Isabel de Cordova
Production editor Maria Elia
Senior production editor Jennifer Murray
Production controller Seyhan Esen
Creative technical support Sonia Charbonnier
Managing editor Penny Warren
Managing art editors Glenda Fisher and Marianne Markham
Category publisher Peggy Vance

Every effort has been made to ensure that the information contained in this book is complete and accurate. However, neither the publisher nor the author are engaged in rendering professional advice or services to the individual reader. The ideas, procedures, and suggestions contained in the book are not intended as a substitute for consultation with your healthcare provider. All matters regarding the health of you and your child require medical supervision. All participants in fitness activities must assume the responsibility for their own actions and safety. If you have any health problems or medical conditions, consult with your doctor before undertaking any of the exercise suggestions set out in this book. Neither the publisher nor the author accept any legal responsibility for any personal injury or other damage or loss arising from the use or misuse of the information and advice in this book.

First published in Great Britain in 2010 by Dorling Kindersley Limited
80 Strand, London, WC2R 0RL

Penguin Group (UK)

Cover design © BabyCenter LLC and Dorling Kindersley Limited 2010
Text © BabyCenter LLC 2010
Copyright © Dorling Kindersley Limited 2010
BabyCenter is the registered trademark of BabyCenter LLP

2 4 6 8 10 9 7 5 3 1

A CIP catalogue of this book is available from the British Library

ISBN 978-1-4053-4125-7

Colour reproduction Colourscan, Singapore
Printed and bound in Singapore by Tien Wah Press

Discover more at
www.dk.com

Contents

Birth and beyond
Becoming a parent

Labour and birth

Life with your new baby

Foreword

Having a baby will probably be the most wonderful, exciting, joyous and life-changing thing you will ever do. It can also be worrying, at times overwhelming and often downright exhausting.

When you become a parent, your life changes for ever. It's an incredible experience but adapting to those changes can be a real challenge. As a mum myself, I understand that having access to the best information and support makes those changes so much easier to cope with. The moment you become pregnant, your mind is filled with questions: How is my baby developing? Why am I feeling like this? Is this safe? Is that normal? There are also lots of decisions to be made: about your care during pregnancy, where and how you want to give birth, what you need to buy for your newborn and even what you should call your baby when she or he finally arrives.

Having a source of information you can really trust will give you the answers to all these questions and more. It will also give you the confidence you need to make choices that are right for you and your baby. And that's exactly what BabyCentre is all about. BabyCentre is the UK's number one website for new and expectant parents. Since we launched in the UK in 2000, our trusted advice and friendly community have supported millions of mums and dads on their journey to parenthood.

This book, with its in-depth information and beautiful photographs, is an exciting new venture for us. We're delighted to be working with Dorling Kindersley to create such a fantastic publication. It brings together BabyCentre's expert content plus the voices of real mums and dads from our online community in a gorgeous book that takes you from the miracle of conception to those first precious weeks with your newborn baby. You may want to put your feet up (go on, it's good for you!) and read it cover to cover, or dip into it as your pregnancy progresses. Whether this is your first pregnancy or you are adding to your family, BabyCentre Pregnancy will be your perfect companion.
Have a wonderful pregnancy.

Sasha Mil

Sasha Miller, Editor
www.babycentre.co.uk

Introduction

BabyCentre Pregnancy is designed to accompany you all the way along your incredible journey into parenthood, from the moment when you make the decision to start a family through to those first precious weeks with your newborn.

Your pregnancy guide

This book is packed with all the information you'll need throughout your pregnancy, including a week-by-week pregnancy diary, helpful hints and checklists, and tips and advice from mums and dads who've all been there, done it and have the milk-stained t-shirt to prove it.

We at BabyCentre want to be your most trusted parenting resource – that's why we offer practical advice from expert sources, such as doctors, midwives and fellow parents. We've divided the book into the four following sections:

Getting ready for pregnancy

Deciding to have a baby is one of the most momentous decisions you're ever likely to make. It requires a lifetime commitment of love and care, not to mention financial support, both in the early years and for many years afterwards.

In this chapter, we'll give you all the information you need to build the right foundations for a happy and healthy pregnancy and baby, whether it's your first baby or a new addition to your family. We'll also give you the low-down on preparing your body for pregnancy, from eating the right foods and cutting out vices such as smoking and drinking, to managing any pre-existing medical conditions.

Dads take note too – your health and lifestyle can affect your fertility. We'll help you protect your potency and prepare yourself for parenthood.

So, what happens next? There are all sorts of fascinating biological events that take place behind the scenes, from ovulation to conception. We cover them all and help to give you a better understanding of your own fertility.

Staying safe and healthy

Once you're pregnant, you'll have many questions about how best to look after yourself and your baby. What should – and shouldn't – you be eating? How can you stay fit and active without getting hurt? What medicines are safe and which should you avoid? Are there any hazards at work or at home you should be concerned about? Being pregnant can seem like a minefield at times. In this chapter, we'll let you know what is safe and what isn't, and give you advice on how you can protect yourself and your baby.

Being pregnant isn't just about your physical wellbeing. You'll find yourself on an emotional rollercoaster over the next nine months; elated one day, anxious about how your life will change the next. We'll help you cope with these feelings and offer some practical tips, from making the decision to return to work and avoiding isolation after your baby is born, to how your relationship is about to change.

Although you might not feel it in those first nauseous months, being pregnant makes you bloomingly beautiful. We'll outline all the changes that your body will go through, what beauty treatments will enhance your pregnancy glow, and we'll give tips on how you can update your wardrobe to accommodate your growing bump.

Nine months may seem like a long time, but before you know it you'll be holding your tiny newborn. We'll explain how you and your partner can bond with your baby before he arrives. We'll also help you prepare your home for his arrival.

Your pregnancy diary

At the heart of the book is a week-by-week pregnancy diary. Here you can find the information you need, right when you need it. You'll find out about how your baby is developing and the remarkable changes your body is going through. You'll find out about common health concerns, your antenatal care options, exercise for each stage of pregnancy, and information on coping with pregnancy while you're at work.

This section is divided into the three trimesters of pregnancy, each of which is made up of around 12 weeks. Here you'll find stage-based tips on healthy eating and how to get a good night's sleep. You'll also discover what scans and antenatal tests are available and, as you enter the third trimester, you'll find plenty of advice on preparing for the birth. This chapter also includes a comprehensive health section, covering all the common medical pregnancy concerns.

Birth and beyond

Every birth is different but our labour and birth information will help you plan and prepare for the big day. We will guide you through the different stages of childbirth and look at all the options available to you – whether you are planning to have your baby at home, in hospital or at a birthing centre. We'll take you through the process of labour and birth stage by stage, from the first signs of labour, to the moment you hold your newborn.

In this section you'll find out about natural and medical pain relief and positions for labour and birth. You'll also find out all about assisted births, breech births and caesarean sections, and what happens when you're overdue. And in the unlikely event that your labour happens very quickly, we'll let you know how to deal with an emergency home birth.

The first few weeks with your baby can be wonderful, challenging and tiring all at the same time. Here you'll find lots of practical advice on caring for your newborn, including "how tos" on feeding, bathing and holding him and changing his nappy. We'll also help you adapt to your new life as a parent, with information on coping with fatigue and understanding your emotions in these tiring early weeks.

"This **book is packed** with all the **information** needed **to guide you** through **pregnancy**."

Getting ready for pregnancy

Before you start

A child demands a lifetime commitment to provide love, nurturing, nourishment, shelter, education and attention. So before you decide to have a baby, it's important that you and your partner consider your decision carefully. This is a decision that will change your lives forever.

Becoming parents will have a major impact on many aspects of your life. You and your partner should discuss it carefully.

Thinking your decision through

Having a baby won't have just a small impact on your life; it's going to shift the entire centre of your universe. Think about how you'll feel, how you usually cope with change, and how you can prepare yourselves properly.

Some key questions to consider include:

- Are you both truly committed to becoming parents?
- Have you thought through how you'll handle balancing work and family?
- Are you prepared for the possibility that you may have twins or more?
- Are you ready to give up sleeping in on Sundays or to line up a babysitter every single time you want to go out?
- If you have religious differences, have the two of you discussed how these will affect your child?
- Have you thought about how becoming parents may change you and your close relationships with others?

Start early

Giving your baby the best possible start means getting your own life sorted well before you get pregnant. Plan a few months ahead if you can, so that changes to your diet and lifestyle (see pp.16–17) have time to take effect. If you have an existing medical condition, such as epilepsy, asthma or diabetes (see pp.22–3) you may need to make some changes to your treatment before you conceive. Most doctors are happy to give you a general pre-pregnancy health check-up to make sure you're in the best possible health for pregnancy.

Stopping contraception

For some people, stopping contraception is as easy as shoving the condoms or diaphragm to the back of a drawer. If you've been on the pill, the usual advice is to start trying once you've had one normal period. If you've been having contraceptive injections, it may take a while for the effect to wear off (about 12 weeks, according to manufacturers).

To have an intrauterine device (IUD or coil) or intrauterine system (IUS) removed, you'll need to make an appointment with your family planning clinic or your doctor. Your normal fertility will return as soon as you have the IUD removed, but it may take a month or so if you use an IUS because of the effects of hormones in the system.

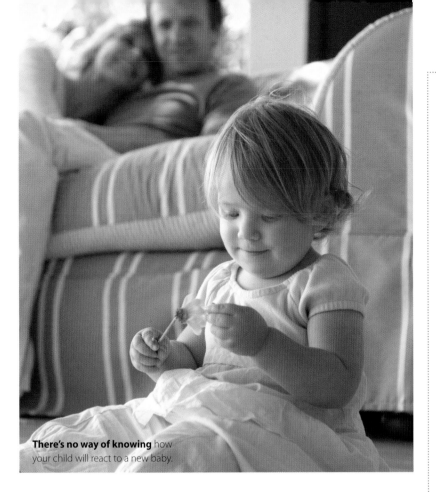

There's no way of knowing how your child will react to a new baby.

Another baby?

When it comes to deciding when is the right time to have another baby, there are no right or wrong answers. Most doctors recommend waiting at least six months after the birth of one child before trying again, and research suggests that leaving a gap of 18 to 23 months before conceiving again is the optimum timing for a healthy baby.

Having said that, there are other factors you'll need to take into account. Sometimes one partner is ready and the other isn't. This is a tough one but the first step is to start talking about your differences. You may not solve anything but at least you'll have a better understanding of the issues involved.

Think about your lifestyle. Do you have good childcare arrangements in place? Are your other children sleeping through the night? Maybe you've gone back to work and you love it. Money isn't everything, but if you're thinking of another baby, you may well need a little extra in your monthly budget before conceiving again.

At the end of the day, you can mull over the pluses and minuses of having another child forever. This is one of those decisions that's best led by the heart, so go ahead and follow yours. If you want another baby, and your partner is happy with that, then there may be no time like the present.

Dad's **Diary**

I'm going to be a dad

"It's a week since we discovered we're pregnant. A week since finding out I'm going to be a father. A dad. Daddy, Pop, Pa. I'm so excited. I'm walking around with the biggest grin on my face. I – OK we – made a baby! I'm scared too, for many reasons.

But mostly I'm daunted. It will be my responsibility to teach our child life skills, to guide him and show him right from wrong. What's my opinion on computer games versus outdoor activities? Should I let him play with guns and toy soldiers?

'Is any of this really worth worrying about right now?' my partner asks, as I price up the cost of buying and owning a pony. Yes. It is. The problem is that I can't help but look at the bigger picture, even if it has yet to be drawn.

'You're going to make a great dad!' she reassures me. But what do I know about being a dad? The only point of reference I have is taking care of Paddy my dog. And of course my own father. I reckon he did a good job. And now it's my time to live up to and pass on that example. It's my turn to be Dad."

Parents**Ask...**

When's a good time to add to my family?

There's no absolute "right" time. If you're worried about your fertility, took a long time to conceive before, or you're over 35, you might want to get moving. On the other hand, if you're in your twenties and have toddler twins, there may be sense in delaying a third baby! Every age gap between children has its pros and cons, and personality factors mean that what works well in one family isn't as successful in another.

Health and lifestyle checks for you

You've decided it's time to start your family. But are you ready? Perhaps you're concerned that you're a little overweight. Or maybe your diet needs a bit of an overhaul. One thing's for sure: by making a few lifestyle changes now, you'll be getting your baby off to the best start.

Systemised mum

If you like to do things by the book, you may want a check-up before trying to conceive.

"I drive my partner and family mad with the way I always want to prepare properly for everything. They say I'm a control freak. Well, maybe I am, but I decided it was worth it when it came to checking out what I could do to improve my chances of having a healthy pregnancy *before* I conceived.

First of all I made sure I'd had a recent cervical smear and I had a urine analysis done, too. I've had urinary tract infections in the past and I certainly didn't want to have one now. I also got checked out for anaemia, with a blood test, and while he was at it, my doctor took my blood pressure, too. My vaccinations were up to date, so no problems there, but my doctor did suggest I get tested for any sexually transmitted diseases, as well as for viral infections like the potentiallly dangerous toxoplasmosis.

I don't take any medications regularly, but if I did, one thing I'd definitely think about would be to check with my doctor they were safe to take during pregnancy. And last but not least, I've started taking folic acid."

Getting your health on track

Now more than ever, proper nutrition is essential. Forget all those fad diets, and learn to eat real food. That means a balanced diet of at least three meals a day, including at least five portions of fruit and vegetables.

Three of the most important nutrients you will need for a healthy pregnancy are calcium, iron and folic acid, so be sure to drink plenty of milk and eat citrus fruits and juices, dark green leafy vegetables, nuts, whole grains, and fortified breads and cereals.

You may also want to cut back on your caffeine. Research linking a woman's caffeine consumption with a lower chance of conception is contradictory but, in general, low levels of caffeine consumption are recommended. By contrast, dads-to-be should feel free to drink an extra cup: caffeine may help to increase male fertility by stimulating sperm motility.

Antenatal supplements

While it's no substitute for a healthy, balanced diet, taking an antenatal supplement ensures that you're getting enough of several important vitamins and minerals. At the top of that list is folic acid, which is a B vitamin that helps prevent neural tube defects in developing babies. Ask your doctor or midwife to recommend a vitamin supplement for you.

Think about your weight

Being underweight or overweight can affect your fertility and pose significant risks to your pregnancy. Now's the time to try to hit a healthy weight if you want to increase your chances both of conception and a healthy pregnancy.

If you're overweight or obese, take it steady. Crash dieting can deplete your body's nutritional stores. Nor is it a good idea to diet while pregnant because you may limit your baby's access to important nutrients. The best route to success is to combine a balanced diet with an exercise programme before you get pregnant. Aim for a safe weight loss of up to 1 kilogram (2 pounds) a week.

If you're underweight, get some meat on you! Your risk of miscarriage is higher if you conceive while underweight. And while skinny women can and do have healthy babies, studies show that underweight mothers are more likely to have low-birthweight babies. Gorging yourself on chocolate won't give you the important vitamins and minerals you need, so try to get your extra calories from a healthy, balanced diet.

Getting your lifestyle on track

A balanced exercise programme is a great place to start when you're preparing for pregnancy. Exercise will give you stamina, strength and flexibility. You'll need all three to lift and carry a baby, run after a small child, and cope with the day-to-day challenges of motherhood. Plus, getting in shape at least three months before you conceive may make it easier to maintain an active lifestyle during pregnancy, not to mention helping you to get through labour. Great exercises to help you get into shape for pregnancy include running and jogging, walking, swimming, bicycling and aerobics.

Stop drinking, smoking, and taking drugs

It doesn't take a rocket scientist to work out that smoking, taking drugs and drinking too much alcohol during pregnancy can harm your baby. Study after study has shown that all three of these are connected to miscarriage, low-birthweight babies, and premature birth. Smoking in pregnancy can increase your baby's risk of SIDS (sudden infant death syndrome), and excessive drinking during pregnancy can seriously affect your baby's development. If you're still partying hard, now's the time to clean up your lifestyle.

Eliminate environmental dangers

There are jobs that can be hazardous to you and your unborn baby. If you stand all day, fly a lot, or are exposed to chemicals or radiation regularly, you may need to make changes before you conceive. Talk to your doctor about it and see if you can come up with ways to avoid or eliminate hazards in your workplace. The government's Health and Safety Executive (HSE) also has some useful information on how you can make your work environment safer.

Get your finances in order

You may never feel that you *really* have enough money to have a baby, but that doesn't mean you shouldn't try to save up a little before you get pregnant. After all, having a baby is expensive, and that expense goes on for 18 years or more! Some other financial issues you may like to consider include taking out life insurance and making a will.

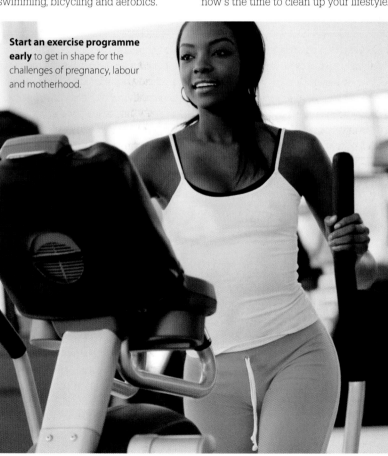

Start an exercise programme early to get in shape for the challenges of pregnancy, labour and motherhood.

Lifestyle readiness

Follow the points in this handy checklist to ensure you get your pregnancy off to a good start:

- Improve your diet.
- Achieve a healthy weight.
- Create (and follow!) an exercise plan.
- If you drink, smoke, or take drugs, then stop as soon as you can.
- Start taking folic acid.
- Get your finances in order.
- Start taking a special pregnancy multivitamin.
- Stop using contraception.
- Eliminate environmental dangers.
- Be sure parenthood is really for you.

Getting ready for pregnancy

Staying safe and healthy

Your pregnancy diary

Birth and beyond

Partners take note

Looking after your health as a prospective father is very important as a there is a host of lifestyle factors that can affect your potency. The good news is, once you become aware of these often hidden threats to fertility, they are fairly easy to avoid.

Father's health and lifestyle

Dads-to-be should aim to maintain a healthy body mass index (BMI) of 20 to 25 while trying to conceive, as having a low or high BMI is associated with a reduction in sperm. It also helps if your diet includes zinc (found in minced beef and baked beans), folates (eat green, leafy vegetables) and vitamin C (citrus fruit is a good source), as all of these help your body to make healthy sperm.

Keep drinking coffee if you like it – studies show that caffeine may improve sperm motility – but cut back on alcohol. An occasional drink (within the government guidelines of three or four units a day) is considered safe, but experts agree that drinking too much will harm the quality of your sperm.

Lifestyle and fertility

Besides food, there are other lifestyle factors that can affect your fertility:

- **Stress** This can sometimes affect men's sperm counts, so simply relaxing may increase your fertility.
- **Medicines** Whether prescription or over the counter, certain medications, such as the antihistamine cimetidine, can affect semen quality. Check with your doctor if you are concerned.
- **Cancer treatment and X-rays** Chemotherapy treatment can induce a permanent loss of fertility, but the jury is still out on whether X-rays have any effect on sperm.
- **Injury to your genitals** This could impair your ability to produce sperm or to ejaculate. If you play contact sports, wear protective gear.
- **Smoking** Men who smoke damage the quantity and quality of their sperm (yet another reason to give up!). Most doctors' surgeries have smoking cessation clinics and there are lots of support services to help you succeed.
- **Recreational drugs** Cocaine, marijuana and anabolic steroids have all been linked with reduced sperm quality.

Dad's **Diary**

Right from the start: counting down to healthy fatherhood

"Claire has given my diet an overhaul since we've been trying for a baby. I thought I was healthy enough, but apparently what you put in your body can really affect the strength of your little swimmers. So, takeaways and fast-food snacks are out, and green vegetables and wholegrains are in. She's even making me eat the skin on my baked potatoes – horror of horrors! The good news is that lean red meat is on the good list, so at least I get a decent steak once a week. And I've not had to reduce my coffee consumption, but the bad news is that I've had to cut down on alcohol – apparently it impairs the quality of your sperm. I bet my workmates will laugh! However, a couple of drinks a week shouldn't hurt. Everything in moderation, as they say. I'm sure a few months of good, clean living will do the trick."

A healthy dad makes healthy sperm, so it pays prospective dads to watch their lifestyle.

Cycling can protect against impotence but limit your cycling to less than three hours a week and invest in a wide, well-padded seat.

Sperm safety

One thing scientists do know is that testicles produce the best-quality sperm when they keep their cool. "The boys" are happiest at 34.5 to 36°C or 94 to 96°F, which is a couple of degrees cooler than normal body temperature. Working in a hot environment or sitting for long periods of time have been linked to an abnormal sperm count or semen quality. Using a laptop on your lap and driving for long periods can also cause overheating, while heated waterbeds and electric blankets are bigger culprits for raising scrotal temperature than hot baths and jacuzzis.

One study showed that men and their sperm are better off wearing loose-fitting boxer shorts than tighter fitting briefs. Another showed no difference in scrotal temperature between men wearing briefs and men wearing boxer shorts, although both types of underwear increased the scrotal temperature compared to wearing no underwear at all. However, this is not an invitation to go commando – more research is needed before you can use this as an excuse.

Cycling rules

Impotence can also be a side effect of too much cycling. A study from the University of Southern California School of Medicine found that while cycling for less than three hours a week has a protective effect against impotence, cycling for three hours or more significantly increases the risk.

Having said that, there are many health benefits from leading an active lifestyle, including preventing heart disease. Besides, impotence can also be developed through inactivity. To avoid developing a problem while cycling, periodically lift yourself off the seat when riding long distances. Better still, invest in a wider, padded bicycle seat, which will spread the load. See a doctor if you feel any numbness or pain or have erection problems after cycling.

Parents**Talk**...

"My job is pretty sedentary and when we didn't conceive after the first few months, I made a big effort to take a break while at work and go for a little walk a couple of times a day – just to make sure there were no 'over-heating' issues going on down there!"
Jules, 27

"As a gardener, I work with pesticides a lot. Then my partner read that they could cause congenital problems in unborn babies, so I made sure that I always washed my hands thoroughly after I'd used them. I know the effects are rare, but I didn't want to take that risk."
Rob, 24

"Working in a factory, I worried that some of the products I was coming into contact with every day would affect both my fertility and my baby's health. I asked my boss if I could be transferred to the office for a few months. I was lucky and they agreed. We now have a healthy daughter."
Jonathan, 31

"I'm a farmer and so come into contact with a lot of pesticides on an almost daily basis. I always take the precaution of following the usage instructions very carefully – wearing the correct protective clothing and showering as soon as I finish work. We're expecting our first child now, and I can't wait to meet him or her."
Paul, 27

You're in this together

Deciding to try for a baby is one of the biggest decisions you'll ever make. A new baby will bring huge changes to both you and your partner's lives, not to mention your relationship. That's why it's so important to make this decision together.

It's important to have discussed how the two of you will cope with the transition from being a couple to being a family.

Working mum

If you've decided to return to work after the birth, it's never too soon to start thinking about childcare.

"I knew that I'd be in for a bit of a juggling act. My partner couldn't stay home with our baby so we had to plan carefully to get dependable childcare. That meant finding a carer that we could both trust. We needed to feel 100 per cent happy that we would be leaving our baby in the hands of the right person, so we put lots of effort into setting things up. The reward? Having peace of mind once we were both back at work."

Are you both committed?

The decision to have a baby is a milestone in any relationship. It can be exciting but also sometimes scary to imagine yourselves as parents. However, you shouldn't forget that, as well as being parents, you will still be partners. Pregnancy and having a baby can bring you closer than you've ever been before. But it can also put pressure on your relationship as you move from being a couple to becoming a family.

So before you take this big step, it's definitely worth both of you thinking about some of the problems that may lie ahead. If you're lucky, you may not encounter any of these problems, but talking them through now, before you embark on parenthood, will mean that you are well prepared in case you do.

The highs and lows

The high excitement of a positive pregnancy test can be quickly followed by a low as you struggle through what can be a difficult first trimester. You'll probably feel tired as you never have before, your hormones will send you on an emotional rollercoaster, and you may suffer from pregnancy sickness that can strike at any time of the day or night. If it's difficult to cope with the symptoms of early pregnancy, living with someone who's experiencing them can be equally hard. Your partner may be wondering what has happened to the woman he loves. He may also feel that he simply doesn't know what he can do to help. If both of you understand why you feel the way you do it will really help you cope as a couple, so read up now on pregnancy symptoms and talk about ways in which you might relieve them.

Pregnancy can also have a dramatic effect on your sex life, though just what this effect will be can be hard to predict. For some couples pregnancy is a time of heightened sensuality when love-making becomes more meaningful and intense. Others find that desire diminishes or disappears altogether. Unfortunately, the two of you won't always feel the same way, so one of you may feel more passionate than ever, while the other wants only to cuddle.

Keep talking

Talking about sex can be difficult but it's much better to discuss these potential problems now than when you are dealing with them for real. You may need to find other ways to express your love and affection during your pregnancy and beyond. If it's difficult to find the energy or desire for sex while

Getting ready for pregnancy

Staying safe and healthy

Your pregnancy diary

Birth and beyond

you're pregnant, it doesn't get much easier in those early, sleep-deprived weeks with a new baby.

Have you thought about whether one of you will give up work after you've had your baby? If that's the case, will the one at home feel trapped? It's easy to become resentful if you miss the mental stimulation of working. Equally, the working partner may feel resentful that they have to go out to work while the other one gets to stay home with the baby. That doesn't mean life will be harmonious if you both go back to work.

Finding good childcare can be difficult and expensive and even the best plans can go wrong. If your childcare breaks down, perhaps because either your baby, or her carer, is sick, who's going to take a day off work to cover? All these are difficult issues that can put a strain on your relationship. At this stage it can be hard to make plans – after all, you may feel very differently after your baby is born. Exploring your options, and all their pros and cons, will put you in a strong position to make these decisions as a couple when the time comes.

Having a family: the financial cost

A new baby brings many things: love, joy, a sense of family – and a large dent in your budget. If you're going to manage financially once your baby is born, it's wise to start thinking about your finances now.

The word budget might fill you with horror. But the financial freedom it could give you can't be sniffed at. Start by reviewing your spending, organising it into categories and deciding what you can give up without changing your lifestyle too much.

Stay on the case

For a budget to work you'll need to sit down once a week or month with pen and paper or a computer program to budget and track your money. The more time you spend on this, the better you'll understand your financial situation. Try to save as much money as possible

before your baby is born. It's sensible advice for everyone to have three months' emergency money up their sleeve and, if you haven't got that amount already, now is a good time to build it up.

Don't forget to tell friends and family you're tightening your belt. This will reinforce it in your own mind and may even encourage them to do the same!

Part of your financial planning can mean shopping around before making a large purchase rather than impulse buying.

Pre-existing medical conditions

Try not to be too concerned if you are trying for a baby and have an ongoing medical condition. Most conditions can now be effectively managed so that you have a safe pregnancy and a healthy baby. Just make sure you see your doctor early on to talk through your options.

Will I have a safe pregnancy?

When you have a pre-existing medical condition, planning your pregnancy can be a little more complicated. If you're on medication, your dosage may need to be altered or you may need to change drugs before you conceive. You'll need to be carefully monitored once you are pregnant. Don't worry too much: your doctor and midwife will be there to give you expert care from the word go.

Underactive thyroid

If your thyroid levels are low you may not ovulate normally, which can make it difficult to get pregnant. Taking the right dose of thyroxine, which is the hormone you lack, can get ovulation back on track and restore your fertility.

A trip to your doctor to get your thyroid levels checked *before* you conceive is very important. If your thyroid levels are low, your doctor will probably suggest that you establish the right level of thyroxine treatment before you start trying for a baby.

As long as you manage it well, having an underactive thyroid does not have a significant effect on pregnancy. By having regular blood tests every four to six weeks, you can make sure that your thyroxine is at the correct level.

Asthma

Most drugs used to treat asthma are considered safe during pregnancy (including salbutamol and beclometasone) and many women carry on with their usual medication. However, if you are trying to have a baby, it's a good idea to review your treatment with your doctor or asthma specialist, as your particular medication or dosage may need to be adjusted. If you're one of those women whose

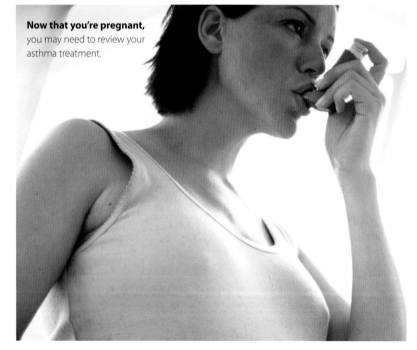

Now that you're pregnant, you may need to review your asthma treatment.

33%
of pregnant women with asthma

experience an improvement in their asthma, according to studies, while for another 33 per cent, their asthma worsened.

Diabetes is manageable in pregnancy but your doctor may suggest changing from oral medication to insulin injection.

asthma improves during pregnancy, you may be able to reduce your dosage, but only under your doctor's supervision.

Diabetes

Whether you have Type 1 or Type 2 diabetes, you are at a higher risk of having a miscarriage or a baby born with a congenital abnormality. You can lower these risks considerably by seeing your doctor or your diabetes specialist before you start trying to conceive.

Your doctor may recommend that you need to change your diabetes treatment, for example from oral medication to insulin. Babies born to diabetic mothers have a higher-than-average risk of birth defects, so it is especially important to take folic acid during your pregnancy. Your doctor will probably advise you to take about 10 times the usual dose of 400 micrograms (mcg). Diet is key, too. Eating a healthy diet and monitoring your glucose levels carefully and frequently will help maximise your chances of having a healthy pregnancy.

Epilepsy

If you have epilepsy and are thinking of having a baby, you should see your doctor, epilepsy specialist or obstetrician

first. Epilepsy and its medication carry some risks in pregnancy, but there are ways to minimise them. Your doctor may advise you to change your medication before trying for a baby. The aim will be to reduce your medication to as few anti-epileptic drugs (AEDs) as possible. Your doctors will probably also advise you to take a higher dose of folic acid than usual because AEDs affect your body's ability to absorb it. Most mothers on anti-epileptic medication give birth to normal, healthy babies.

Irritable bowel syndrome (IBS)

If you are on medication for your IBS, see your doctor before you start trying for a baby so that any adjustments to your treatment can be made before you conceive. Some IBS drugs, such as alverine, mebeverine, and loperamide, are not recommended in pregnancy. Others, such as amitriptyline, can be taken at a low dose.

You might want to use natural remedies such as peppermint oil capsules or fennel tea, but talk to your doctor first.

Lupus

Lupus erythematosus (LE) takes three forms: systemic LE (SLE); discoid LE; and drug-induced LE. SLE is the most common and, when severe, the symptoms (high fever, chest pain, kidney problems) – and some of the treatments – can seriously complicate pregnancy. Women with uncomplicated, mild lupus often have no problems. If you are pregnant and have lupus, your doctor may refer you to a specialist.

Migraine

If you're taking migraine or anti-sickness medication, your doctor may adjust your regime before you get pregnant. If you use injectable drugs,

you'll have to stop using them as there's not enough evidence regarding their safety during pregnancy. Under your doctor's supervision, you should also stop taking preventative drugs. Paracetamol is the painkiller of choice. You can use ibuprofen if paracetamol is not working, but you shouldn't take it after 30 weeks of pregnancy.

Getting ready for pregnancy

Staying safe and healthy

Your pregnancy diary

Birth and beyond

Age and fertility

More of us are waiting longer to start a family than ever before. There are many reasons for this, including financial pressures to work and improved contraception. Don't leave it too late, though, as female fertility starts to decline rapidly after the age of 35.

What happens as we get older

Many more of us are having babies later in life these days – you're likely to know at least one thirty-something first-time mum. But putting off starting a family can have its problems. Fertility falls more sharply for women than for men. As you can see from the chart below, women are most fertile between the ages of 20 and 24. As they grow older the likelihood of getting pregnant falls steeply.

According to the Human Fertilisation and Embryology Authority: "At 35 you're half as fertile as when you were 25; at 40 you're half as fertile as when you were 35". This means that it can take a great deal longer to get pregnant when you hit your late thirties or early forties and you may have problems conceiving at all. Six per cent of women aged 35 years and 23 per cent of those aged 38 will not have conceived after three years of regular unprotected sex.

"At 35 you're half as fertile as you were when you were 25."

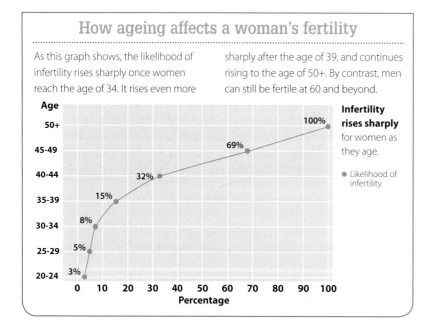

How ageing affects a woman's fertility

As this graph shows, the likelihood of infertility rises sharply once women reach the age of 34. It rises even more sharply after the age of 39, and continues rising to the age of 50+. By contrast, men can still be fertile at 60 and beyond.

Infertility rises sharply for women as they age.

● Likelihood of infertility

Age	Percentage
50+	100%
45-49	69%
40-44	32%
35-39	15%
30-34	8%
25-29	5%
20-24	3%

Fertility factors that change as we grow older include:

● **Fewer eggs** As you get older you have fewer viable eggs left.

● **Menstrual cycle** As women approach the menopause their menstrual cycles can become irregular.

● **Lining of the uterus** The lining (endometrium) may become thinner and less hospitable to a fertilised egg.

● **Mucus secretions** Vaginal secretions can become less fluid and more hostile to sperm.

● **Diseases affecting the reproductive system** Some conditions can damage the reproductive organs as time passes, including endometriosis and chlamydia.

● **Chronic illnesses** Some illnesses can have a negative impact on fertility.

● **Weight problems** Being overweight or obese can make it more difficult to become pregnant.

Effects of age on male fertility

We now know that men have a biological clock ticking away their reproductive years, too. It's thought that the odds on conceiving within a year of trying decrease by three per cent for every year over the age of 24.

As men age, their testes become smaller and softer and the volume, morphology (shape) and motility (ability to move) of their sperm declines. This makes it more difficult for the sperm to fertilise an egg. What's more, there's also growing evidence that the offspring of older fathers run an increased risk of having genetic abnormalities and other long-term health problems.

Improving your fertility

There is plenty you can do to keep your potency in tip-top condition. For a start, you can put yourself on that diet you've been meaning to start. A man's waist size is directly proportional to his testosterone level (a bigger waist means less testosterone). A waist size of 102 centimetres (40 inches) or more is also a risk factor for heart disease in men, which slows blood flow, and that includes the blood flow in your penis.

You may also want to go over other aspects of your lifestyle that could impact on your fertility – consider having an MOT with your doctor or a "well man" check with your practice nurse. Common causes of male infertility include clogged ejaculatory ducts and enlarged veins – called varicoceles – in the scrotum. But do not worry: both conditions are treatable.

Finally, comfort yourself with the fact that, while male fertility may gradually decline with the years, most chaps are still fertile and functioning at 60 and beyond. Compare that with women's fertility freefall after the age of 35. In fact, men in their 70s and 80s can, and do, father children, but a man this age is more likely to take years rather than months to get his partner pregnant.

Lead a healthy lifestyle, keep your weight in check and ask your doctor for a health MOT to maximise your potency.

Parents**Talk...**

"I thought I'd be a lean mean baby-making machine for as long as I wanted – I've already got two kids from a previous relationship, and now I want a baby with my new partner. She's 15 years younger than me, and I thought that even though I'm in my late forties, we wouldn't have any trouble conceiving. We've been trying for over a year, and it turns out it's me, not her, that's the problem."
Mike, 48, dad to teenagers Chris and Samantha

"I'm 44 and my wife's 36. We're trying to start a family but I'm worried we've left it too late. I thought her age would be a bigger issue than mine. But my age might mean that I'd have trouble getting her pregnant even if she were 25 years old!"
Nick, 44, hoping to be a dad for the first time

"After two failed marriages, I found love again. She's 34 and I'm 55. I've got kids from my previous marriages, but I wanted to start a new family with her. It took several months to conceive, which our doctor said was because I'm an older dad. And the fact I'm an older dad may also have played a part in our baby having Down's syndrome – so it turns out it's not just the mother's body clock we need to listen to."
Graeme, 55, dad to Eliott, 13, Stephen, 10, and year-old Jamie

"My partner and I are both 36 and we've been trying for a baby for a year. After various tests our doctor told us that the reason we're having trouble conceiving is a ticking body clock – and that applies to me as well as her."
Alexander, 36

The beginnings of life

We all know how babies are made: man meets woman, they make love and nine months later out pops a baby! But do you know what's really happening when sperm meets egg? Read on to discover the fascinating biological facts behind getting pregnant.

How babies are made

Each month, usually during the middle of your menstrual cycle, between one and three eggs start maturing in one of your ovaries. The ripest egg is released and sucked up by the nearest fallopian tube. This is known as ovulation. The egg lives for about 12 to 24 hours after release, so it has to meet up with a sperm soon if a baby is to be conceived.

Men's bodies, meanwhile, are constantly at work producing millions of microscopic sperm. It takes about 64 to 72 days to create a new sperm cell. Since the average sperm lives only a few weeks, and as many as 300 million are set free with each ejaculation, this sperm factory is kept pretty busy.

The quest to find the egg

When you and your partner make love, your bodies build up tension that you hope will end in orgasm. In men, their orgasm propels sperm-rich semen into the vagina and up towards the cervix at roughly 16km (10 miles) per hour. A woman's climax also aids conception: research shows that the wavelike contractions associated with "the big O" help pull the sperm further into the cervix. While you and your partner are enjoying a relaxing post-romp cuddle, those millions of sperm have begun their quest to find your egg. The fastest swimmers may find it in as little as 45 minutes. If they don't find an egg in the fallopian tubes, the sperm can wait

Female organs

Ovary

Fallopian tube

Uterus

Endometrium

Cervix

Vagina

Female reproductive system The egg from one ovary enters the fallopian tube via the fimbriae. Here it awaits possible fertilisation.

Fimbriae

Male organs

Vas deferens

Penis

Urethra

Glans

Testis

Scrotum

Bladder

Male reproductive system Sperm made in the testis form semen in the vas deferens. The semen leaves the penis via the urethra.

Getting ready for pregnancy

Staying safe and healthy

Your pregnancy diary

Birth and beyond

Sperm swarm over the egg in their attempt to penetrate the egg's outer layer.

The successful human sperm manages to penetrate and fertilise the egg.

there for another 12 to 24 hours, so there is still a chance of conception if you ovulate within this time.

The mortality rate for sperm is so high that only a few dozen make it to the egg. The rest get trapped or lost, or die. The lucky few who get near the egg then have to work frantically to penetrate its outer shell. When the hardiest makes it through, the outer layer of the egg immediately changes so that no other sperm can get in.

What happens during fertilisation

An egg will usually be fertilised within about 24 hours of its release from the ovary. The genetic material from the sperm combines with that in the egg to create a new cell that rapidly starts dividing. But you are not actually pregnant until that bundle of new cells, known as the embryo, travels the rest of the way down the fallopian tube and attaches itself to the wall of your uterus.

Occasionally the embryo implants somewhere other than the uterus, usually in the fallopian tube. This is known as an ectopic pregnancy (see pp.44–5). An ectopic pregnancy cannot grow into a baby, and the embryo has to be surgically removed to prevent the

fallopian tube from rupturing and causing internal bleeding.

The final leg of the trip, from fallopian tube to uterus, takes about three days, but it will be a couple of weeks until you miss a period and suspect that you're going to have a baby.

Once you have missed your period or noticed one of the other signs of pregnancy (see p.36), if you choose to, you can then use a home pregnancy test to find out for sure if you've got a little one on the way. If so, congratulations, and welcome to the start of another incredible journey.

Laid-back mum

You'll try most lovemaking options – within reason! – for a better chance of conception.

"We're now on number three and we've found that the best position for conceiving is that old favourite – the missionary position, with him on top. It allows for really deep penetration so the sperm ends up right next to the opening of your womb.

Another position that's good is with him entering you from behind. He can get closer to your cervix so the sperm is right where it needs to be. Many of my girlfriends tell me they find it easier to orgasm in this position, too, and it turns out that the contractions of orgasm help carry the sperm further into the womb.

I've also tried lying on my back after sex for at least half an hour with my hips raised on a pillow. I've heard this stops the sperm having to swim against gravity. I sometimes lie on my back and bicycle my legs in the air too. That always gives my partner a laugh!"

Parents**Talk...**

"I had no idea that sperm could find an egg in 45 minutes, or wait in the fallopian tubes for up to 24 hours for one to come along. I reckon that means I could get pregnant a whole day after having sex if I ovulate during that time!"
Catherine, 23

"I always knew it. My body is amazing. Each little guy can take up to 72 days to make, and every time

I ejaculate, as many as 300 million of them are set free. That's definitely something to boast about!"
Ben, 24

"Now I know that the contractions during orgasm pull the sperm further into my cervix, I've got a really good reason to make sure my partner understands the importance for me of having an orgasm."
Linda, 28

Your menstrual cycle

If you're trying for a baby, now is a great time to learn a little more about how your body works. Your menstrual cycle indicates when you are fertile, so understanding the changes your body goes through each month can help you to spot any possible problems early on.

Periods and how they happen

Your menstrual cycle is under the control of an array of hormones, and the whole process starts in the brain. The hypothalamus produces gonadotrophin-releasing hormone (GnRh), which travels to the pituitary gland and signals it to release follicle-stimulating hormone (FSH). FSH is carried round the body in the bloodstream and stimulates the ovaries to start ripening eggs. Between 15 and 20 egg-containing sacs, called follicles, then start to mature in the ovaries. One follicle (or, occasionally, two or more) grows faster than all the others.

The role of oestrogen

FSH also stimulates the ovaries to produce oestrogen. This encourages the eggs to mature and starts to thicken the lining of the uterus so that it is ready to support a pregnancy. As oestrogen levels rise, levels of FSH fall temporarily and then rise again, accompanied by a huge surge of luteinising hormone (LH) from the pituitary gland. It is this hormone that triggers ovulation – the moment that the most mature egg in the ovaries bursts out of its sac and away on its journey.

The journey continues

In the ovary, the now-empty follicle collapses and becomes a "corpus luteum". This small yellow mass of cells starts to produce the hormone progesterone. Progesterone acts on the lining of the uterus, which becomes thick and spongy, ready to receive a fertilised egg. As the levels of progesterone rise in your body, your breasts may start to feel stretched and tingly. The pituitary gland stops producing FSH so that no more eggs mature in your ovaries.

ParentsTalk...

"Premenstrual syndrome (PMS) is something so many women experience – and unfortunately I get it really bad. My mood swings take me through a range of emotions which are provoked by the tiniest things. I burst into tears when I spill my tea, I forget to do simple things like take the rubbish out, I get depressed and tired one minute and then angry and irritable the next. And I become very unreasonable – the other day I saw red when my sister popped the foil on my new coffee jar before I could (it's a little obsession of mine). And all this is just the emotional side of PMS – I also get sore boobs, headaches, tummy ache and sometimes nausea, too."
Hannah, 36, mum to William and Tess

"When it's the 'time of the month' I just want to curl up into a ball and hug a hot water bottle for a few days. My period pains are probably fairly normal for most women – not so mild they're barely there or so painful I can't move. I just have a continuous back and tummy ache which makes me feel sluggish and uncomfortable."
Hilary, 37, mum to Joel and Natasha

"I'm now back on the pill (though a different pill than before) so I'm hoping my period pains will calm down now or stop altogether. It was so nice not having any periods while I was pregnant."
Vicky, 27, mum to month-old Nathan

What happens if fertilisation doesn't occur

Early in your menstrual cycle, FSH (see opposite) is released by the pituitary gland and travels in the bloodstream. It stimulates the ovaries so they start to ripen eggs. Ovulation happens when one (occasionally two) of the 15 to 20 egg-containing sacs, or follicles, ruptures and releases its egg. This happens about halfway through the menstrual cycle. The empty follicle then turns into a corpus luteum.

The endometrium

Meanwhile, influenced by oestrogen and progesterone, the lining of the uterus (endometrium) gets thicker and more spongy, ready to receive a fertilised egg. If the egg isn't fertilised, it disintegrates and the corpus luteum shrinks. The thickened endometrium is shed next time you have a period.

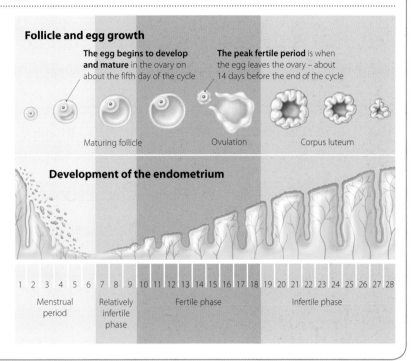

Follicle and egg growth

The egg begins to develop and mature in the ovary on about the fifth day of the cycle

The peak fertile period is when the egg leaves the ovary – about 14 days before the end of the cycle

Maturing follicle | Ovulation | Corpus luteum

Development of the endometrium

1 2 3 4 5 6 | 7 8 9 | 10 11 12 13 14 15 16 17 18 | 19 20 21 22 23 24 25 26 27 28

Menstrual period | Relatively infertile phase | Fertile phase | Infertile phase

If fertilisation occurs, the egg continues to travel to the uterus, where it beds down in the lining. Your progesterone levels will stay high and you may start to feel the very early signs of pregnancy.

If fertilisation doesn't occur, or the egg doesn't successfully implant, it starts to disintegrate and the corpus luteum shrinks. Your oestrogen and progesterone levels drop and the lining of your uterus starts to produce prostaglandins (the hormones which

The lining of your uterus is shed along with the unfertilised egg, and your menstrual cycle starts again.

Your menstrual cycle's length

An average menstrual cycle lasts 28 days – that's counting from the first day of one period to the day before the next. Some women have much shorter cycles, possibly lasting only 23 days, and some have much longer ones, lasting up to 35 days. Cycles that are shorter or

"The **fertilised egg** beds down in the **lining of the uterus**."

can cause cramps). These cause changes in the blood supply to your uterus, breaking up the lining, and stimulating the uterus to contract.

longer than this are probably not normal, and you should see your doctor. You should also see your doctor if you bleed between periods or after sex.

Signs of a normal cycle

If your menstrual cycle tallies with these three signs, chances are that everything's normal.

Signs of a normal menstrual cycle include:

● A cycle that lasts 23 to 35 days. So, for example, a woman with a 28-day cycle starts a period every four weeks while a woman with a 23-day cycle starts hers every three weeks or so. The length of the cycle includes the days of the period.

● Regular periods – if yours are very irregular you may be not be ovulating at all or infrequently.

● No spotting between periods – bleeding between periods should always be reported to your doctor.

Getting ready for pregnancy / Staying safe and healthy / Your pregnancy diary / Birth and beyond

Ovulation calendars

Ovulation is the magical moment that occurs each month when one of your ovaries releases an egg ready for fertilisation. Knowing the signs of ovulation can help you pinpoint those days when you're most likely to conceive and give you a better understanding of your fertility.

Using a basal body temperature thermometer each morning helps predict when you ovulate. You're most fertile a few days before your temperature rises.

What is ovulation?

Ovulation is when one, or occasionally more, eggs are released from one of your ovaries, and it's the most fertile time of your menstrual cycle. It usually takes place 12 to 16 days before the start of your next period. So, for a woman with a 28-day menstrual cycle, ovulation takes place sometime around day 13 to 15.

Possible signs that ovulation is imminent include:

● **Changes in cervical mucus** As your cycle progresses, rising oestrogen levels mean your cervical mucus increases in volume and changes texture. You are most fertile when the mucus becomes clear, slippery and stretchy, rather like raw egg white.

The position and feel of your cervix also changes around this time, from hard, low, closed and dry, to soft, high, open and wet.

● **Lower abdominal pain** About one fifth of women actually feel it when they ovulate. The sensation can range from mild achiness to twinges of pain, and may last anywhere from a few minutes to a few hours.

Other possible signs include:

● **Feeling sexy and flirty** Having an increased libido, being in a better mood and feeling more sociable may all be signs that you're at your most fertile.

● **Looking more attractive** Studies have been carried out showing that both how attractive you feel and how attractive you look to others increases when you near ovulation. You may choose clothes that flatter you and take more care accessorising and grooming.

● **Smelling good** It's been found that women smell more attractive to men just before ovulation. All these signs must be nature's way of helping ensure you mate at the right time!

Following ovulation, your temperature can increase by 0.5 to 1.6 degrees. You won't feel the shift but you may be able to detect it by using a basal body temperature (BBT) thermometer. You can buy one from your chemist.

You're most fertile in the two to three days before your temperature rises. That's why some experts recommend you chart your temperature (taken each morning) for a few months to pinpoint your likely ovulation date. Then you can plan to have sex during the two to three days before your temperature normally rises. However, most fertility experts recommend regular sex throughout your cycle in order to conceive. Regular tends to be defined as at least twice a week.

Ovulation predictor kits

Experts recommend regular sex throughout your cycle as the best way to maximise your chances of conception. Having said that, for various reasons, some couples prefer to identify when they're most likely to conceive and ovulation predictor kits, or OPKs, can help. They give you a quick result and are easy to use. They're available at most chemists and supermarkets without a prescription, and you can also buy them online.

There are two sorts of OPKs:

● A urine-based OPK detects the increase, or surge, of a hormone called luteinising hormone (LH) that occurs approximately one to two days before

for women to use at home. But they are not foolproof. They can measure LH, but since LH can surge with or without the release of an egg, they can't indicate whether you have definitely ovulated after a positive response.

● Saliva-based OPKs test for rising oestrogen levels as you near ovulation, not the hormone that triggers it. A saliva-based OPK is basically a pocket-sized microscope that shows if "salivary ferning" has occurred when your saliva dries on a glass slide. Ferning is more likely to occur in the few days leading up to ovulation. Salivary ferning OPKs can be more economical than urine-based ones, but some experts say they are not as accurate and that ferning

"Ovulation **predictor kits,** or OPKs, give you a **quick result** and are **easy to use**."

ovulation. Depending on the type of urine-based OPK you're using, you'll either collect your urine in a cup or hold a stick in your urine stream. Coloured bands appear on the test card or stick to indicate whether or not the LH surge is occurring. Urine-based OPKs generally provide five to nine days' worth of tests. They are generally accepted as the best method of ovulation prediction available

can sometimes be seen at other times of the menstrual cycle. Also, if your vision is poor these kits may not be the best method for you.

With either type of OPK, it helps to work out when your fertile period is likely to start. It's usually the length of your usual cycle minus 17 days. So, if you have a 28-day cycle, start testing on day 11 and carry on for six days.

Paracetamol and other common drugs don't affect the tests, but contact your doctor if you're taking hormonal medication. Drugs containing human chorionic gonadotrophin (hCG; see p.74) or LH (see p.28) can affect the results, and the fertility drug clomiphene can affect the salivary ferning test.

15-20
eggs will mature each month inside a woman's ovaries but only the ripest egg will be released into the fallopian tube ready for fertilisation.

Systemised mum

If you are trying for a baby, it may suit you to keep track of when you are ovulating.

"When I was trying to get pregnant, I really appreciated the fact that there were things I could buy that would help me to keep track of when I was ovulating and most fertile.

The first thing I invested in was an ovulation predictor kit – they look and work the same way as a home pregnancy test but can predict ovulation 24 to 36 hours in advance. I also monitored my basal body temperature – when you've ovulated, your temperature can increase very slightly, which you'd never be able to feel, but I could check it using a special basal body temperature thermometer. My pharmacist ordered one in for me.

I even bought a salivary ferning kit – there's something in your saliva that helps you predict when you're going to ovulate. I found this quite fascinating, actually – apparently when you're ovulating, you produce more salt, which causes your saliva to crystallise into frost-like ferns when dried and viewed on a slide.

I know that these things aren't for everyone. Some couples might get too stressed using them, and may feel under pressure to have sex only when the gadgets tell them to, but they suited us."

A urine-based ovulation predictor kit detects the very slight increase in LH (see p.28) that occurs just before you ovulate.

Getting ready for pregnancy

Staying safe and healthy

Your pregnancy diary

Birth and beyond

Boy or girl?

For most couples, not knowing whether you're having a boy or girl is one of the most exciting parts of having a baby. Here's how your baby's sex is determined and, just for fun, some traditional ways to bump up your chances of having either a boy or a girl.

X and Y chromosomes

Is it a boy or girl? It's the question we all want to know the answer to. The sex of your baby is actually determined at the moment of conception.

The sex chromosomes are called X and Y. Eggs always contain an X chromosome. If the sperm that fertilises the egg contains an X chromosome as well, then the resulting XX combination equals a girl. If the sperm contains a Y chromosome, the resulting XY combination equals a boy.

You may have heard the old wives' tales: if you carry at the front it's a boy, if you crave sweet foods it's a girl. You may have tried sex predictor methods that involved odd and even days and the numbers of the year. They are fun but none have any facts to back them up.

Scientific studies

Some scientific studies have shown, however, that certain circumstances may influence the sex of the baby.

● How old are you and your partner? There is some evidence that the older you are when you have your first baby, the more likely you are to have a girl. The sex of the baby is partly controlled by the level of the hormone gonadotrophin, and this declines with age. Likewise, it seems that the older a

dad is, the less likely the male sperm are to fertilise the egg and the female sperm win the race. The latest evidence is that older men produce fewer male sperm.

● **Were you newlyweds when you conceived?** If so, you may be more likely to have a boy. The theory is the longer you have been married, the less sex you have and the later in the cycle conception is likely to occur. Late-cycle conceptions are more frequently girls. But it could simply be a matter of age.

● **Do you normally eat a high-calorie diet including breakfast?** If you do,

you may be more likely to have a boy. In a study of 740 British women, 56 per cent of those with the highest calorific intake had boys. In women with the lowest calorific intake, the proportion who had boys dropped to 45 per cent. It has been suggested that our bodies only invest in boys (who are more fragile and statistically less likely to survive) when food is abundant. In times of famine we "play safe" with more robust girls. However, these studies are small-scale and show only minor changes in the likelihood of having a boy or girl.

X and Y chromosomes

Women have two X chromosomes (XX) and men have one X and one Y chromosome (XY). A man can pass on an X or a Y chromosome. The woman's egg always contains an X chromosome.

Dad decides

If the sperm that fertilises your egg contains an X chromosome, that gives the egg two X chromosomes and means your baby is a girl. If the sperm contains a Y chromosome, the egg will have an X and a Y – and it's a boy!

X and Y On the left is the larger X chromosome, with the Y on the right.

The legs and genitals of this 22-week-old male fetus are clearly visible, as is the umbilical cord at the centre top of the scan.

Science and sex selection

Choosing your child's sex is technically possible now, thanks to the many advances there have been in fertility treatments. But the options available in UK fertility clinics are not always effective, affordable or available, and some are unregulated.

Preimplantation genetic diagnosis (PGD)

This is an in-vitro fertilisation technique in which embryos are created outside the uterus and can then be tested for genetic disorders and gender.
Effectiveness Almost 100 per cent.
Cost IVF cycles cost an average of £3,000, not including the costs of the consultations, tests and drugs. PGD adds an additional cost.
Availability In the UK, PGD is strictly regulated and can only be used to help people with serious genetic disorders, such as cystic fibrosis, avoid passing this on to their children.

Ericsson method

This is a sperm-sorting technique that was developed by Dr Ronald Ericsson. Sperm of the desired gender are inserted into your uterus via artificial insemination (AI).
Effectiveness Claimed to be 78 to 85 per cent effective for choosing boys and 73 to 75 per cent effective for girls.
Cost The cost is approximately £4,000 for four attempts.
Availability This is available to anyone who can afford it at private clinics in London and Birmingham in the UK. The technique is unregulated by the HFEA.

Shettles method

This advocates timed intercourse on specific days of your cycle.
Effectiveness Shettles proponents claim the technique is 75 per cent effective.
Cost Nothing.
Availability Anyone can try it.

Whelan method

This also advocates timed intercourse on specific days of your cycle.
Effectiveness Elizabeth Whelan claims that her technique is 68 per cent effective for boys and 56 per cent effective for girls, but many experts dispute this.
Cost Nothing.
Availability Anyone can try it.

Sex-selection kits

These are based on the Shettles theory. Separate girl and boy kits include a thermometer, ovulation predictor test sticks, vitamins, herbal extracts, and douches.
Effectiveness Kit makers claim a 96 per cent success rate, but the American Society for Reproductive Medicine disputes this.
Cost Around £100.
Availability Available from the United States through the GenSelect company.

Getting ready for pregnancy

Staying safe and healthy

Your pregnancy diary

Birth and beyond

Fertilisation and conception

You probably won't know you have conceived yet, but inside your body there's lots of frantic activity going on. Within days of conceiving, the embryo that will grow to become your baby implants in the lining of your uterus where it rapidly starts to grow and develop.

What happens during the first days?

As soon as your egg is fertilised, it goes into action. While it's being wafted gently down your fallopian tube towards your uterus, it begins dividing into a microscopic ball of cells. By the time it reaches the uterus, about three to four days after conception, it has already divided into about 16 cells and looks rather like a miniscule blackberry.

Around day four, this bundle of cells starts to hollow out in the middle and to develop an inner and an outer layer. At this stage, doctors call this hollow sphere a blastocyst. The inner layer expands and presses against the tough outer layer until it gives way and breaks up. This happens around the sixth day after fertilisation. Once the cells of the inner layer are exposed, they secrete an enzyme that erodes part of the lining of the uterus, allowing it to implant. When the blastocyst implants, it is then known as an embryo.

The lining of the uterus

By now the pregnancy hormone progesterone will have stimulated the growth of lots of new blood vessels in the lining of the uterus, ready to nourish the embryo. The outer layer of the embryo carries on breaking down cells in the lining of the uterus, allowing it to burrow further in. It also stimulates new blood vessels to grow, creating the beginnings of the placenta. Ectopic pregnancies (see pp.44–5), where the embryo implants somewhere other than the uterus (this is usually in the fallopian tube), normally occur at around this time.

Around 13 days after fertilisation has taken place, a yolk sac is visible attached to the embryo. This will act as a rudimentary circulation system for the embryo until its own circulatory system is up and running. Different types of cell

---

The first week

You may not even know you're pregnant, but amazing things are happening in that first week.

Step by step

- Fertilisation begins when a sperm penetrates the egg.
- Fertilisation takes about 24 hours.
- The fertilised egg (or zygote) begins to divide into 16 cells.
- It leaves the fallopian tube and enters the uterus.
- Three to four days after fertilisation, it starts to burrow into the blood-rich lining of your uterus.
- At around day eight, the placenta starts to grow.

Parents**Talk...**

"I had my suspicions I was pregnant before I did a test, even though we'd only been trying for a few weeks. It sounds like a real cliché, but the second I saw the line on the test, I just knew that my life was never going to be the same again. And it was an enormous change, but one I've never regretted."

Sinead, 27, mum to two-month-old Lily

"We'd only been trying for two months when I got my big fat positive. I was actually shaking when I saw the blue line. Sam was working away, so I had to keep it a secret for four days. I didn't want to let him know on the phone so I went to meet him at the airport. I sat him down in a coffee shop to tell him."

Jen, 26, mum to Charlie

Getting ready for pregnancy

Staying safe and healthy

Your pregnancy diary

Birth and beyond

are starting to develop in the embryo and these will go on to form the various parts of your baby's body. A stalk is also forming between the developing placenta and the embryo. This will later become part of the umbilical cord.

Next, a thin line of cells, known as the "primitive streak", start to organise themselves down the centre of the embryo. From now on this primitive streak will develop symmetrically on either side of this central line. By the time you would normally be expecting your period, the embryo is just 0.4mm in length – barely visible to the human eye.

Its head end is wider than the tail end and its cells are now organised into three layers that will later develop into baby's organs and tissues. The neural tube – from which the brain, backbone and spinal cord and nerves will sprout – develops in the top layer. The heart and the circulatory system begin to appear in the middle layer. The third layer starts to create the lungs, intestines and beginnings of the urinary system. Strange as it may seem, your doctor or midwife will calculate your baby's gestational age (and your due date) from the first day of your last

period. This is because it's often difficult to know exactly when your egg was fertilised. So, although it's only about a fortnight since you conceived, you are now considered to be four weeks pregnant. In the following days, the embryo's heart, no bigger than a poppy seed, will begin to beat and pump blood.

Gradually the beat will become stronger and more regular. Major organs, will begin to grow, the neural tube that connects the brain and spinal cord will close, upper and lower limb buds will begin to sprout and your baby's facial features will start to form.

Fertilisation and implantation

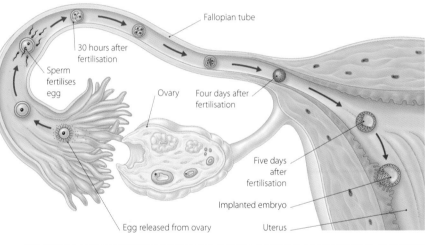

Fallopian tube

30 hours after fertilisation

Sperm fertilises egg

Ovary

Four days after fertilisation

Five days after fertilisation

Implanted embryo

Egg released from ovary

Uterus

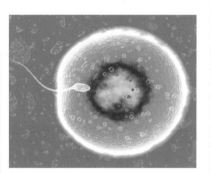

Sperm fertilising egg This egg has left the ovary and entered the fallopian tube where it is being fertilised. The egg starts dividing (see below) and travels to the uterus where it implants itself in the uterine wall.

About 30 hours after fertilisation, this egg is at the two-cell stage and has not yet implanted in the uterus.

Four days after fertilisation, the 16-cell blastocyst is dividing rapidly. It now looks a bit like a blackberry.

Five or six days after fertilisation, the dividing cells break out of the tough outer shell that surrounded the egg.

Am I pregnant?

If you're extremely tuned in to your body's rhythms, you may suspect that you're pregnant soon after conception. But most women won't experience any early pregnancy symptoms until the fertilised egg attaches itself to the wall of the uterus, several days afterwards.

Signs you may be pregnant

For most women, the first sign of pregnancy is a missed period. But there are other telltale signs.

It's a cliché, but food cravings really can be a sign of pregnancy. Don't rely on them, but if you've got other signs of pregnancy, start counting the days from your last period.

You may notice changes in your breasts. They can become tender to the touch, similar to the way they feel before your period, only more so. The skin around your nipples may also get darker.

If you're lucky, nausea and vomiting won't hit you until a few weeks after conception. But as early as a couple of days following conception, you may begin feeling nauseated. And not just in the morning, either – pregnancy-related nausea can be a problem morning, noon or night. You may also notice that your sense of taste changes.

Fatigue is another sign of early pregnancy. High levels of the hormone progesterone can make you feel as if you've run a marathon when all you've done is a day at the office. And you may find that you're running to the loo a lot – this is caused by rising levels of the pregnancy hormone hCG (see p.74).

About six to eight days after ovulation, you may have implantation bleeding – some pinkish, brownish discharge from your vagina – and possibly some cramping. This is caused by the egg burrowing into the lining of the uterus. You might also have spotting around the time you expect your period.

A home pregnancy test is usually accurate once you have missed a period.

All you need now is a positive pregnancy test (see opposite). If you've waited until at least the first day of a missed period and a blue line appears in the test window, congratulations – you're in the family way!

Parents**Talk...**

"The first sign I had that I was pregnant was the nausea and sickness, and it struck any time, day or night. I was constantly exhausted too – I could have happily fallen asleep at my desk at work during the first few weeks."
Vidja, 28, first-time mum

"My breasts were so sore – it was the first thing I noticed. They were tender to the touch, and much bigger too."
Helena, 23, mum to year-old Alex

"Before I took my test, I felt really bloated and needed to go to the loo a lot. I had cramping too, and I wasn't sure if it was period pains or early pregnancy symptoms."
Anne, 28, mum to six-month-old twins

"My first symptoms were light spotting and cramping. Then, when my period didn't arrive, I took a test."
Jo, 31, mum to seven-month-old Barney

Home pregnancy tests

A standard home pregnancy test detects the hormone hCG in your urine. This is first secreted about six days after fertilisation, when the egg implants in the uterus. Levels of hCG build up rapidly, but if you have a negative result when you first test, it may be that the levels of hCG haven't yet reached a level where they can be detected. You may want to wait a few days then test again.

Some pregnancy tests are more sensitive than others and so are usually more expensive. Concentrations of hCG are given in milliInternational Units (mIU). A test with a sensitivity of 20 IU/L is more sensitive than one that has a sensitivity of 50 IU/L.

You can test at any time of day, and as early as the first day of your missed period with most tests. Avoid drinking too much fluid just before testing as this could dilute the hCG in your urine. Over-the-counter medicines, such as paracetamol, should not affect the result, but fertility drugs containing hCG may.

Read the directions carefully, because they vary with different brands. Some ask you to pee in a pot and then, using a dropper, place a small sample into a testing well. With others you pee directly onto a stick. Some change the colour of the urine sample, others show pink or blue lines, reveal a red plus or minus sign, or indicate "pregnant" or "not pregnant" in a little window.

If you follow the directions to the letter, home pregnancy tests are 97 per cent accurate. But mistakes do happen, which is why some kits come with two tests. If the test comes back negative but you still suspect you're pregnant, wait a few days, read the directions carefully, and try again. False positives (when the test says you're pregnant but you're not) are rare.

Your expected date of delivery (EDD)

Find the first day of your last period on the shaded bar. Beneath it you'll see your expected date of delivery or EDD – also called your due date. Your EDD is arrived at by counting on nine calendar months and seven days (40 weeks) from the first day of your last normal period. If your menstrual cycle is shorter or longer than 28 days, your expected date of delivery may be earlier or later. An expected date of delivery based on a dating scan (see p.136) is more accurate than one that is based on your last period.

January	1	2	3	4	5	6	7	8	9	10	11	12	13	14	15	16	17	18	19	20	21	22	23	24	25	26	27	28	29	30	31
Oct/Nov	8	9	10	11	12	13	14	15	16	17	18	19	20	21	22	23	24	25	26	27	28	29	30	31	1	2	3	4	5	6	7
February	1	2	3	4	5	6	7	8	9	10	11	12	13	14	15	16	17	18	19	20	21	22	23	24	25	26	27	28			
Nov/Dec	8	9	10	11	12	13	14	15	16	17	18	19	20	21	22	23	24	25	26	27	28	29	30	1	2	3	4	5			
March	1	2	3	4	5	6	7	8	9	10	11	12	13	14	15	16	17	18	19	20	21	22	23	24	25	26	27	28	29	30	31
Dec/Jan	6	7	8	9	10	11	12	13	14	15	16	17	18	19	20	21	22	23	24	25	26	27	28	29	30	31	1	2	3	4	5
April	1	2	3	4	5	6	7	8	9	10	11	12	13	14	15	16	17	18	19	20	21	22	23	24	25	26	27	28	29	30	
Jan/Feb	6	7	8	9	10	11	12	13	14	15	16	17	18	19	20	21	22	23	24	25	26	27	28	29	30	31	1	2	3	4	
May	1	2	3	4	5	6	7	8	9	10	11	12	13	14	15	16	17	18	19	20	21	22	23	24	25	26	27	28	29	30	31
Feb/Mar	5	6	7	8	9	10	11	12	13	14	15	16	17	18	19	20	21	22	23	24	25	26	27	28	1	2	3	4	5	6	7
June	1	2	3	4	5	6	7	8	9	10	11	12	13	14	15	16	17	18	19	20	21	22	23	24	25	26	27	28	29	30	
Mar/Apr	8	9	10	11	12	13	14	15	16	17	18	19	20	21	22	23	24	25	26	27	28	29	30	31	1	2	3	4	5	6	
July	1	2	3	4	5	6	7	8	9	10	11	12	13	14	15	16	17	18	19	20	21	22	23	24	25	26	27	28	29	30	31
Apr/May	7	8	9	10	11	12	13	14	15	16	17	18	19	20	21	22	23	24	25	26	27	28	29	30	1	2	3	4	5	6	7
August	1	2	3	4	5	6	7	8	9	10	11	12	13	14	15	16	17	18	19	20	21	22	23	24	25	26	27	28	29	30	31
May/June	8	9	10	11	12	13	14	15	16	17	18	19	20	21	22	23	24	25	26	27	28	29	30	31	1	2	3	4	5	6	7
September	1	2	3	4	5	6	7	8	9	10	11	12	13	14	15	16	17	18	19	20	21	22	23	24	25	26	27	28	29	30	
Jun/July	8	9	10	11	12	13	14	15	16	17	18	19	20	21	22	23	24	25	26	27	28	29	30	1	2	3	4	5	6	7	
October	1	2	3	4	5	6	7	8	9	10	11	12	13	14	15	16	17	18	19	20	21	22	23	24	25	26	27	28	29	30	31
July/Aug	8	9	10	11	12	13	14	15	16	17	18	19	20	21	22	23	24	25	26	27	28	29	30	31	1	2	3	4	5	6	7
November	1	2	3	4	5	6	7	8	9	10	11	12	13	14	15	16	17	18	19	20	21	22	23	24	25	26	27	28	29	30	
Aug/Sept	8	9	10	11	12	13	14	15	16	17	18	19	20	21	22	23	24	25	26	27	28	29	30	31	1	2	3	4	5	6	
December	1	2	3	4	5	6	7	8	9	10	11	12	13	14	15	16	17	18	19	20	21	22	23	24	25	26	27	28	29	30	31
Sept/Oct	7	8	9	10	11	12	13	14	15	16	17	18	19	20	21	22	23	24	25	26	27	28	29	30	1	2	3	4	5	6	7

Getting ready for pregnancy

Staying safe and healthy

Your pregnancy diary

Birth and beyond

Pregnancy following IVF

Discovering you have a baby on the way is a hugely emotional moment for any couple. But for couples who have been through IVF, joy at finally being pregnant can be mixed with anxiety about the next nine months. For now, just look after yourself and take each day as it comes.

ParentsTalk...

"I know that everything is OK with my pregnancy now but I'm so over protective. I'm worried that being on my feet all day could hurt my baby. I keep telling myself that it's our one and only baby so it's probably normal to be this crazy."
Gemma, 28, pregnant after IVF

"I have to go back in at 32 weeks to discuss my birth plan. I know I want a natural active birth as I'd like something in this pregnancy to be natural."
Leah, 31, pregnant after IVF

A positive pregnancy test is all the more welcome if you have been trying for a baby for a while, but it can cause concern, too.

Pregnant at last

A positive pregnancy test after IVF can seem like a miracle. But for many couples, the joy of conceiving can be quickly replaced with more worry. Am I really pregnant? Is my baby OK? You'll probably feel anxious about every twinge or change in symptoms. For you and your partner, nine months will probably feel like a very long time.

Reassurance

The first scan will help to reassure you. You should have an ultrasound between six and 11 weeks to confirm that the embryo has implanted. From seven weeks onwards a heartbeat will be visible but it may be detected as early as six weeks. As tiny as your embryo is, seeing it for the first time on a scan with its heart beating, will probably do more than anything to put your mind at rest.

At your booking appointment, your midwife will explain to you when you will have your antenatal appointments. For most women who have had an assisted conception, care will be just the same as if they had conceived naturally. It can feel very strange to have quite long periods between appointments after the busy schedule you had during your IVF cycle. Remember, you can always call your midwife or doctor between appointments if you have any concerns or questions at all.

If you had any complications in a previous pregnancy, or if you have any pre-existing health problems (see pp.22–3), you will be monitored more closely during your pregnancy, and if your IVF has resulted in a twins pregnancy, you will also see your doctor or midwife more frequently.

Looking after yourself is important in any pregnancy and you may feel that you want to be particularly careful. Make sure you follow a healthy diet with plenty of fresh fruit and vegetables. Experts are divided about safe levels of caffeine and alcohol in pregnancy, so you may feel you want to err on the side of caution and cut them out altogether.

Most importantly, try to relax and make the most of your pregnancy. You've probably battled hard to get to this point. You deserve to enjoy it.

Fact: One in every 80 babies born in the United Kingdom is conceived using IVF, according to the HFEA, which monitors fertility clinics. Thousands of IVF babies have been born worldwide since 1978.

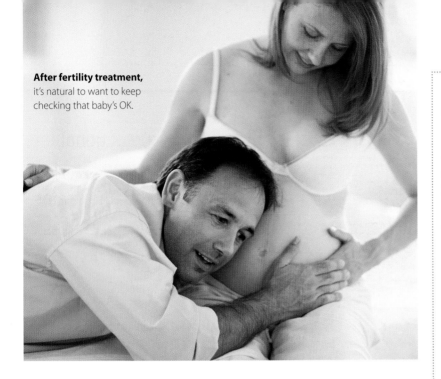

After fertility treatment, it's natural to want to keep checking that baby's OK.

The risks

One of the first things you will probably worry about when you find out that you are pregnant following IVF is the risk of miscarriage. Miscarriage is no more common after IVF than after a natural conception, but it's also no lower. Sadly, about 15 per cent of known pregnancies end in miscarriage, usually in the first 13 weeks of pregnancy (see pp.42–3).

Multiple pregnancy

If you've had more than one embryo placed in your uterus, you'll have a higher than usual chance of having twins or triplets. Around one in four couples will have twins after successful IVF, compared with approximately one in 80 of the general population. Though many couples consider this a blessing, multiple pregnancies do increase your risk of miscarriage and other complications such as premature labour, pre-eclampsia and pregnancy-induced high blood pressure.

IVF also puts you at increased risk of having an ectopic pregnancy, where an embryo implants in your fallopian tube or your abdominal cavity. This is more likely to happen if you have had any problems affecting your fallopian tubes previously. Your first scan will confirm that your embryo has implanted in your uterus and not in your fallopian tube. If you haven't yet had a scan and you have any vaginal bleeding or stomach pain, call your doctor.

Unfortunately, the fertility drugs used to stimulate egg production themselves can have severe side effects. You will need to be closely monitored while you are taking them to ensure you do not develop ovarian hyperstimulation syndrome (OHSS). This is potentially a dangerous condition, which can go on for weeks into early pregnancy. It can mean that you will have to stay in hospital while your over-stimulated ovaries settle down.

 Active mum

Waiting those first few weeks can be difficult after IVF, especially if you're used to a carefree life.

"We've waited so long for this pregnancy; I really want our beanie to stick. I've been having a few cramps and some vaginal discharge, but it's white – no blood or anything so that makes me feel better. I'm just terrified that the clear stuff will change and I'll see blood. The clinic says there's nothing to worry about but I can't help it. I've tried to get a scan but my doctor says there's no point until six weeks. I even tried to go privately but they said the same thing. What's reassuring me is that I've got swollen and sore boobs, some nausea and headaches. I know those are all good signs, but I won't feel better until I go for that six-week scan and see a heart beating on the screen."

Is it twins (or more)?

If you're expecting twins, you're certain to have lots of questions and probably some worries, too. We'll answer your concerns on everything about a multiple pregnancy, from conception and antenatal care, to how your pregnancy will differ from a singleton pregnancy.

How twin/multiple births occur

In the UK about one in 80 births resulting from natural conception is of twins or triplets. Non-identical, or fraternal, twins start off from two different eggs that are fertilised by two different sperm. Identical twins are rarer. They start off as one fertilised egg, which then splits into two.

Influencing factors

There are various factors that can increase your chances of having a multiple birth. Your age is important.

If you're in your 30s or older you have a greater chance of having twins or more. As you age, you naturally produce more ovulation-stimulating hormones, which may trigger your ovaries to release several eggs at once instead of one.

Heredity is another important factor. Non-identical twins tend to run in families, usually – but not always – on the mother's side. If twins run in your mother's family, you're more likely to have a set yourself. They also occur more often in African ethnic groups.

Identical twins, which are the result of a single fertilised egg splitting, don't tend to run in families.

Size matters, too. A US study showed that there was a significant increase in non-identical twin births to mothers who had a BMI of 30 or above, or to those who were in the top 25th percentile for height.

Nowadays, most women who give birth to multiples have undergone some type of fertility treatment, although one treatment – IUI (intrauterine

---

How twins are conceived

Identical twins are formed from one egg that has been fertilised by a single sperm and then has split in two.

Non-identical twins are formed from two eggs released at the same time and fertilised by two different sperm.

There are two types of multiple pregnancy: identical (or monozygotic) and non-identical (or dizygotic). Twins can occur for a number of different reasons:

● In the case of identical twins – the rarer type – the fertilised egg splits in two during the first 14 days. As the twins come from a single egg, they each share the same genetic make-up and may share the same placenta.

● In the case of non-identical twins or multiples, more than one egg is released and each is fertilised by different sperm. Each has its own placenta.

insemination), where sperm are injected into a woman's uterus – doesn't increase the risk of a multiple pregnancy unless you're also taking fertility drugs.

If you're taking a fertility drug, prepare for the possibility of twins. The drugs stimulate your ovaries, increasing the odds that you'll release several eggs at the same time. Up to 13 per cent of women taking the fertility drug clomiphene have a multiple pregnancy.

Newer fertility techniques, such as ICSI (intracytoplasmic sperm injection) and GIFT (gamete intrafallopian transfer), also increase the chances of a multiple pregnancy. Like IVF, these can involve more than one embryo being put into a woman's uterus or fallopian tubes.

The rate of identical twins also increases after IVF for reasons that aren't fully understood, but the vast majority of IVF twins are non-identical.

Twins may provide extra work and you'll need more rest before they arrive, but they'll also give you extra joy and excitement.

What's different about a multiple pregnancy

Early on in pregnancy you may suspect you are having twins if you have gained a lot of weight, your uterus is big for your due date or you are suffering a lot from nausea and vomiting. As your babies grow, you will probably become tired easily and need extra rest. And you will carry more weight than women who are pregnant with one baby, so you might get fed up with feeling so big.

Digestive problems

Nausea and vomiting can be more of a problem if you are expecting twins because you have higher levels of the pregnancy hormone hCG (see p.74), which triggers nausea and vomiting. In the early stages, higher levels of the hormone progesterone can make you feel short of breath. You might also be more likely to have constipation or suffer from wind and bloating.

Later in pregnancy

Later in your pregnancy there is more of a strain on your muscles because you are carrying additional weight, so back pain might be a problem. Anaemia is more common with twins and it can make you feel very tired. Make sure that you eat iron-rich foods and take iron supplements if they are recommended.

The danger signs to look out for are the same as in any pregnancy. You do need to be alert to any unusual or worrying symptoms, though, because the risk of some complications, such as premature labour and pre-eclampsia, is higher when you are expecting twins.

Trust your instincts and, if you're not sure about a symptom, or just don't feel right, call your midwife or doctor.

Get as much rest as you can, ask people for help at home, and remember to enjoy the little things in life. You will need lots of energy both during your pregnancy and after your babies are born, so it's a good idea to get into the habit of looking after yourself now.

ParentsAsk...

I'm expecting twins. Will I have extra antenatal care?
You'll be offered extra scans to see how your babies are positioned, how well they are growing or whether any complications are developing. Regular blood pressure and urine tests are important too.

How much weight will I gain?
You're likely to gain more weight than mothers of one baby. As in any pregnancy, try to eat a healthy, balanced diet.

What are the risks?
Premature birth (before 37 weeks) occurs in about half of twin pregnancies. Call your midwife if you think you are in labour or go straight to hospital. Pre-eclampsia is also more common with twins. This potentially dangerous complication is usually detected by blood pressure and urine tests, but symptoms include severe headaches, vision problems, and sudden swelling of your feet, ankles, face and hands.

Will my labour be induced?
Some doctors argue that it's safer to plan for your twins' birth at about 37 to 38 weeks of pregnancy, either by induction or by planned caesarean. But the choice is yours. If you do want a natural labour, discuss your options with your midwife.

Getting ready for pregnancy

Staying safe and healthy

Your pregnancy diary

Birth and beyond

Miscarriage

Sadly miscarriage is all too common, affecting about 15 per cent of pregnancies. But that doesn't make it any easier to bear if it happens to you. Here's how to reduce your risk of pregnancy loss and how to spot the signs if the worst does happen.

Miscarriage can be heartbreaking but you can take action to prevent it happening to you and can learn to recognise the signs.

ParentsTalk...

"We held out until 10 weeks to tell friends and family our thrilling news, but a week later I miscarried. We were heartbroken – and what was worse was that we'd allowed ourselves and our friends and family to get excited about it."
Julia, 30, pregnant for a second time

"It takes time to get back on your feet after a miscarriage. I went back to work after a week, then had to take a month off to recover properly."
Louise, 28

What is a miscarriage?

Miscarriage is the loss of a baby in the first 24 weeks of pregnancy. Sadly, it's common; about 15 per cent of known pregnancies end in miscarriage. About 98 per cent of women who miscarry do so in the first 13 weeks.

The risk factors

Research suggests that you are more likely to miscarry if you smoke, drink more than four cups of coffee a day or drink a lot of alcohol. You also have a higher risk of miscarriage if you:

- Have had more than one miscarriage in the past.
- Have fibroids (non-cancerous growths of the uterus).
- Have an abnormally shaped uterus.
- Have lupus.
- Have diabetes, kidney disease or thyroid disease (if these conditions are well managed by you and your doctors, the risk of miscarriage is much lower).
- Have an infection in early pregnancy, such as rubella, listeria or chlamydia.

Age also plays a role. Older women are more likely to conceive babies with chromosomal abnormalities, and these pregnancies are more likely to be lost.

Why miscarriages happen

Doctors still don't know why miscarriages happen. Probably at least half of all miscarriages in the first

---

If you think you're miscarrying

If you think you may be miscarrying, ring your doctor, midwife or hospital. **Do not hesitate to contact your doctor, midwife or the hospital immediately if:**

- The bleeding is very heavy.
- You begin to feel feverish and generally unwell.
- You have severe, one-sided abdominal pain – this may be a sign that you have an ectopic pregnancy.

To help cope with the strong period-type pain, rest, take painkillers and use a hot water bottle on your tummy or lower back to ease the cramping.

If the bleeding isn't that heavy, or if there is no pain, then you don't need to rush into hospital, but it is a good idea to contact your doctor anyway. They may want to see you at an antenatal clinic the next day, to examine you to check that you are physically all right.

trimester are the result of chromosomal abnormalities. Miscarriages that occur after 20 weeks may be the result of an infection, an abnormality of the uterus or placenta, or a cervix that is not strong enough to keep the uterus tightly closed.

The signs

The most obvious signs of miscarriage are period-like pains, cramping and bleeding (which may include blood clots). Some miscarriages are only discovered by chance during a routine antenatal visit, when the doctor or midwife cannot find the baby's heartbeat.

Sometimes you may have some spotting – losing very small amounts of blood from your vagina. Spotting in early pregnancy is common and usually nothing to worry about. Often, it's simply "breakthrough" bleeding when your period would have been due, caused by the hormones that control your menstrual cycle; or "implantation" bleeding – when the fertilised egg implants in the wall of the uterus.

With any spotting, bleeding or severe pain, you should ring your doctor or midwife. It could be a sign that you are going to miscarry.

Reducing the risk

By far the best way to reduce your risk of miscarriage is to give up smoking before you become pregnant (see p.118). This may be the hardest thing you've ever had to do, but it will certainly reduce your risk.

Caffeine and alcohol

Even if you're pregnant already, it's still very worthwhile quitting smoking, and cutting down on caffeine and alcohol, both of which are possible additional factors in miscarriage. The Food Standards Agency (FSA) recommends that pregnant women should not have more than 200 milligrams (mg) of caffeine a day as caffeine consumption is linked to miscarriage as well as to low-birthweight babies.

There is also research that links even low levels of caffeine to miscarriage, so if you are really concerned, you may want to cut out caffeine altogether, just to be on the safe side. Although the research isn't absolutely clear, it also seems possible that drinking more than one to two units of alcohol once or twice a week may increase your risk of miscarriage.

If you've had a miscarriage before, your doctor or midwife might suggest that you try to rest as much as possible during the first couple of months of your pregnancy. You might also be advised to avoid sex, again for the first few months, until your pregnancy is well established. If you think this is going to cause problems with your partner, ask your midwife to talk to the two of you together so that he can understand why it's necessary.

If you know you have a weak cervix because that caused a previous miscarriage, you may be able to have a stitch put round it to keep it closed until your baby is ready to be born. This is called a Shirodkar suture or cerclage.

Sadly, there is not much that can be done to prevent a miscarriage once it is underway. Coping with it is very hard, but it may be some comfort to know that most women do manage to get pregnant again, and go on to have a normal, full-term pregnancy.

200mg is the maximum amount of caffeine that pregnant women should have a day, according to the FSA. That means no more than two mugs of coffee, four cups of tea or five cans of cola. Many women find anyway that their fondness for a cup of coffee evaporates when they're pregnant.

 Active mum

If you love your sport, take extra care when you're exercising to protect your baby.

"I've led a really active life ever since I was a child. I love the great outdoors and often go on activity holidays. When I found out I was pregnant, though, I knew I'd have to make some changes for the safety of my baby.

I've had to give up the horseriding; it's been a long time since I fell off a horse, but I don't want to take the risk because I know that it could cause a miscarriage. Plus, I know that my centre of gravity will change as my baby grows, which will increase the risk of a fall.

But because I've always exercised regularly, my doctor says it's safe for me to carry on with my more pregnancy-friendly pursuits. I love going on really long walks, and I've started to swim more often. I'm thinking of joining a yoga class for pregnant women too.

Most importantly, though, I listen to my body and I stop exercising if I feel too tired or too out of breath."

Ectopic pregnancy

Ectopic pregnancy affects roughly one in 100 pregnancies in the United Kingdom. Sadly, it always ends in pregnancy loss, but most women who are affected will later go on to have healthy pregnancies. Here's how to spot the signs early.

Signs of ectopic pregnancy

Most affected women experience symptoms of an ectopic pregnancy about two weeks after missing a period. Signs to watch out for include:

The first signs

● Unusual vaginal bleeding. The blood is often different from your normal period – some people describe it as like "prune juice".

● One-sided pain in the lower abdomen that is severe and persistent. If you have these symptoms and could be pregnant, see a doctor.

When the fallopian tube ruptures

If an early diagnosis is not made, the tube may rupture and you may have the following symptoms:

● Sudden, severe pain gradually spreading out across the abdomen.

● Sweating, feeling light-headed or faint; diarrhoea or blood in your stools.

● Collapse or shock as a result of severe internal bleeding.

● Shoulder-tip pain, which is also a sign of internal bleeding.

If you have any of these symptoms, see your doctor immediately or go straight to hospital.

What's going on?

An ectopic pregnancy is one that develops outside the uterus. It happens in roughly one per cent of all pregnancies in the UK.

Almost all ectopic pregnancies implant in one of the fallopian tubes. As the pregnancy grows, it causes pain and bleeding and, if it's not recognised that you have an ectopic pregnancy, the fallopian tube can rupture, causing internal bleeding. Ectopic pregnancy is a life-threatening emergency. In rare cases it can be fatal. The pregnancy itself never survives as it has to be removed completely.

Symptoms often start about two weeks after a missed period. The most common reason for an ectopic pregnancy is when the fallopian tube has been damaged. This causes a blockage or narrowing, which prevents the egg from reaching the uterus. Instead, it implants in the wall of the tube.

Risk factors

You are more likely to have an ectopic pregnancy if:

● You have tubal endometriosis, which increases the risk of scarring and adhesions in the tubes.

● You've had any abdominal surgery.

● You've had pelvic inflammatory disease (PID) – this can cause scarring to the fallopian tubes (there are signs of PID in about half of all ectopic pregnancies that occur).

● You are pregnant following IVF.

● You have been fitted with an intrauterine system (IUS – also sometimes called a coil or IUCD) or if you are taking the mini-pill.

● You smoke.

● You've had a previous ectopic pregnancy (your risk increases from one in 100 to one in 10).

● You're an older mum.

Pregnancy sac with embryo

In most ectopic pregnancies the blastocyst (see p.34) implants in the fallopian tube. Once diagnosed, the pregnancy must be removed.

Symptoms

It can be difficult to recognise if you are having an ectopic pregnancy, as it may begin with the sort of signs you associate with your period starting or a threatened miscarriage, such as cramping and slight bleeding. Early symptoms of ectopic pregnancy include unusual vaginal bleeding (some women describe the bleeding as looking rather like prune juice). You may also have severe, persistent one-sided pain in the lower part of your tummy.

You might also experience some shoulder-tip pain, which can be felt where the shoulder meets the top of the arm. This can happen if there is internal bleeding which will irritate other internal body organs, such as the diaphragm. If the ectopic pregnancy isn't diagnosed early enough and the fallopian tube ruptures, you may feel sudden, severe pain gradually spreading out across your tummy. You may also start sweating and feeling faint and you may find you have diarrhoea or blood in your stools. If the internal bleeding is severe, you may collapse. This is an emergency and you should call an ambulance or go straight to hospital.

How it is treated

If you've got a suspected ectopic pregnancy, you'll probably be referred to an early pregnancy unit at your hospital. A blood test will measure the levels of the hCG hormone (see p.74) in your blood. If the levels are lower than in a normal pregnancy, it can be a sign of ectopic pregnancy.

Further tests

You may have a vaginal ultrasound examination, as the pregnancy may not show up using an abdominal scan. If this does not confirm what is happening, you will probably be taken to theatre for a laparoscopic examination. This is where a narrow viewing instrument is put into your abdomen.

If an ectopic pregnancy is discovered, the surgeon can sometimes use laparoscopy (keyhole surgery) to remove the pregnancy, leaving the tube intact if at all possible. If the tube has ruptured, though, doctors usually recommend that the woman has full abdominal surgery, because this is the quickest way to stop blood loss.

Whether the tube and pregnancy are removed altogether, or the pregnancy is removed and the tube repaired depends on how damaged the tube is, the health of your other fallopian tube and your desire for future pregnancy.

In a few cases where the tube has been saved, the pregnancy continues to grow and needs treatment with the drug methotrexate, which terminates pregnancy. Otherwise you may need further surgery to remove it.

Methotrexate can sometimes be used to treat an ectopic pregnancy instead of surgery. This is most effective in very early pregnancy. Methotrexate can also be used where there is no bleeding and the tube has not ruptured.

Occasionally, where an ectopic pregnancy has been identified very early on but its exact location isn't known, no treatment will be offered. This is called expectant management or "wait and see". This is because lots of ectopic pregnancies miscarry naturally. Surgery is only needed in about a quarter of these cases.

Getting ready for pregnancy

Staying safe and healthy

Your pregnancy diary

Birth and beyond

Staying safe
and healthy

Healthy eating for you and baby

Now that you're a mum-to-be, it's important to make sure that you and your developing baby are getting all the nutrients you need. That means eating a healthy, balanced diet that's rich in vitamins and minerals. You'll also need to avoid certain foods that could be harmful.

During pregnancy, eating your recommended five daily portions of fruit and vegetables is even more important.

What should I be eating?

Although you're pregnant, don't think that you have to eat for two. The average woman needs only about 200 extra calories per day for the last three months of pregnancy.

Recommended diet
The Food Standards Agency (FSA) recommends that, to keep you and your baby well nourished, you eat:
- At least five portions of fruit and vegetables a day – fresh, frozen, tinned, dried or a glass of pure fruit juice all count.
- Plenty of starchy foods, such as bread, pasta, rice and potatoes – choose wholegrain versions if possible.
- Foods that are rich in protein, such as lean meat or chicken, fish (aim for two servings of fish a week, including one of oily fish, see p.53), plus iron-rich eggs, beans and lentils.
- Plenty of fibre – this helps prevent constipation and is found in wholegrain bread, pasta and rice; pulses and lentils; and fruit and vegetables.
- Calcium-rich dairy foods, such as milk, cheese and yoghurt.

As far as snacks are concerned, try a banana rather than chocolate, or frozen fruit sorbet instead of full-fat ice cream. And if you fancy the occasional biscuit, don't feel guilty – just enjoy every bite!

ParentsAsk...

Do I need a supplement?
While you are pregnant a varied, well-balanced diet should suffice. But if you are suffering badly with nausea and vomiting or are low in iron, your doctor or midwife may advise a supplement especially designed for pregnant women.

What should it contain?
A good one will contain more folic acid, iron and calcium – vital for your baby's development – than a general multivitamin.

It will also contain the plant-derived form of vitamin A (betacarotene). The animal form, retinol, can be harmful to unborn babies in large doses.

Should I take probiotics?
Two studies found that probiotics taken during pregnancy may help to prevent atopic eczema developing in babies. More research is needed, but if you have a family history of allergies you could ask your doctor for advice.

 Active mum

If you're a more than usually active pregnant mum, you should eat when you're hungry.

"Despite all those stories about 'eating for two', it turns out that you don't need any extra calories for the first six months of pregnancy. But as I do a lot of sport, my midwife said I should eat when I'm hungry and that plenty of fruit and vegetables and lots of water would help keep my energy levels up."

Getting ready for pregnancy

Staying safe and healthy

Your pregnancy diary

Birth and beyond

Iron-rich eggs are a healthy choice during pregnancy, but make sure omelettes and frittatas are all well cooked.

A vegetable stir-fry can give you several of your "five a day". Stir-fries are a healthier, less fatty choice than deep-fried foods.

When choosing a dessert, keep sugar to a minimum as it's full of "empty" calories with no nutritional value. Honey's a better choice.

Appetite fluctuations

Your own appetite is the best indication of how much food you need to eat. You may find your appetite fluctuates as your pregnancy progresses:

● In the first few weeks your appetite may fall away dramatically and you may not want proper meals, especially if you are suffering from nausea or sickness.

● During the middle part of your pregnancy your appetite may be the same as before you were pregnant or slightly increased.

● Towards the end of your pregnancy your appetite will probably increase, but if you suffer from heartburn or a full feeling after eating you may find it helpful to have small frequent meals.

Healthy weight gain

Weight gain varies from woman to woman and depends on many different factors. Women are no longer routinely weighed at antenatal clinics, but the average weight gain during pregnancy is between 8kg (18lb) and 15kg (33lb). Most women gain the least weight during the first trimester, then steadily increase, gaining most weight during the third trimester when the baby is growing the most.

Although you may be tempted, dieting during pregnancy isn't good for you or your baby. Diets can leave you low on iron, folic acid, and other vitamins and minerals. Remember, weight gain is one of the most positive signs of a healthy pregnancy. Just eat a healthy diet (see opposite), and try to keep your fat and sugar intake low.

Small frequent meals

Even if you're not hungry, chances are your baby is, so try to eat every four hours. And if nausea and sickness, food aversions, heartburn, or indigestion make eating a chore, you may find that eating five or six small meals, rather than three larger ones, is easier.

Folic acid

The B vitamin folic acid is particularly important during pregnancy. Lack of it has been linked with neural tube birth defects, such as spina bifida (see p.215) . The Department of Health (DH) recommends that women should take 400 micrograms (mcg) of folic acid in a supplement from the time they start trying for a baby until the 12th week of pregnancy. You also need a good intake of the naturally occurring form of folic

acid, folates, from the food you eat. Leafy green vegetables, such as cabbage, broccoli and greens, are all good sources. Other useful sources include black-eyed beans, bran flakes, papaya, and baker's yeast.

Tips for safe eating out

There is no reason why you can't eat safely in a restaurant. Here are a few pointers as to what to choose:

Starters Avoid raw fish and go for cooked dishes, such as grilled sardines or prawns. Pâtés and terrines could contain listeria, so are best avoided.

Main courses Steak tartare, sushi and other raw meat are risky. Opt for meat or fish that is cooked thoroughly.

Desserts Soufflés, mousses and chilled chocolate "pots" may contain raw eggs. Tiramisu often contains raw egg white as does home-made ice cream. Crème brulée and caramel custard are fine, because the eggs have been cooked.

Pregnant and vegetarian

With careful planning, a vegetarian diet during pregnancy can provide all the healthy nutrients you need.

Iron and calcium

Your body requires a little more protein during pregnancy, and this is easily provided by following a healthy, varied

vegetarian diet. However, vegetarians should take extra care to ensure that they have an adequate intake of iron and calcium. Both are very important during pregnancy (see p.121).

Vegetarian mums-to-be should be particularly careful to include plenty of iron in their diet as vegetable sources of iron are not as well absorbed as iron that is found in meat. Good sources include pulses, green vegetables, dried fruit and fortified breakfast cereals.

Try to have some food or drink containing vitamin C, such as a glass of fruit juice, with any iron-rich meals as this helps your body to absorb the iron. Avoid drinking tea with iron-rich foods as this contains tannin, which reduces absorption. If your iron levels become low, your doctor or midwife may advise you to take iron supplements.

The best sources of calcium are dairy foods, such as milk, cheese and yoghurt. Aim to have three servings per day.

The vitamin C in salads helps your body absorb all-important iron from other foods.

Vitamin D is essential for calcium absorption and can be obtained from sunlight, margarine and dairy products. You may want to consider taking a vitamin D supplement.

There are some non-dairy sources of dietary calcium, such as dark green vegetables, sesame seeds and some fortified soya products. Generally, calcium is not as well absorbed from these foods so, if you do not eat dairy foods, it's a good idea to take a calcium supplement. (If you are vegan, you will find more information about healthy eating for pregnancy on the Vegan Society website.)

During the last three months or so of your pregnancy you will need to eat about an extra 200 calories a day to support your rapidly growing baby. You can bump up your calorie intake by eating more cereals, pulses, nuts, seeds, dairy products (unless vegan) and starchy vegetables, such as potatoes. The Vegetarian Society is a good source of information about healthy vegetarian diets during pregnancy.

Parents**Ask...**

Can I diet when I'm pregnant?

Dieting to lose weight during pregnancy isn't advised, but you should follow a healthy low-fat, low-sugar diet. It might help to see a registered dietitian with experience of working with pregnant women to find out how to eat well without loading up on calories.

How many calories do I need?

Your daily calorie requirement depends on how active you are, but most pregnant women need 1,800 to 2,100 calories per day. In pregnancy you only need extra

calories for the last three months and then only about 200 extra per day.

Can vitamin B6 help relieve my morning sickness?

Vitamin B6 helps some women, but no-one really knows why. You can get it from food sources such as bananas, brown rice, lean meats, poultry, fish, avocados, whole grains, corn and nuts, as well as from a supplement. The Food Standards Agency recommends taking no more than 10mg of B6 each day as a supplement. Talk to your midwife or doctor about how much to take and when.

 ## Single mum

There are plenty of ways to save money on your shopping bill and make good food go further.

"I've got a good salary but I still need to watch what I spend. I find it helps to make a shopping list and stick to it. I eat a mainly vegetarian diet as it's cheaper, but I treat myself to some good, lean meat a couple of times a week. I also tend to go for the supermarket's own brand. I really can't taste any difference."

Pregnant and plus-sized

Your weight may not have any effect at all on your pregnancy or your baby's birth, but being overweight or obese could put you at higher risk of certain pregnancy complications. Some of the most common of these are:

- gestational diabetes
- gestational hypertension (high blood pressure)
- pre-eclampsia
- premature labour
- a large baby (macrosomia)

When it's time to give birth, having a high body mass index can mean you are more likely to have:

- an assisted birth (by forceps or ventouse)
- a caesarean section
- shoulder dystocia (where the baby's shoulders get caught on the mother's pubic bone during birth)

Preventing problems

Most of these health conditions and situations are manageable though, and some are preventable. Ideally, you should lose weight before you get pregnant as research has shown an association between dieting during the first three months of pregnancy and babies born with neural tube defects, regardless of the mother's size. But if you are pregnant, there's still plenty you can do to help yourself and your baby.

Exercise

Regular exercise is one of the most effective ways to manage your weight, particularly when combined with a healthy diet.

As long as you get the go-ahead from your midwife or doctor, you can engage in mild to moderate exercise. Stick to low-impact activities like walking or swimming. Keep workout sessions short and stay well hydrated by drinking plenty of water.

Also talk to your doctor about your individual risk factors. Do you have a history of high blood pressure, or of diabetes? Once you know your risk factors, you can work with your doctor and midwife to give yourself the best chance of having a healthy baby.

Healthy eating for working mums

However busy your job, you can make time to eat well at work by following some simple steps.

- Keep some healthy nibbles and drinks in your desk drawer to satisfy hunger pangs throughout the day: try fruit, crackers, organic no-added-sugar cereal bars, seeds and nuts. Bread rolls, cartons of fruit juice, mineral water and strips of carrot or cucumber are also great workday snacks.
- If you can, take your lunch into work so you can be sure you're eating a balanced meal. Transform your usual sandwich into something more interesting by using different breads every day, and fresh fillings such as watercress, rocket and grated carrot.

Or try a salad – pasta and couscous give you a prolonged release of energy. Add vegetables and salad ingredients for added nutrients. For a hot meal, try soup, made fresh or ready made, with a granary bread roll. Baked potatoes are great fillers, too – eat with salads or baked beans.

Getting ready for pregnancy

Staying safe and healthy

Your pregnancy diary

Birth and beyond

Keep a box filled with healthy snacks in your desk drawer for those odd moments when you have an attack of the munchies.

Making your own healthy sandwiches to take into work ensures you'll always eat a balanced meal at lunchtime.

A salmon parcel is a quick, easy and healthy meal to make for dinner when you get home after a long day at work.

What's safe to eat?

It sometimes feels as though the list of foods you can't eat when you're pregnant grows longer every day. Try not to worry too much. Just remember that the risks to you and your baby are low and you can avoid them altogether by taking a few sensible steps.

Cheese is an important source of calcium when you're pregnant, but you should take care which you choose.

Laid-back mum

It may never occur to you before you get pregnant that some foods can be bad for your baby.

"Finding out what I could and couldn't eat when I was pregnant was a revelation. Now I make sure any meat I eat is thoroughly cooked – no more rare steaks for me! Or soft-boiled eggs. And I try not to eat too much oily fish, though I never ate more than a couple of portions a week. Cheese is a tricky one – I've cut out all the mouldy cheeses. But I don't worry too much. As long as you're careful, food-related infections are quite rare."

Why what you eat may be bad for your baby

Confused about which cheeses are safe in pregnancy? Or whether you can drink alcohol? Here's all you need to know to keep you and your baby safe from harm.

Alcohol

Heavy drinking, particularly binge drinking (five or more units of alcohol in one go), during pregnancy can seriously affect your developing baby. The risks of drinking much less, however, are not clear cut. Even so, some experts recommend not drinking during the first three months; others advise staying teetotal for the whole pregnancy. If you do drink, you should not have more than one or two units of alcohol, and no more than once or twice per week.

Caffeine

If there is too much caffeine in your diet your risk of miscarriage (see pp.42–3) goes up and your baby could have a lower birth weight.

Artificial sweeteners

Although there have been several scares about the safety of some sweeteners, overall research suggests that they are safe for most pregnant women to use.

Raw or undercooked meat

Raw, rare, cured and undercooked meat or poultry of any kind is best avoided. It may contain salmonella bacteria, which can cause severe food poisoning, or the toxoplasmosis parasite, which can be harmful to your unborn baby.

Raw or undercooked eggs

Eating soft-boiled or raw eggs is not recommended because of the risk that the eggs may carry salmonella bacteria. To stay safe, boil a medium-sized egg for at least seven minutes, fry eggs on both sides and poach eggs until they are completely set.

Cheese and dairy products

Cheese is an important source of protein and calcium for pregnant women but certain kinds need to be avoided:
● Soft, mould-ripened cheeses, such as Brie or Camembert.
● Blue-veined cheeses, such as Danish Blue and Stilton.
● Soft, unpasteurised cheeses, such as goat's or sheep's cheese.

These cheeses provide a perfect environment for harmful bacteria, such as listeria, to grow. However, thorough cooking should kill any listeria, so it's safe to eat these cheeses in well-cooked food. All hard cheeses, including feta, Gruyère and Parmesan, are considered safe to eat. Yoghurts, probiotic drinks, fromage frais, soured cream and crème fraîche are also safe.

Prepared salads

These are very convenient, but you should take care to wash them again thoroughly before using them. This is because there is a small chance that they may carry the toxoplasmosis parasite or listeria bacteria.

Liver and pâté

Experts recommend pregnant women should not eat liver or any liver products, such as liver sausage or pâté, because they contain high levels of the retinol form of vitamin A, which can harm your developing baby.

Ready meals

Cooked chilled ready-to-eat meals and pre-cooked poultry may potentially be contaminated with listeria bacteria or the toxoplasmosis parasite. Listeria germs can still multiply inside a supermarket chill cabinet or your fridge. However, thorough cooking at high temperatures can kill both of these food bugs and ensure the food is safe to eat.

Seafood

Most fish and shellfish are safe to eat, provided they have been thoroughly cooked. Raw shellfish are a common cause of food poisoning so avoid them completely while you are pregnant.

Oily fish

Seafood is sometimes contaminated with environmental pollutants so it's recommended that pregnant women avoid eating too much oily fish, as it tends to contain more pollutants than white fish. You should eat some, though, so that you and your baby can benefit from the omega-3 fatty acids and other vitamins and nutrients it contains. Just limit your intake to no more than two portions a week. Choose from salmon, trout, mackerel, herring and sardines.

You should avoid eating shark, swordfish and marlin altogether because of their high levels of mercury, which could harm your baby's developing nervous system. You also need to limit the tuna you eat to no more than two fresh steaks a week or four medium-size cans, as this may also contain relatively high amounts of mercury.

Parents**Ask...**

Is it safe to eat sushi when you're pregnant?

Yes, it's safe as long as it's been frozen beforehand to kill any possible parasites. Sushi that uses cooked fish, such as steamed crab and cooked eel, is also fine. Most supermarket sushi is bought in ready-made. This should be safe to eat, because it has to have been frozen at –20ºC (–4ºF) for at least 24 hours. But if a shop or restaurant makes its own sushi, check that the fish has been frozen beforehand. If you make your own sushi, freeze the raw fish for at least 24 hours before using.

Herbal teas

All herbal preparations bought as tea bags from supermarkets and which contain common ingredients, such as camomile and lemon, are thought to be safe for use in pregnancy. However, steer clear of unfamiliar ingredients; black cohosh, pennyroyal, and mugwort are all best avoided in pregnancy. And don't drink raspberry leaf tea until the last two months of pregnancy because of its stimulating effect on the uterus.

Getting ready for pregnancy

Staying safe and healthy

Your pregnancy diary

Birth and beyond

Foods to avoid when you are pregnant

Working out what you can and can't eat when pregnant is confusing to start with.

Just follow these simple rules.

● **Cheese** Steer clear of blue-veined cheeses or soft, mould-ripened cheeses such as Brie or Camembert. Unpasteurised soft cheeses are also best avoided.
● **Eggs** Avoid raw or undercooked eggs. All salad dressings that you buy in supermarkets, such as mayonnaise, are safe. Be careful about eating "home-made" products, such as chocolate mousse, as these may contain raw egg.
● **Pâté** Avoid all pâté, whether made from meat, fish or vegetables.
● **Meat and meat products** Make sure meat is cooked thoroughly. Cured meat products, such as salami, also carry a risk and are best avoided.
● **Oily fish** This is good for you and your baby as it gives you all the benefits of omega-3 fatty acids, but limit your intake to a maximum of two portions a week to cut the risk from the pollutants.

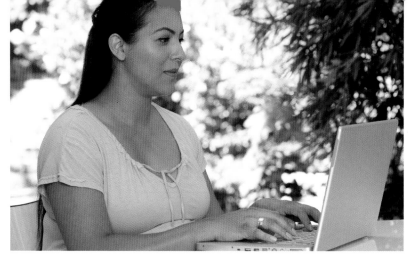

If you are worried about a food scare, you can search for reliable information online.

Food hygiene in pregnancy

During pregnancy, it is especially important to avoid the germs responsible for food poisoning:

- **Personal hygiene** Washing your hands before and during food preparation (especially if you are handling raw meat or poultry) prevents the spread of bacteria.
- **Keep foods at the right temperature** Take bought chilled and frozen foods home quickly and put them straight into the fridge (below 5ºC/41ºF) or freezer (below –18ºC/0.5ºF).
- **Store food safely** Store raw and cooked foods separately in the fridge. Put raw meat on the bottom shelf, where it can't drip onto cooked food.
- **Cook foods thoroughly** Cook until food – especially meat and poultry – is piping hot with steam coming off it.
- **Beware of cross-contamination** Clean work surfaces with soapy, hot water before preparing food, and after contact with raw meat or poultry.
- **Eating out** Look out for dirty public areas, staff with dirty hands or an obvious runny nose, or raw foods displayed next to ready-to-eat foods.

Always wash your hands before and after you prepare food to reduce your risk of getting food poisoning.

Food scares: how to tell the good from the bad

The papers are full of scare stories and lots of them are about food. Remember the "sausages give you cancer" story? Stories like this are worrying, but you should take many of them with a pinch of salt. Next time you see a worrying headline, you should ask yourself the following questions:

- **Is the advice backed up by a trustworthy organisation?**
The DH (Department of Health) and the FSA, for example, issue new guidance from time to time. In order to check, visit the relevant website or look for links from reliable news websites.

- **Is the report based on a true account of the facts?**
Sometimes the media pick on one aspect of a much larger topic. Editors often publish an unbalanced view of an issue that hasn't really been proven yet.

- **What is the source of the story?**
From time to time, companies issue press releases that support the use of their products. These may not give a truly balanced picture of a certain issue. Also, experts sometimes have an investment in the findings of a research study. If the findings are shown in a certain light, it could help sell a drug or product he or she has just patented.

- **Is the story really based on conclusive evidence?**
Experts around the world often report their research findings in specialist journals and at conferences. Sometimes the media reports the findings of very small research studies when, in fact, evidence from much larger studies is needed before the issue can be accepted as fact.

- **Is it really new?**
Sometimes the same old issues are paraded out again and again. For example, the media may report an inquiry into an issue. There isn't any new evidence yet, but the same panic-inducing headlines are released without adding anything new.

If you have asked yourself all these questions and you are still not sure what to do, don't be afraid to ask for some advice. Perhaps a visit to your midwife or doctor may help.

Parents**Talk...**

"I'm never entirely sure if I'm eating something that the government might suddenly decide is bad during pregnancy. I was sticking to the 300 milligrams (mg) of caffeine a day rule (three mugs of coffee) during my pregnancy – but when I was 32 weeks the rules changed to 200mg a day. I panicked, thinking I'd just spent the first 32 weeks of my baby's life impairing his growth. But I was assured by government advice that no harm would have come to my baby. So why did the rules change?

Maybe it's that the guidelines are often overly cautious to compensate for those mums who like things in excess!"
Bel, mum to two-month-old Adam

"We have a history of food allergies in our family and I decided to cut out peanuts altogether when I was pregnant – even though the advice says it's probably OK to eat them. They're difficult to avoid though – they seem to crop up as an ingredient in more foods than you might think."
Jennifer, 30, mum to Max and Cameron

"Having followed the advice to the letter with my first son, only to discover he has a peanut allergy, I decided to carry on eating them when I was pregnant with my second baby and he is fine. I don't know whether eating the peanuts helped or not, but the advice is so vague it's difficult to know what to do sometimes."
Madeleine, 37

If there are allergies in the family

Some experts believe that avoiding allergens, such as peanuts, during pregnancy may reduce your child's risk of allergies. However, there's no evidence to back this up.

Precautions during pregnancy

An allergic reaction is when the body over-responds to some substance causing breathing problems, wheezing, rashes and other, sometimes dangerous, symptoms. Allergic conditions include eczema, asthma and hayfever, plus allergic responses to certain foods. Non-food substances, such as pollen, house dust mites and bee or wasp stings, can also trigger allergies.

Before an allergy can develop, a child first has to be sensitised by contact with a trace of an allergen, such as peanut. Some believe that this may occur during pregnancy, when a tiny amount of the allergen crosses the placenta. However, there's no definite evidence yet.

A review of studies of high-risk pregnant women who avoided common allergens, such as eggs and cow's milk, during pregnancy found that this was unlikely to reduce the risk of allergies in children. On the other hand, exclusive breastfeeding for the first six months of your baby's life does help to lower her risk of allergies.

It's fine to eat peanuts while you're pregnant. The DH states that there is absolutely no evidence that eating or not eating peanuts while you are pregnant will affect your baby's chances of developing a peanut allergy.

Despite this advice, you may still feel reluctant to eat peanuts, and that's completely understandable. Talk to your doctor or midwife if you have a family history of allergies and are worried about the effect eating peanuts will

have on your baby. It's also worth remembering that, as long as you're eating a healthy balanced diet during your pregnancy, excluding peanuts from your diet will not do you or your baby any harm.

If you have food allergies in your family, you'll probably want to check food labels.

Fitness during pregnancy

Staying active has lots of benefits, both during your pregnancy and when it comes to giving birth. Whether you were a regular gym bunny before you got pregnant, or more of a couch potato, we've got tips on how to exercise safely with a bump.

Stretching tones muscles and gives you flexibility, both of which will help you to cope better with pregnancy and childbirth.

Staying active

Why exercise in pregnancy? One reason is that exercise strengthens your cardiovascular system, so you don't tire as easily. Staying active will also:

● **Help prepare you for the rigours of childbirth** Giving birth requires stamina. The better shape you're in, the stronger you'll be to enable you to cope with childbirth.

● **Reduce stress and lift your spirits** Exercise can boost your levels of serotonin, a brain chemical linked to mood, which puts you in better spirits.

When you're feeling a little blue, try putting on your favourite CD and kicking up your heels in the living room, or sign up for a low-impact dance class (make sure you let your teacher know that you are pregnant).

● **Reduce pregnancy discomfort** Exercise stretches and strengthens your muscles, which will help your body to cope better with the various aches and pains of pregnancy.

● **Fend off the pregnancy blues** By the sixth or seventh month, pregnancy can become downright tedious. Finding a new healthy activity appropriate for pregnant women may be the answer.

● **Help you sleep better** When you are carrying all that extra weight, finding a comfortable position to sleep in at night can be a real challenge. Exercise will help to lull you into a deeper, more restful slumber.

● **Improve your self-image** Although you know it's for a good cause, watching the scale creep its way up to numbers you've never seen before can be disheartening. Staying active can make you feel less frumpy.

● **Help you get your body back faster after birth** For many of us, this alone is reason enough to embark on a pregnancy exercise regime.

Tips for a safe workout

To keep you and your baby safe while you're exercising:

● Check with your doctor or midwife before starting an exercise programme.

● Wear loose-fitting, breathable clothing and supportive shoes, and make sure your maternity bra is doing its job.

● Warm up before exercising to avoid straining your ligaments.

● Keep moving – standing motionless can cause blood to pool in your legs, making you dizzy.

● Drink lots of water before, during, and after exercising – to make sure you don't become dehydrated.

● Don't do deep knee bends, lunges, or full sit-ups in case of ligament strain.

● Avoid overdoing it – slow down if you can't comfortably carry on a conversation.

● If you feel uncomfortable or are in pain, stop immediately. You're working your body, not punishing it.

● Avoid exercising while flat on your back after the first trimester – besides being uncomfortable, this position can affect the blood flow to your uterus.

● Get up from the floor slowly – getting up quickly can make you dizzy.

● Cool down to give your heart a chance to return gradually to its normal rate.

Swimming is a great exercise during pregnancy. You get a cardiovascular workout while the water supports your body weight.

Active mum

If you've always exercised, it should be safe to continue your pre-pregnancy exercise routine.

"I've always been heavily into athletics and weight training, so I was so happy to learn that healthy, well-conditioned women who exercised before pregnancy can continue throughout pregnancy without it affecting their baby's health or development. And what was even better, I read that weight-bearing exercise throughout pregnancy can reduce the length of your labour and decrease birth complications. What's not to like about that? So I plan to keep up my exercise routine and I'm looking forward to a shorter labour! It must be better than the marathon I ran last year."

What exercise is safe when you're pregnant?

The following exercises are fairly safe for expectant mothers, although some of them may not work for you during the last few months of your pregnancy. To be safe, do consult your doctor or midwife before embarking on any of these activities.

● **Walking** One of the best cardiovascular exercises for pregnant women, walking keeps you fit without jarring your knees and ankles. It is a safe exercise to do throughout the nine months of pregnancy and can easily be built into your day-to-day schedule.

● **Jogging/Running** Going for a jog is the quickest and most efficient way to work your heart and your body. You can tailor it to your schedule – running 15 minutes one day when that's all you can fit in, and 30 when you have more time.

● **Yoga and stretches** Yoga and stretching can help maintain muscle tone and keep you flexible with little, if any, impact on your joints. Be careful not to overdo it though. You will be more supple as a result of the effects of the hormone relaxin (see p.75), so don't hold the stretches for too long or try to develop your flexibility too much.

● **Swimming** Swimming is ideal because it exercises both large muscle groups (arms and legs), provides good cardiovascular benefits, and allows you to feel blissfully weightless.

● **Aquanatal classes** Exercising while standing in water is gentle on your joints and can help lessen swelling in the legs, which is a common symptom in late pregnancy.

● **Pilates** This can be useful in pregnancy because it targets the tummy and pelvic floor muscles and these muscles can weaken during pregnancy. Many Pilates exercises are performed in a "hands and knees" position. This helps to take a lot of stress off your back and pelvis and, towards the end of your pregnancy, can help to position your baby ready for delivery.

● **Low-impact aerobics** One good thing about joining an aerobics class is that it gives you a consistent time slot when you know you'll do some exercise. If you sign up for a class specifically designed for pregnant women, you'll get to enjoy the camaraderie of others just like you, and can feel reassured that it's safe for you and your baby.

● **Weight training** If weight training is already part of your exercise routine, there's no reason to stop, although you will need to avoid using heavy weights and assuming certain positions.

● **Dance** Dancing will get your heart pumping, but steer clear of dance movements that call for you to leap, jump or twirl, and avoid sudden changes of direction. If you sign up for a class, do tell your instructor you are pregnant.

Relaxation during pregnancy

Pregnancy brings its own stresses, including worries about whether or not your baby is OK, how the birth will go and how your relationship with your partner will change once your baby is born. Discover below why it's important to relax, plus some tips for a chilled-out pregnancy.

Why relaxation is important

Feeling stressed and nervous is not unusual in pregnancy. The odd periods of stress we all experience from time to time do not harm your baby but some experts believe that prolonged, severe stress in early pregnancy can increase your chances of complications, such as pre-eclampsia and premature birth. Research has also shown a link to hyperactivity in pre-school children when the mother had long-term anxiety and stress during pregnancy, so seek help and support if you have a problem.

Talk to your midwife about how you are feeling. Or, if you haven't had your booking appointment yet, see your doctor. They can rule out the possibility that an illness is causing your problems or can arrange for you to see a counsellor if you need to talk through your worries.

Joining a support group in your area might help, too. The National Childbirth Trust (NCT) can put you in touch with other mums-to-be near you and you'll meet new parents-to-be when you start your antenatal classes.

Getting the sleep you crave

Pregnancy often brings with it a multitude of sleep disturbances. To help make your nights more serene, make your bedroom inviting and relaxing, keep it cool and reduce light and noise as much as possible.

When you get home from work, aim to have a leisurely evening meal and do something quiet, such as reading or relaxing in a warm bath. If you have a "to do" list, complete what you can by dinnertime, then leave the rest for the next day so that you have time to unwind before heading for bed. And avoid exercising in the evenings, as exercise too near to bedtime can cut down on deep sleep. If you're troubled by nausea or loo trips at night, see p.199 for some advice on how to avoid these pregnancy problems.

Finally, if you really can't sleep, listen to soothing music or read a magazine until you're drowsy enough to go back to bed. Or you may want to try some self-help – guided imagery, deep breathing, or muscle relaxation.

Stress survival tips

It is best to do all you can to avoid long periods of stress when you are pregnant. These tips show you how:

- Make time to rest.
- Try deep breathing – it really helps.
- Find a friendly ear to talk through your concerns.
- Relax with a massage or reflexology.
- Get clued up about the birth to give you a sense of control.
- Share your relationship worries with friends with young babies.
- Start or finish work earlier to avoid rush hour, or try and work from home a couple of days a week.
- Get your finances in control to avoid worrying about them (see p.21).
- Eat foods that increase your levels of the anti-stress hormone serotonin.
- Treat yourself to the occasional trip to the cinema or weekend break.

If you have trouble sleeping at night take every opportunity for a daytime nap – even if you can only manage it at weekends.

Sideways stretch (left) Place your hands behind your head. Inhale and stretch to the left, keeping your back straight and your elbows back. Repeat on the other side.
Back stretch (above left) Inhale, sit upright and extend your arms to the sides. Exhale and turn your hands upwards in a receiving gesture. Hold for a few minutes.
Groin stretch (above) Sit in front of a chair and bring the soles of your feet together. Lean back onto the seat. Place cushions under your back for support if needed.

Yoga – ideal for relaxation

Yoga combined with a cardiovascular exercise such as walking, can be an ideal way to maintain fitness when you're pregnant, though antenatal yoga classes aren't recommended before 12 weeks of pregnancy. When you stretch or do yoga, you're toning your muscles and limbering up with little, if any, impact on your joints – good news for pregnant women.

Yoga is also great for breathing and relaxation, which can help you adjust to the physical demands of labour, birth and motherhood. One of the first things you learn in a yoga class is how to breathe fully. Yoga breathing techniques require you to take in air slowly through your nose, filling your lungs entirely, and then exhaling completely until your abdomen compresses.

Learning how to do yoga breathing primes you for labour and birth, because it trains you to stay calm when you most need it. When you're afraid – during labour, for example – the body produces adrenaline and shuts down the production of oxytocin, a hormone that makes labour progress. Yoga training will help you fight the urge to tighten up when you feel the pain, and will show you how to breathe, instead.

As with any other exercise in pregnancy, you must always take care. Avoid any movements that involve lying flat on your back, as this decreases blood flow to the uterus. Also avoid movements that over-stretch the abdominal muscles. The pregnancy hormone relaxin, which allows the uterus to expand, also acts on other connective tissue, so you might tear or strain a muscle. If you find you have pain in your back, hips or pelvis, you should modify your postures.

Try to find a specialist pregnancy yoga class. If you choose to go to a general class, tell the teacher that you are pregnant and ask if she is trained to teach pregnant women. To find an antenatal yoga class near you, ask your midwife if there's one in your area, or contact the British Wheel of Yoga.

 Green mum

Massage and aromatherapy are great for helping you to relax when you are expecting.

"I love having a massage even if it's just one from my partner at the end of a long day. I'm definitely going to make time for a few while I'm pregnant. I'm sure my baby will appreciate it too.

In fact, for my birthday my mum gave me a voucher for a treatment at a spa that offers special massages just for women who are pregnant. I'm really looking forward to that. And if they do aromatherapy massage, I might book one of those as well. I've heard that some oils aren't suitable during pregnancy (see p.95), so you need to go to someone who's qualified and knows which oils are OK."

Safety at home

When you're newly pregnant it's natural to be wary of the cleaning products and toiletries you normally use without a second thought. Is it safe to clean the oven now? Can you still use aromatherapy oils? Here's how to keep you and your baby safe around the house.

How safe is my home?

While we usually see them as places of safety, it can feel as though your home is full of potential hazards once you're pregnant. Here are some dos and don'ts:

Cleaning products

In general these are safe. Just make sure you have good ventilation and wear gloves. Avoid cleaning the oven, though, as it's hard to get good ventilation in such a tight space. If any fumes make you feel nauseated, choose products that are environmentally friendlier, such as vinegar and bicarbonate of soda.

Paint

Painting exposes you to many chemicals, but it's difficult to know the exact risks. It's safest to let someone else do any painting, but if you do decide to do it yourself:

- Limit the time you spend doing it.
- Keep the windows open and don't sleep in a newly painted room.
- Wear gloves, long trousers, and a long-sleeved shirt to protect your skin.
- Don't eat or drink where you work: that way you won't accidentally take in any chemicals.

Aerosols and air fresheners

Recent research found that pre-school children whose mothers used aerosols and air fresheners most frequently during pregnancy were more likely to wheeze persistently in early childhood. While the researchers don't recommend chucking out the aerosols and air fresheners just yet, they do recommend:

- Wearing gloves when using indoor aerosol products.
- Reducing your aerosol use.
- Opening windows whenever you are using aerosols.

ParentsAsk...

Is it safe to use cat litter?
Cat faeces can carry the toxoplasmosis parasite, which may harm your developing baby, so experts recommend you avoid emptying the cat litter tray. If you have to do it, wear rubber gloves and wash hands and gloves afterwards.

Are aromatherapy oils safe?
These may be natural, but there are some you shouldn't use while pregnant. Rather than using them in the home, you may want to go to a professional aromatherapist so you can be sure the

oils used are safe (see p.95). Ask around for a personal recommendation for a registered practitioner who is experienced in working with pregnant women.

Are electric blankets safe?
Probably, although some studies show that raising a pregnant woman's body temperature to 38.3°C (101°F) or higher for an extended period can increase the risk for miscarriage or neural tube defects. But it's very unlikely that a heated blanket would elevate your body temperature high enough to endanger your baby.

 Green mum

Safety in pregnancy is an added reason to use "green" household cleaning products.

"I've always played it safe when it comes to cleaning products, but now I'm pregnant I make sure I stick to old-fashioned things – white vinegar for cleaning glass and unblocking showerheads and sinks, lemon juice instead of degreasers and bleach, and bicarbonate of soda for everything from removing stains on the carpet to cleaning the toilet seat."

Can I take that medicine?

If you have, or develop, any of the following conditions during pregnancy, check out whether the over-the-counter or prescribed medicines used to treat them are safe for you and your baby.

- **Headaches and other pains** You'd be lucky to get through pregnancy without a single headache or back pain, but you're limited in your choice of pain relief. Aspirin should be avoided, as it has a blood-thinning effect, and ibuprofen isn't recommended in pregnancy as it may affect your unborn baby and prolong labour. Paracetamol is considered safe as long as you stick to the recommended dosage and only use it occasionally.
- **Acne and spots** Benzoyl peroxide and salicylic acid are the main

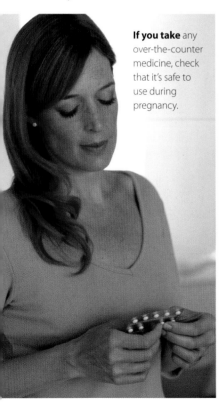

If you take any over-the-counter medicine, check that it's safe to use during pregnancy.

ingredients in over-the-counter spot treatments and these are safe to use in pregnancy. However, if you're taking oral treatments for acne you must be sure that you check with your doctor that these are OK during pregnancy.

- **Asthma** Not only is using asthma inhalers safe during pregnancy, it's recommended to keep your asthma under control. Uncontrolled asthma can result in too little oxygen getting to your baby, increasing the risk for low birthweight and other problems.
- **Colds** Avoid decongestants. Many contain ephedrine, which can raise the blood pressure and should be avoided in pregnancy.
- **Constipation** Laxatives are best avoided in pregnancy. Instead, increase the fibre content of your diet and drink more fluids.
- **Coughs** Speak to your pharmacist before taking a cough medicine, as they tend to contain several different ingredients, some of which aren't recommended in pregnancy.
- **Cystitis** Over-the-counter remedies that contain sodium citrate and sodium bicarbonate aren't normally recommended for use in pregnancy because of their high salt content. See your doctor, who can prescribe a remedy that's safe to use.
- **Diarrhoea** Treatments such as loperamide aren't recommended in pregnancy, but your doctor can prescribe rehydration salts and isotonic drinks, which will replace lost minerals.
- **Eczema** Emollients, plus hydrocortisone cream to calm an occasional flare-up, are safe to use. But if you get a skin infection you'll need to see your doctor, who can prescribe a safe antibiotic.

- **Flu** Check with your pharmacist as many flu remedies contain ingredients, such as codeine, that might not be suitable for you. If you're thinking about having a seasonal or swine flu vaccination, talk to your doctor early.
- **Hayfever and allergies** Speak to your doctor to find out which antihistamine is best to take, as some may raise your blood pressure.
- **Heartburn and indigestion** Try simple remedies first such as drinking a glass of milk or peppermint tea. If this doesn't help, antacids that contain aluminium and magnesium can be taken occasionally. Check with your doctor first.
- **Threadworms** You should always see your doctor for advice as some of the over-the-counter remedies, such as mebendazole, can be harmful if you use them during pregnancy.
- **Thrush** Although anti-fungal creams and pessaries can be used safely in pregnancy, your pharmacist will refer you to your doctor before selling you one. Your doctor needs to check you don't have a more serious infection that could affect your baby, and if you're suffering recurrent thrush, you may need to have a test done to rule out the possibility that you are suffering from gestational diabetes (see p.229). Oral thrush remedies shouldn't be taken in pregnancy.

Fact: An uncontrolled asthma attack is more dangerous to your baby than the risks of taking asthma medication during pregnancy. Uncontrolled asthma can result in your baby getting too little oxygen.

Getting ready for pregnancy

Staying safe and healthy

Your pregnancy diary

Birth and beyond

Safety at work

For most pregnant women, there's no reason why you shouldn't continue working for as long as you are able. But your employer must make sure that the kind of work you do, and your working conditions, won't put your own or your baby's health at risk.

How safe is my workplace?

If your pregnancy is uncomplicated or low-risk, and you work in a safe environment, you can work until close to your due date. Safety regulations protect new and expectant mothers and their babies in the workplace. Employers must be aware of, and if necessary remove, any risks or hazards.

Your rights and choices

Once you have notified your employer in writing that you are pregnant, they are required to:

● Carry out a risk assessment at your place of work.

● Do all that is reasonable to remove or reduce the risks found.

● Give you information on the risks and the protective measures.

● Alter your working conditions or hours of work if the risks still remain, as long as it's reasonable for them to do so. If they can't, or the risk is unavoidable, your employer must offer you a suitable alternative job. If this also isn't possible, your employer must then suspend you on full pay for as long as is necessary to avoid the risks.

If you are refused any of these rights, consult your trade union, a law centre or a Citizens' Advice Bureau (CAB).

Health and safety issues also cover things such as mental and physical fatigue, movements and postures, noise, and travelling. So the risk assessment should include these, too. Your employer must repeat the assessment at different stages of your pregnancy or if your work changes, as what may not be a risk early on might become one later.

Legally, you can work as long as you want it's your choice when to start maternity leave. The only exception is if you are sick with a pregnancy-related illness in the last four weeks before your due date. In this case, your employer can start your maternity leave at once.

Some occupations pose a special risk to you and your unborn baby. Make sure your employer carries out a risk assessment.

 Single mum

If you need to work as long as possible for financial reasons, do ensure that you're safe at work.

"Being a single mum and needing to earn, I'm planning to work for as long as I can – right up until the week my baby's due if possible! I'll have to change my duties at work, though. I often help out in the warehouse and sometimes end up having to lift things. Luckily, my boss has made arrangements for me to remain on desk duties until my maternity leave."

If you do develop complications, talk things over with your doctor. You may be advised to stop if you've previously given birth to more than one premature baby, have either diabetes or high blood pressure, have a history of miscarriage, or are expecting twins.

Towards the end of your pregnancy, you may get tired very quickly, so take it as easy as possible. If you can afford to start your maternity leave a week or two before your due date, you might consider using the time to rest, prepare, and indulge yourself. Remember: this may be the last quality time you have for yourself for a while.

Make sure your workplace is comfortable and that you can take regular breaks. And do accept any help your workmates offer.

Staying comfortable at work

Coping with nausea and vomiting at work can be difficult. If you are prone to vomiting, keep wipes and mouthwash in your desk drawer. If no one knows your news yet, you could come up with a few convincing lines about "food poisoning".

Practical tips

During the first and third trimesters, you may have other symptoms like tiredness and absent-mindedness. It might help you to talk to a colleague who has been through this too and can support you. If there is a working parents' group in your workplace, join it to get some support.

Your pregnancy, though visible, can still be private. You may welcome the interest from colleagues and enjoy the opportunity to talk about your growing baby. On the other hand, you may prefer to keep your pregnancy personal and not to discuss it at work.

To make sure you stay comfortable throughout your working day:

● **Put your feet up** Keep a box or stool under your desk.

● **Wear comfortable shoes** You might try maternity or support tights, too.

● **Dress comfortably.**

● **Seek the support of fellow mothers.**

● **Take breaks** Stand up and stretch if you've been sitting; sit down and raise your feet if you've been standing.

● **Drink a lot** Keep a tall water glass at your desk, and refill it often. (This will also give you a chance to take a break.)

● **Evaluate your office space** Working at a computer won't harm your baby, but pregnant women are more susceptible to carpal tunnel syndrome (numb, achy fingers), so try to make your workplace as comfortable as possible.

● **Rest, rest, rest** Don't over-exert yourself at home or at work.

● **Eat properly** Keep a supply of healthy snacks in your drawer (see p.51).

● **Reduce stress** If you can't eliminate stress at work, find ways to manage it, such as deep-breathing exercises, stretching, or simply taking a short walk.

● **Accept help** If your colleagues offer to help, make the most of it!

(see opposite)

Your rights at work

You have certain rights at work designed to ensure that you and your baby have a healthy pregnancy.

● Ask your employer for a health and safety risk assessment (see opposite).

● If your workplace isn't safe, your employer is legally obliged to offer you alternative work or time off on full pay (see opposite). The same is true if your doctor decides that you have to ease up at work.

● You cannot be dismissed, treated unfairly, or made redundant for any reason connected with pregnancy, childbirth, or maternity leave.

● You have the right to take time off for antenatal appointments if they take place during working hours.

● If you have a strenuous job, discuss it with your doctor. If she thinks you must reduce your activities, your employer is obliged to offer you a suitable alternative or to suspend you on full pay for as long as necessary (see opposite).

● Employers must, if possible, find a suitable place for you to take a break.

Parents**Ask...**

Is it safe to use a computer?

It's impossible to prove that using a computer in pregnancy is 100 per cent safe, but research has so far failed to find any evidence of harm. So you can be pretty confident that it's safe to use a computer while you are pregnant. However, when you do, make sure you look after your general health and comfort. Take regular breaks and adjust your chair and monitor so your forearms are roughly horizontal, your back is well supported and your feet are flat on the floor or a footrest.

Getting ready for pregnancy

Staying safe and healthy

Your pregnancy diary

Birth and beyond

Rights and benefits at work

As a working mum-to-be, you're entitled to extra rights and benefits during pregnancy and beyond. Don't leave it to chance, though. Make sure you swot up on what rights you're entitled to. You also need to know about the money you might be able to claim.

What are my rights?

It's always a nerve-racking moment telling the boss you're pregnant. But it's well worth doing it sooner rather than later. Once you've told your employer, it is against the law for them to dismiss you, treat you unfairly, or make you redundant for any reason connected with pregnancy, childbirth, or maternity leave. It doesn't matter how long you have worked for them or how many hours you work.

Working mum

If you're in paid employment, you must tell your employer you're pregnant by the correct time.

"To be sure I gave my employer the correct notice, I checked things out and found I had to let her know about my pregnancy by the 15th week before the week that my baby was due. You work this out by going to the Sunday before your due date and counting back 15 weeks. I was thrilled to find that I could choose when to start my maternity leave. I wanted to leave it as late as possible to enjoy more time at home with my baby after the birth."

Before taking maternity leave
To take maternity leave you should inform your employer no later than the end of the 15th week before the week your baby is due (called the Notification Week or Qualification Week):
- That you are pregnant.
- The week in which you expect to give birth.
- When you would like your maternity leave to start.

Your employer must then let you know within 28 days the date on which your maternity leave will end.

Maternity leave
If you are a pregnant employee, under British law you are currently entitled to 26 weeks' Ordinary Maternity Leave, (OML) followed by a further 26 weeks' Additional Maternity Leave (AML) – one year in total. As long as you give the correct notice to your employer, you can take this amount of leave regardless of how long you've been working with that employer, how many hours you work or how much you are paid.

You can also choose when you want to start your maternity leave. Usually this can be any date from the beginning of the 11th week before the week the baby is due. Legally, you can change this date as long as you give your employer 28 days' notice.

Antenatal appointments
You should be also able to take time off for your antenatal appointments, including parentcraft and relaxation classes, without loss of pay. After the first appointment, your employer is allowed to ask to see your appointment card as well as a certificate signed by your doctor, midwife, or health visitor saying that you are pregnant.

During maternity leave
Your employer is allowed to make contact with you (and vice versa) while you are on maternity leave, as long as the amount and type of contact is not unreasonable. It can be, for example, to discuss your plans for returning to work or to keep you informed of any important relevant developments at your workplace. Your employer should also keep you informed of any promotion opportunities or job vacancies that arise in your company while you are on leave.

What you can claim

Babies can cost a small fortune, but you may well find that you are eligible for maternity pay or, failing that, for maternity allowance.

Statutory Maternity Pay

Whether you are eligible for Statutory Maternity Pay (SMP) will depend on a variety of factors, such as your length of employment and your salary. To qualify for SMP you must have been:

● Employed by the same employer without a break for at least 26 weeks by the end of the 15th week before the week your baby is due. Part weeks count as full weeks.

● Earning an average of £90 a week (the Lower Earnings Limit for National Insurance Contributions) before tax.

SMP is paid for up to 39 weeks. For the first six weeks you will be paid 90 per cent of your average weekly earnings with no upper limit. For the remaining 33 weeks, you will be paid a standard rate of £117.18 per week or the equivalent of 90 per cent of your average weekly earnings (whichever is lower).

You may find that your company has its own maternity policy, which is better than the legal minimum, outlined above. So your entitlements could differ to those of your colleagues or friends who work for other companies. You should find out exactly what you might be entitled to by contacting:

● The human resources or personnel manager where you work.

● Your trade union representative.
● Your local Jobcentre or your Benefits Agency.

You should also look in your contract of employment to check your company's maternity policy.

Claiming SMP

You must provide your employer with evidence of when your baby is due: maternity certificate MATB1. The earliest that this certificate will be issued by your doctor or midwife is 20 weeks before the week in which your baby is due (around the 21st week of your pregnancy).

You will also need to tell your employer when you want your maternity pay to start. You should do this by the 15th week before your baby is due. You can change your mind but you must still give your employer at least 28 days notice of the new SMP start date.

Maternity Allowance

This benefit is usually awarded to you if you've changed jobs during pregnancy, are self-employed or have been unemployed during pregnancy. If your employer decides you don't qualify for SMP, they will give you form SMP1, explaining why. In this situation, you should be able to get Maternity Allowance by sending your SMP1 to your local Jobcentre Plus/social security office together with your Maternity Allowance (MA) claim form.

Systemised mum

You need to be organised to be sure of claiming all your pregnancy rights and benefits.

"I soon found that there are so many forms and procedures to sort out when you're pregnant that it can be quite confusing. To minimise the stress, I made a list of all the forms I needed and where I could get hold of them. Then I ticked off each one as I went along.

Many of these procedures are kick-started by other people, so I was happy to find that it wasn't as stressful as I feared it was going to be."

Telling your boss you're pregnant may be a bit nerve-racking, but is essential to ensure you get all the maternity benefits available.

Getting ready for pregnancy

Staying safe and healthy

Your pregnancy diary

Birth and beyond

"You should be able to **take time off work** for your antenatal classes, parentcraft and **relaxation classes** without any **loss of pay**."

Environmental hazards

Everyday things can suddenly have you worrying about safety when you are pregnant. We round up some of your most common safety worries so that you can feel clear about what does pose a risk to you and your baby, and what doesn't.

Water filters claim to reduce harmful contaminants such as chlorine and lead in tap water.

Playing safe

You can't be expected to live in a sterile bubble throughout your pregnancy, so start thinking about how to protect your developing baby and minimise the risks of exposure to chemicals and radiation. Talk with your doctor and read the Health and Safety Executive booklet *New and Expectant Mothers at Work*.

Lead and mercury

Various chemicals in our environment can cause birth defects. These are known as "teratogens" and include lead and mercury. How poisonous or harmful a teratogen is depends on different factors, including the amount you're exposed to and when in the pregnancy you are exposed.

You may be exposed to lead if your work or hobbies include ceramics, jewellery-making, print-making, stained glass, electronics, or glassblowing. Lead exposure can also happen during home redecorating if old paint is removed.

The most common way for people to be exposed to mercury is by eating contaminated fish. The highest levels of mercury are found in large fish at the top of the food chain, such as swordfish, shark and marlin.

Insect repellents

Mosquito repellents often use diethyl-3-methyl benzamide (DEET), but little information is available on any harmful effects in pregnancy. A 2001 study carried out in Thailand showed no adverse effects to mother or baby when moderate amounts were used in the second and third trimesters. But because DEET is considered toxic in high doses, it's still recommended that pregnant women either avoid such repellents or use only small amounts.

As a natural alternative try using an oil that contains citronella, as this is considered safe for pregnant women.

Parents**Ask...**

Is it safe to use mobile phones?
The short answer to this question is that mobile phones probably are safe to use in pregnancy. Research suggests that there is no risk to health from mobile phones in the short term, but no one is certain of their long-term effects yet.

Mobiles emit low levels of "non-ionising" electromagnetic radiation as do televisions, computers, and microwave ovens. Experts agree that this radiation is unlikely to harm a developing baby. However, if you want to err on the side of caution, you can reduce your exposure from your mobile phone by keeping your calls short or by sending a text or using a landline instead.

Is it safe to walk through airport screening machines?
The metal detectors in airports use a low-frequency electromagnetic field to look for metal objects. This exposure is considered safe for everyone, including pregnant women. The same holds true for the wands that are sometimes passed over individual passengers.

X-rays

Most diagnostic X-rays (dental X-rays, for example) do not expose your baby to high enough levels of radiation to cause a problem. While fetal exposure over 10 rads (a rad is the unit of measurement for absorbed radiation) may increase the risk of learning disabilities and eye abnormalities, it's rare for a diagnostic X-ray to exceed 5 rads.

Experts still recommend that women postpone getting unnecessary X-rays until after giving birth. However, if your doctor feels X-rays are needed for your particular medical situation, it may ease your mind to know that the amount of radiation your baby receives will most likely be well within the safe range. On the day of the test, make sure the radiographer knows you are pregnant so she can shield you properly.

If your work involves you being around radiation, you should talk to your supervisor about ways to reduce or eliminate your exposure. You may want to discuss the possibility of wearing a special kind of film badge that monitors the amount of radiation you receive. If you're concerned that your employer isn't addressing safety issues, you should contact the Health and Safety Executive, the government agency responsible for overseeing safety in the workplace.

Dry-cleaning chemicals

Worries about dry-cleaning chemicals often stem from research that suggested dry-cleaning machine operators had a higher rate of miscarriage than other women. The risk did not apply to other dry-cleaning workers or to women who had their clothes dry cleaned.

The risk occurs because the organic solvents used in dry cleaning can pass through the placenta. Perchloroethylene (perc), a commonly used dry-cleaning fluid, has also been associated with male fertility problems.

Tetrachloroethylene is another solvent sometimes used in commercial dry cleaning. Several studies have found an association between inhalation of tetrachloroethylene and an increased risk of miscarriage and infertility.

If you're pregnant, you'd be wise to minimise your exposure to organic solvents at work. Ask your employer to change your job for the duration or carry out a risk assessment at your workplace.

 Laid-back mum

Feeling anxious when pregnant is natural, but it helps to find a way to deal with your worries.

"You know what they say about a trouble shared being a trouble halved? Well, my mum reminded me of that when I was worrying about whether or not our baby was going to be healthy after I had a small show. I'm not usually a worrier, but I couldn't help thinking something was horribly wrong or that I was about to have a miscarriage. So I talked about my concerns to Ian and it turns out he was worrying about the same thing.

Once we'd talked about it together, we agreed that the best thing was to go and see our doctor to try to arrange a scan, just to be sure. I know they say that a scan can't detect every possible problem, but they arranged for us to have one within a few days. I must say, just seeing that fuzzy outline of our growing baby on the screen made us feel a whole lot better!"

Parents**Talk...**

"We both decided to cut down on smoking before we started trying for a baby. It was really tough at first. But as soon as we found out I was pregnant, it gave us both a very good reason to stop altogether."
Julia, 34, mum to seven-month-old Zoe

"In the early weeks, I have to admit to having the odd sneaky cigarette when my partner wasn't looking. She'd smell the smoke on me, though. In the end I realised that it wasn't fair to her when she was doing so well at quitting."
Leon, 29, dad to four-month-old Zac

"Quitting smoking was a whole lot easier for me – I found even the smell of it made me feel sick in first three months anyway. And once I'd banned smoking in the house, it was easier for Ben to give up too!"
Hannah, 28, pregnant for the second time

"I knew the risk to the baby of smoking during pregnancy – and we didn't want our baby to be exposed to smoke once he was born, either. There's no better incentive."
Kallie, 29, mum to two-month-old Dan

"Stopping smoking when there's a baby on the way is simply a no-brainer. Giving up was much easier with each other's support."
Frances, 27, mum to month-old Sam

The body beautiful

After the first trimester, lots of women start to "bloom" and enjoy glowing skin, thick shiny hair and strong nails. Others aren't so lucky and find themselves struggling with unmanageable hair and blotchy skin. Here are the changes to expect as the weeks pass.

Your skin, hair and nails

Your appearance changes when you are pregnant, often for the better. However, you may also have to adjust your beauty regime as you cope with niggles related to your skin, hair, nails and teeth.

Your new skin

Glowing skin is one of the great beauty bonuses of being pregnant. However, other, perfectly normal, skin changes may not do as much for your looks. The good news is that they generally clear up soon after your baby is born. Here's an idea of what to expect.

Stretch marks

Thin reddish or brownish (depending on your skin colour) lines of stretch marks usually appear on the abdomen, breasts and thighs. They affect between 75 and 90 per cent of pregnant women and may appear as you put on more weight and cause the skin to stretch. Higher levels of hormones also disrupt your skin's protein balance, making it thinner.

After pregnancy, the pigmentation in the stretch marks gradually fades, and the streaks become lighter than the surrounding skin. This takes time.

Some lucky women have more elastic skin than others, meaning they won't get stretch marks, but for most of us they are simply a fact of pregnancy. Try to minimise them by avoiding putting on weight too quickly, rubbing oil or cream rich in vitamin E over your abdomen to keep it supple, and eating a healthy diet that is rich in vitamins E and C, and in zinc and silica, to help keep your skin healthy. A research review of creams for preventing stretch marks found only one study, based in Spain, which showed creams to be of

---

Real mummy vs yummy mummy

Are you a real mummy or a yummy mummy when it comes to beauty treatments? Read on to find out.

On hair

We: put off going to the hairdresser for fear of scaring him with our wild manes.
She: enjoys a weekly trim and blowdry at a posh salon, reading *Tatler* and *Vogue* while her highlights are touched up.

On pregnancy pampering

We: feel grateful to have 10 minutes of peace in the bathroom with a gossipy magazine and a splash of bubble bath.
She: thinks that "low-maintenance" means going a week without a facial and massage at the country club spa.

On skincare

We: ditch any pretence of having a cleansing, toning and moisturising routine in favour of an extra 10 minutes in our cosy bed.
She: is soooo inspired by her fabulous "glow" that she dreams up her very own skincare range and pitches it to an upmarket skincare manufacturer.

Keep the skin of your abdomen supple and reduce stretch marks by rubbing with a cream or oil that is rich in vitamin E.

Parents Talk...

"With my second pregnancy, the hair on one side of my head, just above my ear, started to go curly! After having my second baby, I had my hair cut shorter, hoping that would calm it. But that just made it worse and curly all over! I've finally found a hairdresser that can make it straight, so I'm off to buy some hair straighteners!"
Claire, 35, mum to Mabel and Joelly

"I had problems with my hair. Imagine already having thick hair – and it just getting thicker and thicker! It was also really dry and I looked awful. I kept getting it cut but it didn't make any difference. Not long after having my baby my hair returned to normal and I got it thinned."
Amy, 29, mum to six-month-old Laura

"My hair with my first baby was great! My sister-in-law decided she'd update my look halfway through my pregnancy, and gave me a great crop, a la Posh Spice (short and spiky). But as my bump grew bigger, I looked like a weeble, with a tiny pea-head on top!"
Mel, 34, mum to Lucy and Freddie

benefit. This involved massaging with a cream called Trofolastin, containing the active ingredients centella asiatica extract, alpha tocopherol (vitamin E) and collagen-elastin hydrolysates. This cream is currently unavailable in the UK.

Chloasma

Also known as the "mask of pregnancy", chloasma is the appearance of brown patches of pigment on the neck, cheeks, and forehead. Darker-skinned women have lighter patches. They are caused by the increased production of melanin, the tanning hormone that protects the skin against ultraviolet light.

Exposure to sunlight will darken the patches, making them more obvious, so protect your skin with a high-factor sunscreen (SPF15 or more) and a hat when you go out (see pp.96–7). Sunlight will also make it more likely to reoccur with any subsequent pregnancies. If you feel that the patches look unsightly, use

a tinted foundation to blend them with your skin. They will begin to fade within three months of your baby's birth.

Linea nigra

A dark, vertical line, up to 1cm (½in) wide, appears down the middle of your stomach, often crossing the navel. This is the linea nigra and it tends to appear around the second trimester. It is caused by changes in the skin pigment where your abdominal muscles stretch and slightly separate to accommodate your baby as it grows. The line may darken in sunlight, so you should use a high-factor sun lotion (SPF15 or more) or avoid the sun completely, especially during the hottest part of the day. The line will fade within a few weeks of your baby's birth, although it may need a gentle rub to remove any dry skin. Other areas with pigmentation – such as your nipples, moles and freckles – may darken too, but these will also fade.

Glowing skin

The "bloom" or "glow" of pregnancy is not just a saying. Your skin retains more moisture during pregnancy, which plumps it up, smoothing out any fine lines and wrinkles that you may have. The pinkish glow that makes you look radiant is due to increased amounts of blood in your body. This may make you feel slightly flushed sometimes.

Another downside is that you may look a little bit puffy from water retention and, unfortunately, any red patches that you already have on your face may become more visible.

The solution is not to cut down on drinking water to counteract the fluid retention – your body needs fluids – but to rest as much as you can. Any red patches will calm down once you've given birth, but meanwhile if you want to hide them, you could try using a tinted moisturising foundation.

ParentsTalk...

"I use a commercially available oil for stretch marks and soak in a baby oil bath every night."
Emma, 25, mum-to-be

"I didn't use anything more special than an ordinary baby oil. Listen to your body and take note of areas of skin that are getting a bit tight, then moisturise those parts – several times in a day if you can manage it. Making sure that the skin is elastic will help."
Phoebe, 29, mum to month-old Jake

"I've heard and read that drinking plenty of water is good for preventing stretch marks. I certainly plan to give it a try."
Jenny, 26, mum-to-be

"My stretch marks didn't show until the end of my pregnancy. I used cocoa butter on my hips and belly twice a day, which may have helped, but personally I wouldn't worry about them too much. They fade eventually."
Safa, mum to nine-month old Josh

Spider veins

Small, thin veins that lie close to the surface of the skin may become more noticeable in pregnancy. They tend to run in families and, sadly, don't usually go away after the birth. They can be just faint red lines or else develop as a circle rather like a spider's web, hence the name spider veins. The good news is they aren't harmful, and are reasonably easy to cover with make up.

Laser treatment can successfully remove spider veins in the legs – but you shouldn't have this done when you're pregnant. Some complementary therapists say that eating a diet rich in vitamin C will help strengthen capillaries, and that taking extra vitamin E might help, too. However, no studies support either of these suggestions.

Acne in pregnancy

Pregnancy can sometimes trigger acne, which many of us have not experienced since being a teenager. Higher levels of certain hormones can encourage the production of sebum – the oil that keeps our skin supple – and too much sebum causes pores to become blocked, resulting in greasy skin and spots.

Cleanse your facial skin regularly with a gentle cleanser and use an oil-free moisturiser. If you prefer to avoid using skin products, keep your skin fresh and clean by patting it dry rather than rubbing, so that you minimise the irritation to the acne.

Don't use acne creams or treatments unless your doctor advises you to do so – some of them cannot be used during pregnancy. A few weeks after your baby is born, your skin should return to its pre-pregnancy condition.

Oral medications containing retinoic acid (Roaccutane) are used for treating severe acne. Roaccutane is one drug that is definitely not safe to take during

Your hair may look better than ever now that you're pregnant. Pregnancy hormones help to reduce the rate of hair loss.

pregnancy because it's known to cause birth defects. Experts associate it with an increased incidence of miscarriage. Topical treatments containing tretinoin are also not safe for use in pregnancy.

Your hair

During the second trimester, you might notice that your hair looks super healthy and full. This isn't because you are growing more but because, thanks to the pregnancy hormones, you're just losing less.

Some women worry about using hair dyes in pregnancy. The chemicals in both permanent and semi-permanent hair dyes have been around a long time. No research shows they harm unborn babies, so colouring your hair during pregnancy is probably safe.

If you apply the dyes safely (using gloves in a well-ventilated room, and not leaving solutions on for long periods of time), you don't absorb much of the chemicals into your system. However, you may like to wait until after the first trimester, just to be on the safe side.

Another option is highlighting, painting, or frosting your hair. You absorb hair colouring agents into your system through your skin (scalp), not through your hair shaft. So any process that puts less of the chemical in contact with your scalp reduces your exposure to the compounds in dyes.

Vegetable hair dyes are another alternative to chemical dyes when you are pregnant. However, many of these dyes also contain some of the same synthetic chemical compounds that the major cosmetic companies put in their permanent and semi-permanent dyes. Pure henna, a semi-permanent vegetable dye that is available in a number of colours, is the exception. This dye is considered to be very safe.

If you like to use an eyelash or eyebrow tint, have a patch test to test for sensitivity, even if you've had the treatment before without a problem.

Once your due date is approaching, it's a nice idea to book yourself in for a consultation and cut with a really good stylist. You'll be starring in lots of photos alongside your baby over the next few weeks, and there won't be time to have your hair done once she's born. Your stylist will be able to help you find a lower-maintenance style that will see you right through those first few weeks of living with your baby.

Your nails

Around the fourth month, your nails may start to grow faster than usual. This is due to the effects of pregnancy hormones. Your fingernails may become softer or more brittle than usual, and you may notice tiny grooves forming along the base of the nail. Don't worry; they should return to normal within a few months after giving birth.

Pregnancy hormones can make your fingernails more brittle, so always file them gently to prevent them breaking.

Handy make-up camouflage tips

Pregnant women are beautiful, but their skin can also become blotchy, prone to acne, and dry or oily. You don't have to grin and bear it, though, thanks to the wonders of make-up.

● Adjust your skincare regime. Add more moisture to combat dryness or change to oil-free products if your skin is feeling greasy.

● Apply corrective concealer with a brush to cover hyper-pigmentation. Then lightly spread foundation or tinted moisturiser over the whole of your face.

● When you're lacking a healthy glow apply a pretty shade of blusher or a light touch of bronzer over your face.

● If your eyelashes appear a little sparse, invest in a good pair of eyelash curlers. Finish by applying lots of lengthening and thickening mascara.

● Apply a shimmery highlighter over your cheek- and brow-bones for an extra sparkle.

● Keep your beauty routine simple – you'll need it for when you don't have so much time to beautify!

Your dental health

Gum problems are a common concern in pregnancy. You may find that your gums bleed when you brush or floss them. This is because the hormone progesterone softens your gums and your increased blood supply makes them more likely to react to the bacteria in the plaque that forms on your teeth.

Take good care of your teeth in pregnancy, partly to avoid bleeding gums (gingivitis) developing into a more serious condition called periodontitis. One study has shown that infection can progress from your gums into your teeth and jaw bones, and may possibly cause premature labour in some mothers.

Brush your teeth thoroughly but gently. If you brush them too vigorously you can damage your fragile gums. Make sure you brush your teeth at least twice a day. You could try to brush after every meal, preferably within 20 minutes of eating or drinking anything, but this is not essential. Use a brush with soft bristles or, better still, an electric or battery-operated toothbrush. Use fluoride toothpaste, and floss at least once a day. Eat a well balanced diet and avoid fizzy or sugary drinks.

Remember that dental care is free for pregnant women and until your baby is one year old, so take advantage of this.

Getting ready for pregnancy

Staying safe and healthy

Your pregnancy diary

Birth and beyond

Pregnancy weight gain

Piling on the pounds during pregnancy is difficult for the body-conscious among us, but it's a sign that your pregnancy is progressing well. Too much weight gain, though, isn't good either for you or your baby, so try not to indulge too often in comforting sugary snacks.

Don't pile on the pounds

First and foremost, it is important to accept that you are going to put on weight during pregnancy! You are meant to because your body is growing and changing to give your baby the best possible start in life.

By the end of pregnancy you will weigh about 11kg (24¼lb) more than you did before you became pregnant. This is an average weight gain but, of course, you're not an average woman. The amount of weight you should gain will depend on how heavy you were before you became pregnant. Or, more accurately, on what your body mass index (BMI) was.

It's now recommended that your midwife calculates your BMI when you have your booking appointment. In order to calculate your BMI, your midwife needs to know how tall you are in metres and how heavy you are in kilograms. If you would like to have a go at doing it yourself, here's how it's done:
1. Multiply your height in metres by your height in metres. If you are 5 feet 3 inches, your height in metres is 1.6m. So multiply 1.6 by 1.6 which gives you 2.56.
2. Then divide your weight in kilograms (kg) by this figure. So, if you weigh 60kg, your BMI is 60 divided by 2.56 = 23.43.

Here's how your BMI is classified:
BMI less than 18.5 – Underweight
BMI 18.5 to 25 – Ideal
BMI 25 to 30 – Overweight
BMI 30 to 40 – Obese
BMI greater than 40 – Severely obese

What makes up your pregnancy weight gain

Your weight at the end of pregnancy compared to what it was before you became pregnant is considerable. Here's where the extra weight comes from:
● At birth, your baby will weigh approximately 3.3kg (7¼lb).
● During pregnancy, the muscle layer of your womb (uterus) grows dramatically and weighs an extra 0.9kg (2lb).
● The placenta (afterbirth), which keeps your baby nourished, weighs around 0.6kg (1¼lb).
● Your blood volume increases and weighs an extra 1.2kg (2¾lb).
● Your breasts are busy creating milk-producing tissue and, at birth, will weigh an extra 0.4kg (¾lb).
● You have extra fluid in your body, and amniotic fluid around the baby, weighing 2.6kg (5¾lb).
● Plus, you will lay down some fat during your pregnancy to provide you with extra energy for breastfeeding. This comes to about 2.5kg (5½lb).

These are only average figures. The actual amount of weight you should gain will depend on how heavy you were before you became pregnant. Your age, race and height will also influence how your body will change over the next nine months.

This chart shows at what stage of your pregnancy you will put on weight, and what percentage of your total pregnancy weight gain should occur when.

Accept that you will gain weight during pregnancy, but eat a healthy, well-balanced diet to protect yourself and your baby.

ParentsTalk...

"I think the reason I was getting so depressed was because so much of my sense of identity lay in my self image. I really had to pull myself together and realise that the first of my many sacrifices as a parent had to be my figure for a few months. It's worth it for a baby. I'm now trying to just stay healthy rather than slim by going swimming twice a week to keep my fitness levels up."
Kate, 25, mum to two-month-old Bea

"One thing that drives me mad is when you see someone that you haven't seen for a while and the first thing they say is, 'Wow, you're massive'. Like I hadn't noticed! I feel like saying, 'I do have another person growing inside of me you know. What's your excuse?'"
Emma, first-time mum-to-be

"I knew I was overeating early in my pregnancy so I started walking, swimming and basically doing whatever I could to keep active. I've come to accept the weight gain and now I simply plan to get back to my normal weight within a year after the birth. I am sure I can do it!"
Polly, mum to four-month-old Daisy

In the 1990s, the Institute of Medicine in the United States recommended that women should aim for a weight gain that is related to their BMI before they became pregnant:

- If your BMI was less than 19.8, you should aim for a weight gain of between 12.5 and 18kg (28 to 40lb).
- If your BMI was between 19.8 and 26, you should aim for a weight gain of 11.5 to 16kg (25 to 35lb).
- If your BMI was above 26, you should aim for a weight gain of 7 to 11.5kg (15½ to 25lb).

The 1-2-3 rule summarises this in a way that is easy to understand:
- If you were overweight before you became pregnant, you should aim for a weight gain of around one stone (6.3kg).
- If you were a normal weight, you should aim for a weight gain of around two stone (12.7kg).
- If you were underweight, you should aim for a gain of around three stone (19kg).

If you were younger than 20 years old when you became pregnant, you should aim for a weight gain at the top end of the range for your pre-pregnancy BMI.

Limiting your weight gain
UK doctors agree that women with a high pre-pregnancy BMI should try to limit their weight gain. Putting on a lot of weight could increase your risk of getting high blood pressure (see pp.229–30), gestational diabetes (see p.229) and having a big baby.

Don't try to diet, though. Research shows that, for a pregnant woman who is overweight – or who has put on a lot of weight in the first half of pregnancy – a low-calorie diet does not reduce your chances of developing high blood pressure or pre-eclampsia.

Instead, get some advice from your midwife or doctor about how to eat a sensible, nourishing diet that doesn't pile on the pounds, but which still keeps you and your baby happy and healthy. It's far better to stick to a normal, well-balanced diet (see pp.120–21, 148–9 and 182–3) and just cut out things

such as biscuits, sweets and ice-cream, which are loaded with calories and are low on nutritional value. All you really need to do is to eat sensibly, bearing in mind that a pregnant woman needs approximately 2,500 calories a day.

If you are underweight, you risk having a small baby and small babies sometimes have lots of problems. If you are already pregnant, do speak to your midwife, doctor or practice nurse, and ask them for advice on the best diet for you and your baby.

In 2002, the American Association for Cancer Research reported a study showing that women who put on a lot of weight during pregnancy and don't lose it again afterwards are at increased risk of developing breast cancer after the menopause. Experts recommend that women should pay attention to their lifestyle during pregnancy and especially to taking regular exercise. They also recommend women try to lose any excess "baby weight" after having their baby and before the menopause.

Getting ready for pregnancy

Staying safe and healthy

Your pregnancy diary

Birth and beyond

Hormones in pregnancy

Hormones play a vital role in maintaining your pregnancy and kickstarting labour. From telling your body that pregnancy has begun, to relaxing ligaments so that your baby can pass through the birth canal, here's how your body's chemical messengers do their amazing job.

What do the hormones do?

Hormones are substances formed in our body and carried in the blood to other parts of the body to make them perform specific tasks. They are vital in pregnancy, creating a variety of physical and mental effects. We blame everything from mood swings to swollen ankles and varicose veins on "hormones", but which hormones are responsible and what do they do?

Human chorionic gonadotrophin (hCG)

Your body makes large amounts of the hormone hCG in early pregnancy (see p.36). This hormone plays a key part in your baby's development, makes your periods stop and maintains the high levels of progesterone that are needed for a healthy pregnancy.

It is also thought that hCG is the hormone that is responsible for nausea and vomiting.

Fact: Around 8 out of 10 women feel sick in pregnancy, and about half actually vomit. The cause is unknown, but it's thought to be connected to the hormone hCG. Other hormones, such as oestrogen and thyroxine, are also thought to be responsible.

Human placental lactogen (hPL)

Made by the placenta, this hormone may help to prepare your breasts for breastfeeding. The hormone hPL also ensures your body uses less glucose, which leaves more for your baby. This hormone can block the action of insulin in your body. Your pancreas usually creates more insulin to compensate, but occasionally it doesn't, which can result in gestational diabetes (see p.229).

Oestrogen

Your oestrogen levels increase tenfold during pregnancy. Among other effects, oestrogen ensures that the uterus can receive and maintain a fertilised egg. High levels mean that some women find their skin improves during pregnancy. Oestrogen makes your breasts swell and makes your vagina extra sensitive. It also makes your blood clot more easily. Obstetric cholestasis (see pp.230–31) is a rare condition related to a liver problem. It's believed to be associated with high levels of oestrogen.

Progesterone

When you become pregnant your ovaries produce more progesterone, which helps keep the lining of your uterus thick for implantation of the fertilised egg. Later, the placenta produces progesterone, which causes your blood vessels to relax or soften. This can make your gums swell and become inflamed, which leads to frequent, easy bleeding, especially when you floss or brush.

Progesterone also swells your nasal passages, can lead to varicose veins, and may raise your core body temperature, so you feel hot. It can also affect your gut, causing bloating, indigestion, heartburn and constipation.

Both progesterone and oestrogen are thought to be partly responsible for

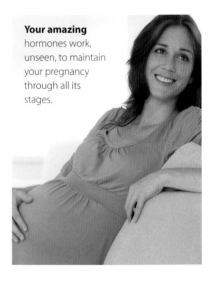

Your amazing hormones work, unseen, to maintain your pregnancy through all its stages.

pregnancy mood swings, but general stress and tiredness, coupled with the fact that you're going through a major life change – also play a large part.

Relaxin

During pregnancy you produce a hormone called relaxin, which softens your ligaments, allowing the joints in your pelvis to open so your baby can be born. Sometimes, however, relaxin can cause problems where the joints open up too far, and become unstable, causing back and pelvic pain. Higher levels of relaxin in your body can also make you more prone to injury, which is why it's not a good idea to start a strict exercise regime when you're pregnant.

Melanocyte stimulating hormone (MSH)

This hormone, together with oestrogen and progesterone, is responsible for some skin changes during pregnancy. For example, it produces the linea nigra, a dark, vertical line down the middle of your stomach (see p.69). The line usually appears around the second trimester where your abdominal muscles stretch and separate a little, to make room for your growing baby. The line fades within a few weeks of your baby's birth.

MSH may also affect pigmented areas, such as freckles, nipples and moles, which may darken. You may also get chloasma, the "mask of pregnancy" (see p.69). This is brown patches of pigmentation that appear on your forehead, cheeks, and neck. All these conditions usually fade a few months after your baby is born.

Oxytocin and endorphins

Oxytocin and endorphin levels rise in pregnancy. These hormones help us to feel happy, and help us deal with stress and pain. They rise sharply during labour – preparing you for birth. Oxytocin triggers contractions and stimulates the flow of breastmilk.

Hormonal changes

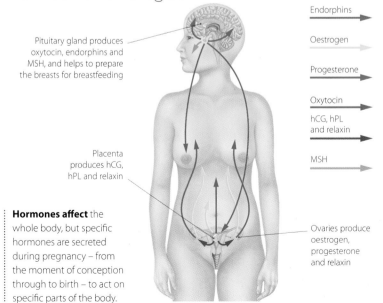

Pituitary gland produces oxytocin, endorphins and MSH, and helps to prepare the breasts for breastfeeding

Placenta produces hCG, hPL and relaxin

Ovaries produce oestrogen, progesterone and relaxin

Endorphins

Oestrogen

Progesterone

Oxytocin

hCG, hPL and relaxin

MSH

Hormones affect the whole body, but specific hormones are secreted during pregnancy – from the moment of conception through to birth – to act on specific parts of the body.

Getting ready for pregnancy

Staying safe and healthy

Your pregnancy diary

Birth and beyond

Staying positive

You've taken the pregnancy test and shared the good news with everyone. They all say, "Congratulations! You must be so happy." Yes, you are glad you're expecting, but you're downright unhappy sometimes. Don't worry – these ups and downs are a very normal part of pregnancy.

Emotions and mood swings

Are you fine one minute and in tears the next? Welcome to the club – it's quite common to have major fluctuations in your emotions during pregnancy.

Progesterone and oestrogen, the hormones that regulate the reproductive cycle (see pp.28–9), are thought to be partly responsible, but much of your moodiness is simply because pregnancy is a time of tremendous change. You may be overjoyed at the thought of having a baby one day, then just as quickly begin wondering what on earth it is that you've got yourself into.

Even when a baby is very much wanted, many ecstatic mothers-to-be find that concerns about the future momentarily cloud their happiness. You may be worried about how your relationship will be affected, the health of the baby you're carrying and how you'll handle future financial challenges. Some of the minor problems of pregnancy, such as heartburn, fatigue and frequent urination, can also be a burden.

You may also find that your dreams seem more bizarre than usual, filled with images of sex, talking animals, and huge, towering buildings for example. This is completely normal. Such dreams may provide a way for your subconscious to deal with any fears and insecurities you may have about pregnancy and motherhood. Or they may just be sleep disturbances caused by indigestion, hormones, or aches and pains.

For a few women, pregnancy mood swings can turn into depression. You're more vulnerable if there are aspects of your life that aren't going well. For instance, you are more likely to suffer from depression if you aren't getting along well with your partner, or you don't have a partner living with you. If you feel you may have depression, do speak to your doctor or midwife.

Pregnancy is a life-changing experience so it's perfectly normal for you to feel up some days and down on others.

Single mum

Being a mum on your own is a real challenge, so you need to find ways to stay upbeat.

"There are days when I wonder what the hell I'm doing and others when I'm so happy that I'm pregnant. Maybe I would be like this even if I wasn't on my own but I'm sure it's making the worry worse. I try to keep busy and I've started writing my worries down. It helps to stop me from going over the same thoughts again and again. Then when I've written it down I put it away and get on with something else.

My main worry is that my little girl will grow up not having a daddy or a name on her birth certificate. My doctor offered to sign me off from work for a week but I think that would make me feel even more isolated."

Managing your mood swings

Mood swings tend to be most pronounced in the first 12 weeks of pregnancy. However, they should gradually diminish as you sort things out and as your body adapts to the hormonal onslaught.

If you're down in the dumps, do something that makes you feel good. Take a nap, go for a walk or see a film with a friend. Talk through your feelings with your partner, friends and family or, if you prefer, with your midwife or doctor. Talk therapy is one of the best antidotes. Don't be hard on yourself. Pregnancy is a life-changing event. It's bound to make anyone – even a mum who's wanted a baby for years – feel overwhelmed and anxious sometimes.

Talking to a good friend about your anxieties can help you deal with them.

If you feel like your mood swings are more than run-of-the-mill, it may be a good idea for you to see a counsellor. About 10 per cent of expectant women battle mild to moderate depression throughout their pregnancies. If you often or consistently feel blue, you may fall into this category.

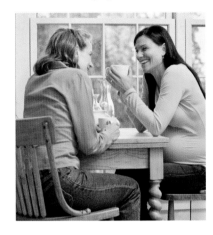

Dad's **Diary**

More than baby blues

"My wife had postnatal depression after our first son was born. Sarah had enjoyed her pregnancy – and was so excited about becoming a mum. But after we brought Harry home, she got anxious and irritable. She'd cry over the slightest problem. We'd read about the baby blues and thought that, with some rest and time, she'd be soon be back to normal. But things only got worse. It took a while to convince her that she needed help. I don't think she would have gone if I hadn't offered to go with her. The doctor prescribed some drugs and I took a couple of weeks off to help look after Harry, do housework, and just generally be there for her. That helped her – and it helped me feel like I could actually do something to support her."

Need professional help?

Pregnancy is usually a positive time, but not for every woman. About one in 10 women suffers from bouts of depression during pregnancy.

There isn't a simple set of symptoms which add up to depression; it varies from person to person. Some people have a low mood all the time, others feel irritable and tearful, or feel useless and want to withdraw from life. Possible triggers for depression include:

- stressful life events
- low income
- problems with the pregnancy
- complications that you've had in a previous pregnancy
- infertility or previous pregnancy loss
- abuse – past or present
- having a family or personal history of depression

To ward off antenatal depression, or to manage it once you have it:

- **Take it easy** Read a book, have breakfast in bed, or meet up with a friend. Don't feel guilty: taking care of yourself is an essential part of taking care of your baby.
- **Get active** Exercise can help lift your mood and is a recognised therapy for mild and moderate depression.
- **Talk it out** Keep the lines of communication between you and your partner free and clear.
- **Consider therapy or counselling** If you've tried everything for two weeks to snap yourself out of a low spell, but nothing seems to work, seeing a therapist or a counsellor may help. You should talk to your doctor or midwife about this.

Knowing when you need help

These are just some of the symptoms that you may have if you're suffering from depression:

- inability to concentrate
- anxiety
- extreme irritability
- sleep problems
- extreme or unending fatigue
- a desire to eat all the time or not wanting to eat at all
- a sense that nothing feels enjoyable or fun any more
- difficulty making decisions
- persistent sadness

If you're feeling suicidal, or disoriented, unable to handle your daily responsibilities, or if you're having panic attacks, talk to your doctor or midwife immediately.

Getting ready for pregnancy

Staying safe and healthy

Your pregnancy diary

Birth and beyond

First-time parents

If this is your first baby, no doubt you're incredibly excited, but also a little nervous. Try to relax and enjoy your pregnancy. Your midwife is there to support you throughout and you can learn everything you need to know about giving birth at your local antenatal classes.

Your antenatal classes

For first-time parents, pregnancy, and the arrival of your baby, is a giant step into the unknown. Antenatal classes can help. They come in various forms, but all have the same aim – to help prepare you for labour, birth, and early parenthood. Those run by midwives or at your local hospital don't cost anything, but you may have to pay for others, such as those run by the NCT.

You may find it helpful to go to more than one type of class. Just remember when attending classes other than those run by your hospital or health centre to check that the teacher is properly trained.

Antenatal classes not only help you focus on your pregnancy and forthcoming labour and birth, but they're a great place to meet other parents-to-be. After everyone's births, you'll have a ready-made network of friends whose babies are the same age as yours.

Your midwife or doctor can tell you about the free classes in your area. These are usually run by midwives with some input from health visitors and physiotherapists. They can vary considerably – for example, they may be between three and six sessions of different lengths in the afternoon or evening, or the course might take place over a weekend. They can get very booked up so ask about them early on.

The classes should include some of the following:
- Information about the process of labour and childbirth.
- What-to-expect details of medical procedures and interventions.
- Advice on relaxation techniques.
- The opportunity to learn about and experiment with different birth positions.
- A guide to pain relief choices.
- The chance to learn and try out massage skills and breathing techniques.
- Time to ask questions and to rehearse the variety of decisions you may have to make during labour.
- Some indication of the changes you might experience after the birth and in early parenthood.

Classes may include a tour around the labour suite of your hospital. This gives you the chance to get familiar with the layout and to find out how things are done there.

Whatever class you decide to attend, the idea is that both you and your partner will acquire the necessary skills and the confidence you need to make birth and the early days with your baby a positive experience.

Your local antental class will help prepare you for the next few months, and it's a great place to meet other mums-to-be.

ParentsAsk...

How will we ever manage on a single income?

When crunch time comes and that second income vanishes, parents often find it financially easier than they had expected. If you add up the cost of your working wardrobe, commuting, lunches, coffees and more, you'll be amazed at how much you can save. And remember, too, that if you do decide to go back to work after you've had your baby, childcare will probably eat up a large part of your salary.

The challenge of giving up work

Whichever way you do it, babies are expensive. If one of you decides to stay at home you lose one salary or, if you both work and you're not lucky enough to have family or friends caring for your baby, you have to pay for childcare.

But money isn't the only factor when making your decision. In general, modern society encourages mothers to return to work – all your friends may be returning and you may feel pressure to do the same. Yet running a family home and caring for children is far harder work than many other jobs so working may be an attractive option. Around half of all mothers have returned to work by the time their child reaches the age of one.

Decisions about whether to return to work are often made by looking back on our own childhood. It may be that we don't want to give up as much as our mothers gave up for us, or maybe our mother held down a responsible job and wasn't around that much for us.

Flexibility is an issue, too. Some jobs are flexible, while others are more difficult to adapt to family life. If you work in an office, for example, and your company has a rigid approach to overtime and early morning meetings, there's a risk that you will be resented by colleagues if you have to leave at 5pm to pick up your children each day.

For some women there's the need to know that they are financially independent and can continue up the career ladder. Staying on at work can also provide insurance for the future. Although life may be more difficult short term, the long-term prospects are better.

Staying at home with your baby is not always easier than the job you were doing before, so try not to feel pressurised to return to work if you don't want to.

The role of dads

During those early weeks, it can be hard for dads to work out how to get involved. Here are our top tips for being the best possible dad from the word go:

● **Educate yourself** Read all you can on pregnancy and babies. It isn't rocket science, but you've got homework to do.

● **Practise, practise, practise** Learn how to do it just like mum. So get in there and change that dirty nappy, give your baby a bath, and do your best to comfort him when he's grizzly.

● **Take the time** Once you're back at work, make spending time with your baby a regular part of your evening and weekend routine.

● **Step in** It's vital for your baby, and for your partner's sanity, that you take over some of the chores.

● **Stand your ground** If your partner criticises your attempts at helping – which she will, without realising it – gently remind her that you can handle it, as long as she gives you the chance.

● **Be a breastfeeding partner** If your partner is breastfeeding, bring your baby to her for feeds and, once breastfeeding is well established, you could give the occasional bottle of expressed milk. Your partner will be eternally grateful and you'll get some baby-bonding time.

● **Get physical** Fathers interact differently with their baby to mothers: dads' high-energy physical play is the perfect counterpoint to mums' gentler, nurturing care. So don't hesitate to offer a game of airplane, horsey or other time-tested dad-and-baby pastimes.

Dad's **Diary**

Coming to terms with fatherhood

"In the final months of my wife's pregnancy, people would corner me in the lift at work and say things like, 'So, are you enjoying your last days?', as if I had terminal cancer. A lot of people fear parenthood as the death knell of their creative ambitions.

I started compiling a mental list of activities that I'd never done and now would never get around to doing. Joining the foreign legion, joyriding, going on a Club 18–30 holiday, attending a hard house night! I quickly realised that all these things actually sounded rubbish, and I found the idea of dividing my spare time between 'Bear In The Big Blue House' and a box of Lego quite appealing. All those dreams – that best-selling novel! That winning goal in the World Cup final! – time to let go!"

Getting ready for pregnancy

Staying safe and healthy

Your pregnancy diary

Birth and beyond

Meeting other mums *(above)* who have babies the same age as yours can be a social lifesaver during that first year.

Making time for each other *(left)* and involving dad in the care of your baby can help solidify your new family.

Is there life after baby?

Yes! But it won't be the same as the life you have now. You and your baby will be on a round-the-clock cycle of feeding, nappy changing and comforting and there just won't be a moment for anything else. A typical newborn sleeps for between 16 and 20 hours in a 24 hour period, but that will be in bits and pieces throughout the day and it will never feel like enough time to get anything done. As time goes on, and your baby begins to settle into a routine, you should be able to carve a little space for yourself in his days. Until then, it's really important to give yourself time to adjust and don't expect too much of yourself. If you have fed your baby, changed his nappy and cuddled him you will have done enough. So what if you haven't got dressed!

The feeling that your time is not your own is one of the hardest things to get used to when you're a new parent but there are lots of other adjustments to be made, too. You and your partner will have to get used to each other as parents and that can be a difficult process. He may feel jealous of the attention you give to your baby and if you've given up work, even if only temporarily, you may feel jealous of his life outside the home. On the plus side, you will see a whole new side of each other as you grow together as a family.

You may think that having a baby means the end of your social life but that need not necessarily be the case. However, if going out used to mean going for a drink after work you'll find you need to make some new daytime friends. Mums with babies the same age as yours will be a lifeline during your baby's first year and there are lots of classes and activities you will be able to take your baby to. Far from having no

social life you may find that you're busier than ever – even if big nights out are a thing of the past. If you're planning to go back to work when your maternity leave finishes you may find you feel differently after your baby is born. You may want to work part-time or you may decide that you want to embark on a new career altogether. So there is undoubtedly life after having a baby, but perhaps the best approach is to keep an open mind as to what that life will be.

76% of new mums go straight back to work part-time

after their maternity pay runs out, although most new mums are entitled to an extra six months' unpaid leave from their jobs. Of course, whether you take this is up to you.

Avoiding isolation

During those early days with your newborn you can feel quite isolated. Just getting out of the house can be hard enough; the thought of being sociable and making new friends can seem impossible. Don't worry, there are lots of ways of meeting new "mum friends". And the great thing about meeting other new mums is that they know just how you feel.

The first obvious port of call is your health visitor. She can put you in touch with other new mums who live near you. Some health visitors run breastfeeding or postnatal groups where you can chat, ask questions and generally enjoy a bit of company.

Another good source of new friends are mother-and-baby groups. These drop-ins are often run in village or church halls, or in Sure Start Children's Centres. Some have visiting health visitors which gives you an opportunity to get support with any problems you may be having.

Keep an eye open for baby-signing classes, baby music groups and mother-and-baby swimming sessions, as well. Some cinemas now have special mother-and-baby showings of the latest film releases, and lots of libraries do story times for babies and toddlers.

You might also enjoy going to the NCT groups for new mums. Unlike many mother-and-baby drop-ins, you'll need to pay for these, but lots of women make firm friendships through them. If you have any health concerns, such as postnatal depression, the NCT Experiences Register can also put you in contact with other mums who are in the same position.

Getting some help

It can be hard to get the help you need in those first few weeks with a new baby. You feel like you're suddenly trying to juggle 100 things at once, while being the most exhausted you have ever been. Visitors will ask you what they can do to help. Don't be afraid to tell them.

The truth is that your visitors are there to see your baby. Take advantage of this and leave them billing and cooing over your little one while you use the time to take that relaxing bath you've been craving or have a sleep. When visitors phone to say they're on their way, don't dash around putting the kettle on and tidying up. They'll be only too glad to help out with those things when they arrive.

If you know that visitors will be arriving in the next few days, phone them and ask them to stop off at the supermarket on their way over to pick up any shopping that you need. It may feel cheeky asking, but it will be a lifesaver until you feel able to face the scrum at the supermarket yourself.

Even better, put out the word that you would appreciate a few ready-cooked meals. When you're a new mum (or any mum for that matter!), there's nothing better than tucking into a delicious meal that someone else has gone to the trouble of cooking.

If mum is coming to visit, ask her to bring some essential food shopping with her.

Working mum

It's perfectly normal to worry about how having a baby might affect your career.

"I'm still unsure if I'll go back to work after my baby's born. I know I'll definitely take at least six months maternity leave, but I haven't decided whether I'll go back to work part-time, full-time – or at all.

The idea of us living on just one income is something I'm struggling to get my head round, although I'm sure there are lots of savings we can make. If I stay home I'll be doing without my coffee-shop run every day for a start, and we could spend less on holidays.

But it's more than just the money. I've worked very hard to get where I am today and I worry that, if I don't go back to work, it'll take me years to get my next promotion. My company has a fairly child-friendly policy, and I've got the option to go back part-time, but I feel you have to be seen to be totally committed to the job.

I guess I'll have to wait until after the baby is born and see how I feel then."

Getting ready for pregnancy

Staying safe and healthy

Your pregnancy diary

Birth and beyond

Coping with a sibling

Those first weeks with a newborn are always hectic, but even more so if you already have a toddler. Make your new baby's entrance into the world easier by preparing your toddler in advance for her arrival. With luck this will help to keep sibling rivalry at bay.

Encourage any interest your toddler shows in your developing baby. It can help him deal with any jealousy he will feel.

Be prepared

Once you've told your toddler he's going to have a sibling, let him decide how much he wants to talk about it or be involved in the preparations.

He may be curious about what the baby is doing in there: "Is she moving around?". Let him feel the baby kicking once her movements are strong enough. Also consider taking him to an ultrasound scan so he can see the baby. It will help to make it more real for him.

Keep your talk about the new baby light and positive. If you want to explain your tiredness, for example, you could say, "Growing a baby is hard work. I sometimes felt tired when you were growing inside, too". Toddlers like to hear about themselves and learning about any similarities will help him to feel closer to the baby. You can also tell your toddler stories about what he was like when he was a baby. Explain how excited you were when he was born so he understands that he was once the baby who got the special attention.

As you get more focused on the impending labour, your toddler may become clingy, develop new fears and even regress slightly. This is all perfectly

Top tips for coping with more than one

● Prepare as much as possible – for example, cook and freeze meals while you're still pregnant so you will have a supply of nutritious food to see you through the early post-birth days.
● Lower your expectations – it doesn't matter if the dusting doesn't get done, if there are crumbs on the floor or you wear un-ironed clothes.
● Help your toddler feel included – let him play with the baby's things and unwrap presents that arrive for her.
● Regularly reassure your toddler that you love him and that having the new baby hasn't changed your feelings toward him.

Parents**Ask...**

How should I break the news to our toddler?
When you're ready to tell him about the pregnancy, keep the language positive and simple. For example, "There's a baby growing inside Mummy. You are going to have a little sister or brother next year." Perhaps start reading him stories about babies or siblings or talk about his friends and their little siblings.

Can I leave my toddler alone in a room with my new baby?
It's probably sensible to stay nearby in the early weeks in case your baby is the subject of any misplaced attention. If you have to move out of the room where the children are for more than a few moments, encourage your toddler to come and help you, or distract him from the baby by offering him some activity.

Children like to hear stories about when they were smaller. Telling him how you felt when he was in your tummy helps to make him feel closer to your unborn baby.

Systemised mum

Even the most organised mums need some help when they're expecting a second baby.

"We thought we could manage by ourselves when we were having Tom, but when crunch time came, we realised we'd need some help. Mum had said she'd look after Emma when I went into labour, and fortunately she lives nearby, so as soon as I got a few twinges I called her to warn her. We were determined that we should tell Emma about her new brother, so although Mum was busting to break the news, we made sure she didn't. When I gave the word, she brought Emma to see us in hospital. I like to think Tom was a nice surprise!

My best friend Jo was great, too. She made some meals and put them in the freezer while I was in hospital... and she did a quick tidy-up before I got home. That's what friends are for."

normal. Lots of love and affection will help him to regain his confidence, so try to spend as much time as you can with him during these last few weeks before your new baby is born.

Dealing with jealousy

It can be especially hard for a toddler who thinks he's the centre of the universe to welcome a new baby into his home. Desperate to win your attention, he may react by misbehaving, regressing or even by giving his new sibling a few less-than-subtle pinches, prods or smacks.

Rather than scolding him, acknowledge his feelings by saying something like, "I know you wish I wouldn't spend so much time with the baby, but she needs her nappy changed right now. As soon as I've finished we'll read a story together". Set aside time each day to do something just with him, even if it's only a few minutes drawing or playing. If he is aggressive towards the new baby, intervene right away. Tell him plainly that his behaviour is not acceptable and that it's never OK to hurt the baby. It may help you both to give him a time-out until he is calmer.

Blended families

While marriage breakdown is a sad fact of life for many people, one in two divorced parents goes on to remarry or re-partner. When new partners have a baby together it can be difficult for existing children. They often see it as a signal that their parents will never get back together, and might be jealous of the new baby. To make the arrival of a new baby easier:

● You and your partner should tell your children about the new baby together – it's not a good idea to let them find out from anyone else.
● Once everyone knows, spend plenty of time with your children and stepchildren, reassure them that you still love them and that will never change.
● Decide with your partner how to describe the relationship between existing children and the new baby – will they be half-siblings or just siblings?
● Once baby arrives, give your other children opportunities to help care for him and to choose gifts, names and clothes. Don't force them if they're reluctant – they may need more time.
● In the early days, set aside some one-on-one time each day to spend with your children.

Sex in pregnancy

Nausea and tiredness can put a dampener on your love life during the first trimester of pregnancy. But once you're feeling up to it, there's no reason why you and your partner shouldn't enjoy a normal sex life, even when your growing bump starts to get in the way.

It's perfectly safe to have sex when you're pregnant, but your libido – and his – may fluctuate wildly with every stage.

Where's my libido gone?

During pregnancy, sex is even better for some women, not as good for others. Increased blood flow to the pelvic area can cause engorgement of the genitals and heighten the sensation. But the same engorgement gives other women an uncomfortable feeling of fullness after intercourse ends. Sometimes, women find sex painful during pregnancy.

Also, some women feel abdominal cramps during or after intercourse because orgasm can set off a wave of contractions. This may be particularly noticeable in the third trimester. It can be off-putting but give it a few minutes and the tightening of your uterus will ease; just like it does when you have Braxton Hicks contractions.

The big changes in your body are bound to change your sex life. Some women, finally free from worries about conception and contraception, feel sexier than ever. But others are just too tired or nauseated to make love, especially in the first trimester. Some women find that their libido is at a high in the second trimester but, there is always a wide variety in how women feel and how sexually active couples are.

All these feelings and experiences are perfectly normal – every woman is different, and it's just as normal to experience either more or less desire at the various stages of pregnancy.

It's not uncommon for men to feel just as sexually attracted to their partner in the first two trimesters but then to feel less interested in sex in the third trimester. But don't worry: this doesn't mean necessarily that he doesn't find you attractive anymore. Your partner's desire may be dampened by fear that sex can hurt the baby. Or he may be worried about you and your unborn baby's health, feel apprehensive about the burdens of parenthood, or even feel self-conscious about making love in the presence of your unborn child.

Is it safe?
Sex is perfectly safe during a normal pregnancy, and you can keep on making love right up until your waters break if you feel like it. If you're feeling sexy and well enough, having sex during pregnancy may be good for your relationship now and after your baby has arrived. But do check with your doctor or midwife first if you're having any problems, such as a low-lying placenta (placenta praevia) or bleeding, or if you have a history of cervical weakness. There are situations when sex isn't a good idea (see opposite).

Lovemaking in later pregnancy

Desire sometimes wanes in the third trimester as birth, labour and your belly loom large, or you may simply feel unattractive or worried as to whether your partner is satisfied sexually. Yet it is possible to have an active sex life throughout pregnancy.

As your pregnancy progresses, you may find that the missionary position (man on top) is no longer comfortable. You'll need to be inventive. Below are some time-tested positions and tips for making love late in pregnancy:

- **Lie sideways** Lying partly sideways allows your partner to keep most of his weight off your uterus.

- **Use the bed as a prop** Your bump isn't an obstacle if you lie on your back at the side or foot of the bed with your knees bent, and your bottom and feet perched at the edge of the mattress. Your partner can either kneel or stand in front of you.

- **Lie side-by-side in the spoons position** This allows for only shallow penetration. Deep thrusts can become uncomfortable as the months pass.

- **Get on top of your partner** This puts no weight on your abdomen and allows you to control penetration.

- **Enter from a sitting position** This position is another one that keeps the weight off your uterus. Try sitting on your partner's lap as he sits on a (sturdy!) chair.

Have faith – where there's a will, there's a way. With some experimenting, you and your partner are sure to find a technique that works for you.

Although your bump may get in the way when you try making love later in pregnancy, there's no reason why you shouldn't experiment to find a more comfortable position. And don't worry – making love cannot hurt your baby; he's cushioned in his amniotic sac.

When not to have sex during pregnancy

There are some important circumstances in which you may be advised not to have intercourse. These include if you have experienced:

- bleeding
- abdominal pains or cramps
- broken waters
- a history of cervical weakness
- a low-lying placenta after 20 weeks (placenta praevia)

You may also be advised to avoid sex if your partner has genital herpes. If you catch this for the first time when pregnant, there's a risk it could affect your developing baby.

ParentsAsk...

Will sex harm the baby?
Perhaps the most common reason couples cut back on sex during pregnancy is a fear that they'll hurt the baby. If you're concerned about that, you can stop worrying right now. Your baby is safely cushioned in an amniotic fluid-filled sac and, unless you're having very rough sex, you have almost no chance of injuring anyone. There are some important circumstances, however, when you may be advised not to have sex (see above).

Getting ready for pregnancy

Staying safe and healthy

Your pregnancy diary

Birth and beyond

Style, fashion and comfort

You can still look amazing, even though you're pregnant. In fact, having a bump can give extra impact to your outfits – you'll find that you can try different styles to complement your new shape. Here's how to get that special va-va-voom.

A short-term solution to a tight waistband is to loop a rubber band through the buttonhole then loop it around the button.

Green mum

Don't worry – you can still choose organic clothing when you're buying maternity wear.

"I was concerned I wouldn't be able to find maternity wear in organic fabrics, but I was surprised at the amount of choice. I looked online and found lots of companies that sell organic maternity clothes. They're a little bit more expensive than standard maternity wear, but I've made the most of my existing wardrobe– which includes a few items made from bamboo and hemp – and so only need to buy a few essential things."

Stylish at each stage

For the first three months or so, you'll probably be able to wear your usual clothes. You may have to leave the top button undone on your skirts and trousers, but you can hide that by leaving your shirts untucked. When your waistband gets tight, loop a rubber band through the buttonhole and then wrap it around the button. This will provide a crucial extra bit of breathing room.

If your bust grows quickly, opt for loose tops or wear suit jackets open over a T-shirt or shirt to disguise it. You'll also almost certainly need to invest in a few good maternity bras (see pp.92–3).

Pashminas and wraps are great pregnancy accessories. They drape over your bump and distract attention, so you can go sleeveless or wear something low cut, safe in the knowledge that you can cover up. You can find simple, dressy wraps in the accessories area of most department stores.

Mixing and matching

Once you enter the Awkward Zone – that time in your pregnancy when you're a bit big for your normal clothes, but not big enough for proper maternity wear – it can be quite frustrating. You will usually find you can get round this problem with:

● A few pairs of trousers and skirts with elasticated or drawstring waistbands in a size larger than you usually wear. You could ask your larger friends – discreetly! – if they have anything they could lend you for a week or so.
● Low-rise trousers that will sit nicely below your belly.
● A wrap dress that accentuates your curves and accommodates your bump in its various stages of growth.
● Jumpers, cardigans, loose shirts and pretty floaty tops.

Long tops work especially well at this awkward stage, gracefully hiding your growing tummy without drawing attention to it. If you haven't shared your news with your work colleagues yet, dressing in this way might buy you a little more time.

After the word on your pregnancy is out, you may as well make life easier by dressing the part. Now it's time to hit the shops. You could try buying five items of clothing in similar fabrics and complementary shades: trousers, a skirt, a jacket, a dress and a top. If you shop carefully, these can form the basis of your wardrobe over the next few months and you can even mix and match them with a few non-maternity items to ring the changes.

Accessorising

Beads, bangles, bags, ribbons, scarves, shoes – the possibilities are endless. The most basic maternity wardrobe can be brightened up with accessories. Think belts that sit below your bump, colourful beads to cheer up a plain black dress, an armful of trendy bracelets.

You can dress an outfit up or down, and the best thing about accessories is that you'll still be able to wear them after the baby is born, unlike those enormous pants that suddenly remind you of a military parachute. And it doesn't matter how big you get, you'll never outgrow that must-have handbag.

Perfect footwear

The ligaments that control your lower back are softened during pregnancy, so they are more at risk of being stretched and damaged. The problem with high heels is that they alter your posture and put a strain on this already weakened area. This could contribute to lower back pain, which can be severe.

Flat or low-heeled shoes are therefore better for your ligaments. They will ensure that you are more comfortable and will minimise the strain on your back. To compromise, you could spend part of the day in heels and keep a pair of low-heeled shoes in your bag to change into when you get tired.

Shop around for elegant, flatter-heeled shoes that can be worn with lots of outfits. Ballet-style leather pumps look great with skirts, trousers or jeans, but snuggly suede boots are equally versatile. Retro trainers often look smarter than their sporty cousins and are perfect for walks or weekends away.

All in all, it's best to save your high heels for special occasions. Especially as your feet can get wider in pregnancy, so if you have a much-coveted pair of Manolos, they may stretch and not fit you afterwards. The horror!

Top tips for comfortable clothes

Your changing body shape requires some wardrobe changes. These tips cover the essentials for comfort.

- Good underwear is a must. See our advice on choosing maternity bras on p.93. You may be able to keep wearing regular bras, though, but go for fittings throughout your pregnancy to make sure you're wearing the right size.
- Maternity knickers are brilliant because they stretch as your bump grows. Low-slung hipster pants, or even briefs that can fit under your tummy, are other good options.
- When buying maternity jeans, go by the size you were before you became pregnant. These jeans come in many different styles and fits – choose from those that fit over your bump, on it or under it.

Getting ready for pregnancy

Staying safe and healthy

Your pregnancy diary

Birth and beyond

Low-rise trousers (above) work well, sitting either on top of your bump or below it. **Wearing a long cardigan or coat (left)** and leaving it open – weather permitting! – can save you buying a new coat or jacket. And it looks super-stylish, too.

As your centre of gravity changes and the ligaments in your abdominal area stretch, you'll find that high heels can give you backache. Your feet can get wider, too. Invest in a couple of pairs of flat or low-heeled shoes, plimsolls or trainers.

Maternity wear

Tops are a doddle when you're pregnant, but, as your bump grows, trousers and skirts are a bit more of a challenge. Investing in a couple of pairs of maternity trousers, and perhaps a smart maternity suit, will help you look great at home, at work and when you're out for the evening.

What to look for in trousers

You won't find many women's wardrobes that don't have a pair or three of jeans in them, so why should it be any different when you're pregnant? A well-fitting pair of maternity jeans makes an invaluable addition to your wardrobe. Below are a few tips to remember before you buy them:

● Fittings vary from style to style and from brand to brand so do make sure that you try before you buy.

● Buy your normal size jeans, but make sure they are maternity jeans: don't be tempted just to go for a bigger size jean.

● Don't put style over comfort: go for what you will be happy wearing for at least 12 hours a day.

● There are plenty of styles to choose from, not just leg styles (bootcut, straight leg or boyfit, for example) but also the way the style sits over or under your bump.

● Some styles may fit better at different stages of pregnancy, so think about getting two different styles.

● Go for reasonably priced pairs rather than expensive ones. That way you won't feel too guilty if you get only six months' wear out of them.

At work, you may be able to get away with swapping a jacket for a softer cardigan or tunic top, but good work trousers are essential. When shopping for work trousers:

● There is no need to spend a fortune on maternity trousers. Remember, you will only be wearing them for around six months, although if you have more than one child you may be able to wear them for subsequent pregnancies.

● Choose two different colours of trousers to make your pregnancy work wardrobe more versatile.

Buying a pair of proper maternity jeans is best. You won't find a larger size of your normal jeans nearly so comfortable.

 Laid-back mum

You'll have to get yourself a few maternity clothes, but you don't need to spend the earth.

"After weeks and weeks of declaring that I will never spend money on maternity clothes that I'll only wear for a month, I finally had to give in.

All my tops started to roll up so I could feel a breeze on my belly. I sorted through my wardrobe and had to put most of my clothes in a suitcase because nothing fits. Even my baggy tops don't fit over my boobs. A few weeks ago I was able to wear my trousers and not do up the button, but now the zip can't even do up so I've been forced into buying some new clothes.

Having said that, I still don't want to spend a fortune on maternity clothes. Fortunately, there are lots of reasonably priced – and fashionable – ranges on the high street now, and I've even managed to borrow a few items from some of my friends who've had babies recently.

Besides, as the world and his wife keep telling me, I'll probably have to carry on wearing my maternity clothes for some time after the baby's born, so at least I'll get my money's worth."

Maternity clothes on a budget

You deserve to look and feel good throughout your pregnancy. It's not always easy, though, especially when both your clothes and finances are getting tight. Before you dismiss the idea of clothes altogether and head for the nearest tent shop, below are some top tips for looking great on a budget while you're pregnant:

● **Buy basics** Investing in a few "key" items of maternity wear that can be mixed and matched will take you a long way. Try two pairs of well-cut trousers, a plain skirt or dress, a cardigan or jacket, a plain jumper that can be worn over most outfits, two casual tops and a smarter top for special occasions.

● **Throw a clothes-swapping party** Ban all men from your house and invite round your pregnant friends, plus those who are already mums. The latter should have maternity clothes they feel more than happy to part with, and might like to borrow some of your clothes in exchange. The swap does not need to be permanent, and you could turn it into

a fun evening by sharing stories and even playing silly games.

● **Borrow your partner's clothes** If you're just relaxing at home, raid your partner's wardrobe. His shirts and jumpers may well be big enough, and you can save your own clothes for when people will actually see you. The elasticated waist on men's boxer shorts and pyjama bottoms makes them comfortable to wear in bed – and if you can distract your partner's attention for

long enough, his bathrobe might come in handy too.

● **Get online** If you're a fan of internet shopping, the web is a real treasure trove. Some sites offer exchange services for women who no longer want their maternity clothes, while others sell discontinued lines and ex-catalogue clothing for a snip of their original prices. If you're a fan of auctions, go online for a vast selection of maternity wear at very reasonable prices.

> **Try looking in charity shops for clothes** when pregnant. You can find real bargains while also supporting a good cause.

Real mummy vs yummy mummy

There's nothing that separates the real mums from the yummy mums more than their maternity clothing choices.

On jeans
We: squeeze into our trusty old jeans for as long as possible, even though the top button's popped off.
She: dashes to a posh maternity shop for customised top-of-the range jeans.

On maternity shopping
We: pick up the best bargains from the high street.
She: buys a whole new wardrobe and enlists a team of personal shoppers. How else would she carry all the bags?

On shoes
We: squeeze our swollen ankles into some rather large and clumpy flats.

She: is aware that motherhood means making sacrifices – and reduces the 85mm heel on her Jimmy Choos to a highly unglamorous 65mm...

On underwear
We: abandon thongs in fear of losing them somewhere they shouldn't be(!)
She: plans to wear Agent Provocateur on her big night out at the Portland.

Special occasion wear

Being pregnant doesn't mean you can't look gorgeous. Whether you're after the perfect Little(ish) Black Dress, or something floor-length and fabulous, it really is possible for mums-to-be to look fab on a night out.

Evening wear

For evening wear, keep it simple with trousers or a skirt and a pretty top. Not only will you look great but you can mix the separates with the rest of your maternity wardrobe to give you maximum use from them. Also, a pretty top can be a great way to show off that extra cleavage you have!

A wrap dress can adapt to all the different stages of your pregnancy just by loosening the fastening. Wrap dresses can be quite figure hugging, so be prepared to show off your bump. Try using different accessories to make your outfit really special.

A classic empire line dress has been a wardrobe staple for fashionistas for years. Dresses like this that pull in under your bustline then flare out can really

Try a stunning empire line dress for a big night out. If you don't want to splurge for a single occasion, you could consider hiring.

flatter your pregnancy figure. For best effect, look out for one cut on the bias (across the grain of the fabric).

If you don't fancy buying an outfit you are unlikely to get wear out of, look into hiring a dress. This could be a more economical way of looking fabulous on a special occasion.

Wedding day

If you are getting married, it's time to really push the boat out. Your wedding day is one of the most important days of your life and being pregnant doesn't mean you can't still look the part. Look for dresses that have been specifically designed for pregnant women as they are more likely to be flattering for your bump. You can find beautifully simple ones if you are going for a low-key affair, or classic floor-length gowns for something a little bit more dressy. There are also pregnancy wedding dresses for hire if you prefer.

Parents**Talk...**

"There are no shops in my local town that stock extra-large maternity clothes. I can't keep buying the next size up. Even worse, I've just got back from my holidays to find that nothing fits, other than the shorts I took with me. They're not exactly work wear! Help!"
Louise, 27, first-time mum-to-be

"You should try eBay if you don't want to spend loads of money on new clothes. They always have lots of maternity stuff for sale to suit all shapes and sizes."
Jodi, 27, mum to William and Anna

"I'm a larger lady and was mostly able to get away with my normal clothes. I did need something new to wear for a wedding at the end of my pregnancy though. I went to a

high-street shop specialising in big sizes, and bought a lovely skirt and top. I was so pleased."
Vicky, 26, mum to 11-month-old Alexander

"About halfway through my pregnancy, I couldn't fit into any of my normal clothes and couldn't find a single item to buy. The only option left seemed to be an old smock dress that I found stashed at the back of my wardrobe! What would Gok say?"
Rachel, 31, mum to 18-month-old Hugh

"Luckily, I discovered the plus-size maternity ranges at a couple of high-street chain stores. Finding them saved me from the fashion police! I feel almost human again."
Jackie, 30, first-time mum-to-be

Getting ready for pregnancy

Staying safe and healthy

Your pregnancy diary

Birth and beyond

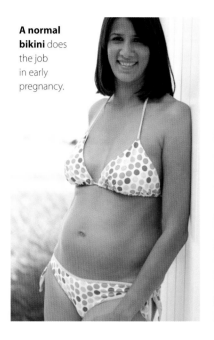

A normal bikini does the job in early pregnancy.

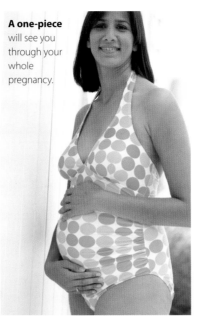

A one-piece will see you through your whole pregnancy.

Active mum

You want sports clothes while you're pregnant? Some ordinary sports clothes adapt well.

"I was disappointed to find that there's not much choice in the shops for sporty pregnant mums, apart from basic stuff like yoga pants and cami tops. So it was a relief to discover that low-slung tracksuit bottoms sat happily under my bump. And they were super-comfortable in the last weeks of my pregnancy. Sports T-shirts with in-built shelf bras helped stop my breasts from taking on a life of their own, too."

Maternity swim wear

Swimming is a great way to stay fit and healthy during pregnancy, so it's definitely worth taking the plunge. If you're planning a last romantic trip before baby arrives, naturally you'll want to look gorgeous on the beach. Normal swimsuits aren't stretchy enough to see you much past your first trimester, so do invest in a maternity swimsuit early on. Below is a list of what's available:

● **The one-piece** Almost always the easiest to find. It's made of a material that stretches as your bump grows, so it can last you your whole pregnancy.

● **The bikini** If the one-piece seems too conservative for you, then why not try a maternity bikini? It allows you to reveal and draw attention to your new cleavage with a supportive, built-in shelf bra, while showing off your bump and legs to boot.

● **The tankini** This is for those who don't like one-piece swimsuits, but feel reluctant to reveal themselves so much in a bikini. Instead of a bikini bra, the tankini comes with a stretchy vest-style top, which will cover most of your bump.

● **The nursing swimsuit** A nursing swimsuit is perfect if you are breastfeeding and want to start swimming with your baby. The clips on the straps let you open and close the drop cups with no fuss. The adjustable straps and shelf bra also make sure that you can stay comfortable and that there's no chance of your breasts making a great escape!

● **The sarong** This is an essential for every woman who feels self-conscious about her bottom, thighs – or any other wobbly bits. Sarongs come in loads of different colours and fabrics and can be wrapped around you at the beach or while you're lazing by the pool. And there's no need to buy a special pregnancy version – one size fits all!

Working mum

In early pregnancy you may well get away with wearing your normal work suit – with a twist!

"I work in PR and need to look smart for meetings with clients and giving presentations. A friend of mine who was pregnant last year gave me a great tip for the office for the first few months of pregnancy. She suggested going for a long-line jacket and wearing it open to cover my bump. Luckily I already had a jacket like that.

Once I began to show, though, I did have to invest in a maternity suit. Some ranges can even be altered to fit. They're expensive, but worth it to make me feel the business. I had a look around, and found quite a few stockists, so they're widely available."

Breasts and bras

A bountiful bust is one of the great things about being pregnant. But your newly expanded bustline needs extra support, so make sure you get measured up for some proper maternity bras. And don't miss our tips for keeping your breasts healthy and comfortable in pregnancy.

Your breasts will change – you'll need one or two maternity bras as soon as your normal bras start to feel uncomfortable.

How your breasts change

Your expanding boobs can be one of the first signs of pregnancy. They'll get bigger and heavier as your pregnancy progresses and, as your breasts have only ligaments and no muscles, they could be stretched if they are not properly supported.

Most mums-to-be experience an expanding bust, and sometimes sore breasts, well before a growing tummy and many outgrow their ordinary bras early in pregnancy. As soon as your normal bra starts to feel uncomfortable you need some maternity bras.

Shopping for a maternity bra?
Look for the following:

● **Support** Look for wide straps, sides, under-bust band and a deep centre at the front. Firm elastic straps eliminate bounce and give you extra support.

● **Coverage** You need as much fabric as possible over the breast area; this will be more comfortable for you as your breasts become more sensitive.

● **Adjustability** A minimum of four rows of back eyes will allow your bra to grow with you.

● **Comfort** Look for bras that are mainly cotton. Many pregnant women find they get hot; cotton lets your skin breathe so you are less likely to sweat.

Make sure you go for professional measuring and fitting either in a store or through a specialist agency whose staff are specially trained to fit women in pregnancy. They can assess your changing shape and size, ensuring you get bras that fit perfectly and give you the support you need. Make sure you get measured every six to eight weeks.

It's especially important to wear a well-fitting, supportive bra if you are planning to exercise since your breasts are heavier during pregnancy. A special exercise bra will give you support and minimise discomfort.

ParentsAsk...

How do I know when I need a new bra?
As soon as your normal bra starts to feel uncomfortable you should start wearing a maternity bra. It's the best way to support your growing breasts.

Are underwires OK?
Some midwives and shops advise against underwired bras, believing that the wire interferes with the natural changes in size and shape of the breast. If you do wear one, make sure the wire doesn't press anywhere on the breast and don't sleep in it.

Will I need a bra at night?
If your breasts become very sensitive, a pregnancy sleep bra – a soft, unrestrictive cotton bra available at maternity clothing stores – will help immensely.

When do I need a feeding bra?
Believe it or not your breasts will get even bigger after the birth, so wait until the last month of your pregnancy, then buy two or three. A good nursing bra needs to be flexible, allowing extra room for when your milk comes in and for when your breasts reduce in size (usually after 12 weeks or so).

Sore breasts

One of the early signs of pregnancy is extremely sensitive, sore breasts. Some women's breasts become so sensitive, in fact, that the sensation of clothing against them is unbearable. This tenderness should get better after the first trimester, once your rising hormone levels have stabilised and your body gets used to them.

A familiar feeling

As your body gears up for the months of pregnancy to come, you produce more of the hormones oestrogen and progesterone, just as you do before each menstrual period. In fact, the tenderness you feel is probably an exaggerated version of how your breasts often feel before your period. Along with the hormone surge, your breasts are beginning to increase in size as the fat layer thickens and you add milk glands and extra blood. These changes, though temporarily uncomfortable, have an important purpose: they're preparing your breasts for feeding your baby.

Though your breasts will continue to grow throughout your pregnancy – it's common to go from a B to a D cup, for example – they'll feel more uncomfortable during your first trimester. The size change is most noticeable in first pregnancies.

Tingling and leaking

You may also notice that your breasts throb or tingle during the initial "excitement" phase of lovemaking. In the first trimester, you may also find that you no longer like having your breasts touched. Any pain or discomfort such as this is likely to subside during your second and third trimesters.

Towards the end of pregnancy, you may also find that your breasts start to leak slightly. This is absolutely normal and nothing to worry about. The leaking is a fluid called colostrum, which is your baby's first milk. This rich, high-protein pre-milk is being produced ready for when your baby is born.

If you're experiencing tenderness, your best bet is to find a good, supportive bra (see opposite). Take the time to get fitted by a specialist, perhaps in a department store or maternity shop. For leakages, you may want to buy some breast pads to put in your bra.

Have a professional fitting for your maternity bras and get yourself re-measured every six to eight weeks as your breasts will keep growing.

Pointers for buying the correct-sized bra

Follow these handy pointers to be sure you buy the right size of bra throughout your pregnancy:

● Make sure the cups fit snugly and smoothly, with no overflow at the top.

● Make sure the centre seam lies comfortably against your breastbone.

● Get fitted more than once during your pregnancy, as you may need to change cup sizes several times as your breasts grow.

● Early in pregnancy, ensure that your bra fastens comfortably on to the first row of eyes, to leave plenty of room for your expanding ribcage.

● Late in pregnancy, buy a bra that fastens comfortably on to one of the last rows of eyes to allow for your imminent reduction in size.

Dad's **Diary**

The breast issue

"As my partner's breasts became larger, it opened up a whole new can of worms. 'Do my boobs look all right?' she'd ask. 'Yes, they look great.' 'But you always told me that you preferred small breasts?' 'No, yours always look great.' 'But are they better when they're big?' 'Err, no. Yes. Whatever.'

Melanie was actually more sensitive about her changing body shape than I was. Even when she'd wail that she was the size of a house and had the belly of a darts champion, I rushed to reassure her that she still looked gorgeous all the time. Why, I'd say, you only have to explore the more extreme titles lurking on the top shelf of any newsagent's to discover just how pregnant women can trigger the strangest carnal impulses in many men…"

Getting ready for pregnancy

Staying safe and healthy

Your pregnancy diary

Birth and beyond

Beauty treatments

If you're a regular at your local beauty salon, the good news is that being pregnant doesn't mean putting your beauty routine on hold. Your skin may be more sensitive, though, so it's wise to use treatments involving inks, electric currents, and creams and lotions with caution.

ParentsAsk...

Is it OK to have a tattoo done while I'm pregnant?

It's not unusual for people having a tattoo to faint or pass out. Most tattooists wouldn't be prepared to take the risk of a pregnant woman fainting. Also, not enough is known about any possible effects that the ink, which may be partly absorbed into the body, may have on your baby. So it's sensible to wait to have a tattoo until after your baby is born.

Is it best for me to take my body piercings out now that I'm pregnant?

That depends on where they are. During pregnancy, your abdomen will expand until eventually your belly button protrudes. At this point you may need to remove your navel ring or swap it for a flexible barbell. When it comes to giving birth, if you have to have a caesarean you will be asked to tape your navel ring or possibly remove it.

You don't need to remove jewellery from pierced nipples during pregnancy unless it begins to feel uncomfortable. However, it will need to come out if you want to breastfeed. Your midwife will probably ask you to remove jewellery from any genital piercings when it comes to giving birth. This is because of the risk of them getting caught during the birth or of that area tearing.

The highs and lows

Fabulous and feminine or fat and frumpy? However pregnancy makes you feel, it's bound to change how you feel about your body. It's all too easy to forget about the joys of impending motherhood when you're feeling sick, exhausted, nervous or just fed-up. As your breasts grow, your abdomen swells and your waistline disappears, you may well long to have your old shape back.

So while you're revelling in being pregnant, you might not be revelling in looking pregnant. A massage or other treatment can lift your spirits and make you feel better. If you've had a breakout of pregnancy acne, a professional facial might improve your skin and give your confidence a boost. Even a manicure or pedicure can help you feel just a little more glamorous and groomed.

However, before you book yourself into your local salon for a pampering session, bear in mind that there are certain procedures that you need to be careful with while you're pregnant. Below is a guide to which are safe and which are best avoided:

Tattoos

Little is known about the effects of the ink used during the tattooing process on mother and baby. There's also a small risk that you could catch an infection, such as hepatitis B, from unclean equipment. It's best to err on the side of caution and wait until after your baby is born to have a tattoo.

Hair-removal creams

There's no evidence about the safety or otherwise of hair-removal creams during pregnancy, but your skin may be more sensitive than usual. If you're using them at home, always read the instructions on the packet carefully first, don't use them on broken skin and always do a patch test first. Remember to tell the beauty therapists you are pregnant if you go to a salon.

Electrolysis

No adverse effects have ever been recorded for electrolysis in pregnancy. However, electrolysists recommend you don't have work done on your breasts or tummy during late pregnancy, as both are very sensitive at this stage.

Bikini and leg waxes

The biggest problem with waxing in pregnancy is that, towards the end, it can be difficult to reach, or even see, certain body parts! This is the time to treat yourself to a full salon treatment.

A relaxing facial or gentle massage at your local salon can be just what you need to make you feel great – as well as giving you some time just for yourself!

Oils to avoid

Here are some commonly used aromatherapy oils that should not be used during pregnancy:

- Aniseed
- Angelica
- Basil
- Cedar wood
- Cinnamon
- Sage
- Clove
- Fennel
- Jasmine
- Juniper
- Lemongrass
- Myrrh
- Parsley
- Pennyroyal
- Thyme

Aromatherapy

Many aromatherapists believe that the essential oils – extracts of certain plants and flowers – used in aromatherapy can balance hormone levels, improve your mood and soothe stress.

There is no doubt that the relaxing effects of many of the oils and massage techniques used in aromatherapy can increase your sense of wellbeing and improve your general health, although there are some oils you shouldn't use while pregnant (see above right).

During pregnancy, it's best to consult a professional aromatherapist to be sure that you are not using an inappropriate aromatherapy oil or technique. Many complementary therapists can be found in the Yellow Pages (often listed under "Clinics"), but try asking around first for a personal recommendation for a qualified registered practitioner in your area. She should be someone who has plenty of experience of giving aromatherapy treatments to pregnant women. Some practitioners believe that a pregnant woman should not have aromatherapy massages during the first or third trimester, while others take care to use only specialised and light massage techniques.

Create your own mini spa

If you fancy a pregnancy pick-me-up, creating your own home spa could be the answer. All you need is a few pampering products.

- **Preparation** Make your bathroom tranquil; dim the lights and put some scented candles on a safe surface. Pour your favourite bubble bath under warm running water and sink yourself into a deep, luxurious bath.

- **Buffing and exfoliating** Buff your body with an exfoliating brush or use a salt scrub to banish all those dead skin cells. Pay special attention to your elbows and knees, which are usually rougher than the rest of your skin. Use an exfoliating facial wash to get the blood rushing to your cheeks, then relax for a few minutes in the bath with a deep cleansing face pack.

- **Grand finale** When you've finished, wrap yourself in a warm, fluffy towel and when you're dry spend a few minutes moisturising your body with a super-rich body cream.

- **Time for sleep** By now, you should be feeling so relaxed and soothed that it's time to blow out all those candles, curl up in bed and drift off to sleep. Sweet dreams!

Getting ready for pregnancy

Staying safe and healthy

Your pregnancy diary

Birth and beyond

Staying safe in the sun

Many women find their skin is more sensitive to ultraviolet radiation during pregnancy. Even so, the temptation to develop a tan may be strong. But is it safe? Here we give the latest advice on the dangers of sunbathing and the risks of using sunbeds, sunscreens and fake tans.

Your skin may be more sensitive now that you're pregnant so always use sunscreen and wear a hat in strong sun.

Is it safe to get a tan?

Many experts advise that getting a tan – whether in a salon or in the sun – isn't a good idea, even if you aren't pregnant. A tan is your skin's protection against the damaging effects of ultraviolet (UV) radiation; evidence suggests that prolonged exposure to UV exacerbates the effects of ageing and also increases your risk of developing skin cancer.

Risks of sunbathing

Many pregnant women find they are more susceptible to sunburn. If this applies to you, slap on the sunscreen (see opposite) and avoid the sun where possible. Pregnant women are prone to excessive skin pigmentation because they have higher levels of melanocyte-stimulating hormone than normal. If you get chloasma (see p.69), your skin may react more strongly to sunlight than usual. Take care: sunbathing may well make it worse.

Also, lying in the hot sun for hours on end increases the risk of overheating and dehydration – neither of which are good for you or your developing baby. Hot weather can make you sweat more, so watch out for the warning signs of dehydration: your nose and mouth may feel dry and your urine may turn dark yellow. However, don't worry if all you want to do is spend a peaceful afternoon in the sun though – just guard against overheating and burning.

The safety of sunscreens

You may find you are more prone to sunburn during your pregnancy, or you

9,500 is the number of cases of malignant melanoma diagnosed in the UK every year. It's a shocking fact that the incidence of malignant melanoma has gone up fourfold since the 1970s.

ParentsAsk...

Supposing I used a tanning bed before I knew I was pregnant?
Regular use of tanning beds is a fairly recent trend and there is little research on their effects in pregnancy. Nor are there any definitive studies about how exposure either to sunlight or to artificial ultraviolet rays affects a developing baby. Some preliminary studies suggest there may be a possible link between exposure to ultraviolet rays and folic acid deficiency. This is because folic acid can be broken down by strong sunlight. In the first few weeks of pregnancy, high levels of folic acid help protect against neural tube defects, such as spina bifida, in the developing baby. While further studies have yet to be done, these studies suggest that intense or prolonged exposure to UV light – as you get on a sunbed – should be avoided around the time of conception and in early pregnancy. After the first 12 weeks, all the developing baby's major organs have been formed so the risks are reduced.

may feel "prickly" after exposure to the sun. That is why it's very important to protect your skin with a high-factor sunscreen (SPF15 or more) and to wear a hat whenever you go out. Sunscreens are generally safe to use during pregnancy, but you may like to use one for sensitive skin for now. Reapply it regularly and avoid the midday sun. Remember that both chemical and physical sunscreens can deteriorate over time, so before you use one, check the bottle or tube for the expiry date. If you can't find a date, or if the product seems to have dried up or changed

"Sunscreens are **generally safe** but you may prefer to use one for **sensitive skin**."

colour or consistency, it's better to be safe than sorry: throw it away and buy some new sunscreen.

Tanning beds are an alternative way to get a tan, but you may want to avoid them (see ParentsAsk, opposite). If you have a skin problem that responds well to controlled light treatment, ask for a

referral to a dermatology department so that your treatment can be properly controlled to keep any damaging effects to a minimum.

If you desperately want to be brown, the current medical opinion seems to be that it's probably safer – and easier – to use fake tanning lotions (see below).

Fake tans may be safer

Fake tans have become more popular recently. The active ingredient of fake tans is dihydroxyacetone (DHA), which only interacts with the cells in the outer layer of the skin and isn't absorbed into the body's system. The British Medical Association (BMA), however, advises pregnant women not to use self-tanning

lotions, as their skin may be more sensitive than usual and may be more prone to an allergic reaction.

If you do decide to use a fake tan, do a patch test first, even if it's a lotion you have used before. If you have any kind of allergic reaction to the product you should stop using it at once.

Tanning pills

If you see advertisements in magazines or websites for tanning pills, don't buy them as the pills can be toxic to an unborn baby. They have also been known to cause hepatitis and eye damage. For these reasons they are banned for cosmetic use in the UK.

Solar UV index

The strength of the sun's ultraviolet (UV) radiation is given as the "Solar UV Index". This system has been developed by the World Health Organization (WHO) and is used in many countries alongside weather-forecast maps. Colour coding on a map warns of the level of skin-damaging UV radiation in an area. Follow the colour coding to make sure you use the correct level of protection.

UV Index		Protect yourself
11+	Extreme	Slip on sun-protective clothing
8, 9, 10	Very High	Slop on SPF30+ sunscreen. Reapply every two hours
6, 7	High	Slap on a broad-brimmed hat and wear sunscreen
3, 4, 5	Moderate	Seek shade and wear sunscreen
1, 2	Low	Sun protection is generally not needed unless outside for extended periods

Getting ready for pregnancy

Staying safe and healthy

Your pregnancy diary

Birth and beyond

Holidays and travel

Once your baby arrives you won't be able to make a move without a mountain of baby gear. That's one good reason to get away for a last romantic break before you give birth. It's usually safe to fly in pregnancy, but do give the scuba diving a miss once you're there!

Before you travel

Taking a holiday when you are pregnant is a great idea, especially if this is your first baby. It's likely to be a while before you'll get another chance to really relax.

The time to travel

As long as your pregnancy is going well, it's safe to go ahead and make travel plans. If you have complications, such as high blood pressure, spotting or diabetes, check with your doctor first.

Most mums-to-be find that the second trimester – weeks 14 to 27 – is a perfect time to travel. With nausea and vomiting behind you, your energy levels high and the chances of miscarriage low, you can relax and enjoy your time away.

As long as you don't have medical complications, aren't carrying twins or more, and haven't had a prior premature birth, you can fly on most airlines until 36 weeks of pregnancy. Travel agents and airlines won't ask if you're pregnant when you book your seat, but you may be challenged at the check-in desk. For this reason, from about 28 weeks of pregnancy, you will need a letter from your doctor confirming your due date and stating that you're unlikely to go into labour on the flight. Check the airline's policy on flying in pregnancy before you leave and don't forget that it applies to your return trip, too.

There's no reason to avoid car travel when you are pregnant – don't forget your seatbelt! However, at the end of your pregnancy you may prefer to let your partner drive as your bump will be very close to the steering wheel.

When you are going on a long drive, you should take a toilet and stretching break at least every 90 minutes. Sitting for long periods can make your feet and ankles swell and your legs cramp. When you are flying, you are at special risk of your feet swelling, so remove your shoes. Keep your blood circulating by strolling up and down the aisle and doing simple stretches and choose an aisle seat so you can easily get to the toilet without disturbing other passengers. Finally, if there happens to be an empty seat next to you on a plane, train or bus, take the opportunity to put your feet up.

Tips for safe plane travel

Following the tips below can help you to enjoy safe travel by plane during your pregnancy:

● **Wear support stockings** Keep your circulation flowing and reduce the risk of thrombosis (blood clots).

● **Do some stretches** Stroll up and down the aisle of the plane occasionally and do some simple leg stretches.

● **Don't wear tights** They encourage the moist conditions that increase your chances of developing thrush.

● **Drink lots of water** The air on planes can be very dry and you may get dehydrated. Avoid coffee and tea.

Packing for a last romantic fling? Travel light and take loose cotton clothes so you stay cool and comfortable.

A beach holiday can be a great way of relaxing before your baby is born, as long as you take a few precautions.

Tips for pregnant travellers

Following these tips can help you travel safely during your pregnancy:

- **Reduce stress** Make sure that you schedule plenty of time for travelling and travel light. Relax by reading or listening to music.
- **Maximise your energy** Build quiet times into your routine. Have a bath, take a nap, read on the beach and spend an evening with room service.
- **Eat smart** Pack healthy snacks in your hand luggage, but if you're flying, remember, these may be removed by security. Drink plenty of extra fluids.
- **Make frequent toilet stops** and carry wet wipes and a hand sanitiser.
- **Avoid thrush** Wear cotton pants and loose cotton layers, especially in hot, humid climates.

Getting ready for pregnancy

Staying safe and healthy

Your pregnancy diary

Birth and beyond

While you're there

Holidays taken while you're pregnant are the stuff that memories are made of, so you'll want your special trip to go smoothly. You will need to take a little extra care to keep you and your growing baby safe and to ensure that your time away isn't ruined by illness or accidents.

Sports like waterskiing, snowboarding, skiing or surfing that carry a risk of falling will have to be put on hold. Scuba diving and other "pressurised" sports are also out, as are amusement park rides.

Wear loose clothes made of natural fibres to help you stay cool, and to prevent rubbing and chafing. Drink

plenty of fluids, especially bottled water. To help prevent tummy upsets, always wash your hands before eating, after a visit to the toilet and when you get back from excursions. And finally, avoid ice and steer clear of hotel buffets that have been left out of the fridge for long periods or food sold on the street.

Parents**Talk**...

"If you're going to take a holiday during pregnancy, go for all-out relaxation. During my first pregnancy I went to Cyprus for a week with my husband – we booked a hotel in a lovely resort right next to the beach, with spa facilities, plenty of places to eat and lots to do and see. Having a week in the sun, taking life at a slow pace and enjoying delicious food and gorgeous surroundings was a truly restorative experience."
Liz, 31, mum to year-old Adam, and two-year-old Shane

"If money's tight, there are plenty of ways to get that much-needed holiday during pregnancy. When I was pregnant with my second baby, we asked my parents to look after our two-year-old daughter for a couple of days and my partner and I had a short break in a country hotel. We visited the spa, went for some gentle walks, wined (for him!) and dined, slept late – and came back feeling refreshed, relaxed and ready to face what lay ahead."
Julia, 34, mum to Paul and Milly

Bonding with your unborn baby

As a mum-to-be it's not hard to bond with the baby inside you. Those little kicks and hiccups give you heart-warming clues to the small person who'll soon arrive. Dads-to-be may take more time, but getting involved with antenatal appointments and choosing names can help.

Single mum

If your partner can't be with you for that first scan, a supportive mum's definitely not second best.

"Mum was with me when I had my first scan. I was so nervous there might be something wrong with the baby, but she kept reassuring me that everything would be OK. It was such a relief to see my fully formed baby on screen with his heart beating strongly. Then he sat bolt upright and that's the picture we got to take home! He'll be her first grandchild. She's been so supportive since I found out I was pregnant, I wouldn't have wanted anyone else there with me."

The importance of bonding

Bonding is the word used to describe the intense attachment that develops between a mum and her baby. Talk about bonding often focuses on the time after your baby is born. But for many mums-to-be, bonding begins much earlier than that, often from the moment you see that line on the pregnancy test telling you you're pregnant.

There are many reasons why bonding with your bump is good for you and your baby. First of all, making healthy choices about your diet or lifestyle becomes easier because you'll remember why you're doing it.

Pregnancy can be hard work. There are times when you'll feel tired, nauseous, sore or just plain huge. Feeling a bond between you and your baby will help you see it's all worthwhile. And it will also get your relationship off to the best possible start when you finally meet for the first time.

In the early days, during your antenatal appointments will probably be when you feel closest to your baby. Hearing your baby's heartbeat or seeing your baby on a scan will make her feel so much more real to you.

When you feel your baby move for the first time, somewhere between 16 and 20 weeks, your relationship will develop even further. As those early fluttery butterfly feelings develop into more powerful kicks and slides, try to spend some time each day relaxing and just focussing on your baby's movements. You'll feel like you're beginning to get to know her personality through all her tiny thumps, jabs and even hiccups.

By this time your baby will be able to feel your touch if you gently rub your hand over your bump. She can also hear your voice and her heart will beat a little faster when she hears it. Some mums find that talking, reading or even singing to their bump is a lovely way to connect with their baby. But don't worry if you

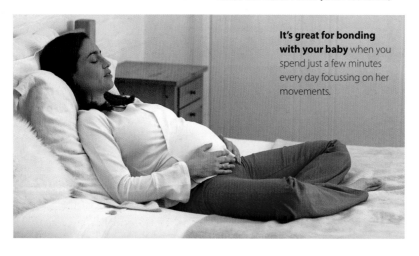

It's great for bonding with your baby when you spend just a few minutes every day focussing on her movements.

don't feel comfortable doing that. Your baby will still hear your voice as you talk to other people.

If you know your baby's sex, giving her a name (or nickname if you haven't yet decided on a name) will help you imagine what she'll be like.

Then, as your due date draws closer you'll spend time preparing the nursery or buying baby clothes. Now you'll probably be imagining her wearing the clothes or sleeping in the cot. And when that finally happens, your relationship will have moved on to its next phase.

Encourage your partner to bond with your baby, too.

Involving dad

It's not unusual for dads-to-be to seem a little detached from their partner's pregnancy at first. After all, he's got a lot of thinking to do. Questions that may be running through his mind include: Will he be a good dad? Will labour go smoothly? Will he love the baby?

No dad can possibly relate to the minute-by-minute reality of carrying a baby. But he can be an active observer. Encourage him to take pictures as your bump grows or maybe give you a back massage when you're tired. When the baby's kicking, put his hand on your bump and let him feel the movements.

Go to antenatal appointments together. Be sure he doesn't miss the chance to get a first glimpse of your baby during an ultrasound. And, of course, you should attend antenatal classes together. By the time your baby arrives, you and your partner will have prepared the nursery, installed a car seat (hospitals won't let you drive baby home without one), settled on boy and girl options for your child's name and decided about breast- or bottle feeding.

Dad's **Diary**

The first scan
"Seeing the baby for the first time at the scan – I have to admit, I was speechless. Literally. Reality hit home in a big way, making everything very real all of a sudden. It finally sank in. I was going to be a dad. There was a real baby in there – one that I'd have to care for and provide for during the next 18 years! I didn't know whether to laugh, cry, smile or what.

Sally was a bit confused by my lack of reaction, but I really couldn't find the words to describe how I felt. Saying I was happy wouldn't have come close to it.

I was surprised by how clear the image was, too. Whenever I'd seen friends' scan pictures, I'd always joked about how all those scan pictures are the same – and how you can't really see what the baby looks like. But seeing my own baby on screen, with his tiny heart beating (strongly thankfully!), his little arms and hands (one hanging onto the umbilical cord), his little legs with his feet crossed and kicking – it was amazing.

It was such a huge relief to know that there were no problems too. Although I know the next scan will be able to tell us more…

We'd decided to wait until we'd had the first scan before we told people our news, so it was great to be able to take our scan pictures and show our tiny baby off to all our friends and family."

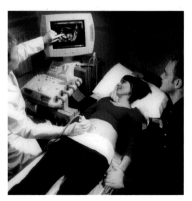

Dads-to-be often find seeing their baby on a scan for the first time very moving.

Preparing the nursery

Planning your baby's nursery is incredibly exciting and it's something you and your partner can enjoy doing together. Make sure you get the basics covered first – a cot, mattress and some bedding – and think about safety, heating and lighting before your little one arrives.

Key nursery needs

Whether your baby's a boy or girl, the basics are always the same. Either sex will need:

● A Moses basket or carrycot and stand – and later on a full-size cot.
● Sheets and blankets or some sleep sacks.
● Storage (a chest of drawers or wardrobe) for clothing, blankets, and toys.
● A changing mat and a safe, well-positioned place to put it.
● A comfortable chair for feeding.
● A baby monitor and a smoke detector.

Not everything needs to be brand new. Having a baby can be expensive, but with a bit of know-how you should be able to save a lot on your purchases. There are some exceptions, though – most recommendations say not to use a second-hand mattress – but there's no harm in using your niece's cot or finding suitable decorations such as mobiles in a second-hand shop. Just keep in mind current safety standards for things like the spacing between cot bars (see opposite) and make sure anything second hand is clean, undamaged and in good working order.

Starting to plan

Becoming a parent can feel vaguely dreamlike until the cot or rocking chair arrives. But the planning should start before that. Begin with the practicalities, such as whether the radiator will need replacing and how to light the room.

You may have no choice about which room to make into the nursery, but ideally it should be near yours and somewhere quiet. If your home is draughty or damp, can you keep the nursery warm and dry, perhaps with new insulation, double glazing or damp-proofing? When your baby starts to explore, he shouldn't be able to open windows, lock doors, play with outlets, cords or wires, or get to the stairs. Can you clean the floors easily and is there a suitable place nearby to store dirty nappies or laundry hygienically?

Then there's storage for all his clothing, blankets and towels, as well as for books and toys. Shelves need to be secured and boxes shouldn't have lids that will slam on little hands or trap your toddler inside. Furniture should be too heavy to tip over if your baby pulls himself up on it, and it shouldn't have loose, sharp or damaged bits. Beware, also, of lead paint; it's dangerous for pregnant women to remove it and for babies to peel and play with or eat.

Cots and mattresses

A cot will probably be your baby's bed until he is two or three years old. It should be strong and sturdy without cracked or broken slats, and with no jagged points or edges. You can use your cot from the day your baby is born if you prefer, although many parents choose a Moses basket, crib or carrycot for the first few months, or have their babies in the same bed as them; babies can look and feel a little lost in a big cot.

Cots can be expensive so you might like to buy one second-hand. They come in many shapes and sizes, including corner-shaped cots that sit neatly in the corner of the room, and oval-shaped cots that can be converted into a junior bed, chair or even a sofa later on. You can also buy bedside cots which can be useful for night-time feeds; they have a removable side so you can put your baby's cot right next to your bed.

Buying a mattress

There are many different types of cot mattresses available so you may be confused at first. You may also be concerned to know which is the best

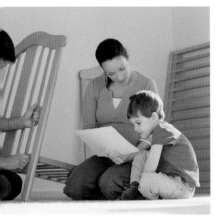

Getting the baby's nursery ready can be exciting and gives you the opportunity to involve the whole family.

and safest mattress to use for your baby. In fact, the Foundation for the Study of Infant Deaths states that it doesn't matter what kind of mattress you use, as long as it's firm, not soft, and doesn't sag or show any signs of wear and tear. Unless you know the history of a second-hand mattress, buy a new one.

- **Foam mattresses** These are generally the cheapest. They often have an easy-to-clean PVC cover. Choose one which is at least 8 to 10cm (3 to 4in) thick, to help support your baby while she sleeps. Some have ventilation holes but the Foundation for the Study of Infant

Deaths says these are not necessary.
- **Spring interior mattresses** These consist of coiled springs covered with a layer of foam and soft cotton fabric. One side is usually covered in cotton fabric and the other in wipe-clean plastic.
- **Natural fibre mattresses** The interior of a natural fibre mattress is usually coconut fibre coated in latex, which is waterproof. The covers are made from soft cotton.
- **Hypoallergenic mattresses** Choose one of these mattresses if allergies or asthma are a concern in your family. They have a quilted top layer that can be detached easily from the body of the mattress, and machine-washed at 60°C (140°F) to kill the dust mites that may cause allergies.

Safety in the nursery

When thinking about your baby's nursery, keep these safety tips in mind:
- All cots sold in the UK should conform to BSEN716. This ensures that the cot is deep enough and that cot bars are less than 45 to 65mm (1¾ to 2½in) apart.
- Check that the mattress fits snugly; there should be no corner-post

extensions and no decorative cut-outs that could trap your baby's limbs.
- Don't use a pillow. For safe sleeping, your baby needs a firm, flat surface.
- When you're not in the room with your baby, make sure that you keep the drop side of his cot up and locked.
- Position the cot away from direct

sunshine, windows, heaters, lamps and wall decorations.
- Avoid curtains and blinds with cords – dangling cords carry a risk of strangulation. If you already have them, make sure that you tie them up.
- Stay with your baby when he is on his changing table.

Too hot? Too cold?

It is a natural instinct for you to wrap up your baby warm, especially during the winter, but do not overdo it as overheating is associated with an increased risk of cot death. A baby will sleep comfortably in a room heated to a temperature between 16°C (60°F) and 20°C (68°F). Our chart will show you how many blankets your baby needs according to the room temperature.

Room temperature	Amount of bedding	Tog rating for the sleeping bag
24°C / 75°F or more	Sheet only	0.5 tog
21°C / 70°F	Sheet plus one blanket, or a 1 tog sleeping bag	1 tog
18°C / 64°F	Sheet plus two layers of blanket, or a 2.5 tog sleeping bag	2.5 tog
16°C / 61°F	Sheet plus three layers of blanket, or a 2.5 tog sleeping bag plus a blanket	2.5 tog

Getting ready for pregnancy

Staying safe and healthy

Your pregnancy diary

Birth and beyond

Credit-crunch nursery

If you're clever about it, you can kit out your baby's nursery for next to nothing – great for young couples or anyone on a strict budget.

- Your baby will eventually sleep in a cot, so you could skip the expense of a Moses basket or crib and go straight for the cot. The cheapest option is to get one second hand, then all you need to buy new is a mattress (see p.103) and bedding.
- You don't need a state-of-the-art changing table – just a basic changing mat which won't cost the earth.
- Brighten up the nursery with a lick of paint and a few fun posters.
- Toys and mobiles don't have to cost the earth – find cheap and cheerful bargains in high-street discount shops.
- If friends and family want to buy your new baby gifts, ask for specific things or set up a gift list with a department store.

Decorating

Now for the fun part. If you have a colour or theme in mind, build it around the furniture and other pieces you must have in the nursery. Window treatments can create a focal point in an otherwise subtly decorated room, or they can just complement the overall colour scheme by pulling together shades or textures that you've used elsewhere in the room. Either way, the window treatment you choose should be able to make the room sufficiently dark for naptime or bright summer evenings and keep the cold out in the winter. Look for materials that won't fade or gather dust, and keep any cords out of baby's reach. You should also make sure that your window treatments – like the bedding or any other fabric in the room – is flameproof.

Why not ask family members for their input on the decorating? Someone may even volunteer to make the curtains or help with the painting!

Colour, movement and music

Infants have limited eyesight at first (they focus best on objects 23cm away), but they love black and white patterns. Some babies are even mesmerized by the black beams that run across the white ceiling in traditional old houses.

Young babies also love mobiles with strong colours, music or nightlights, while pictures or mirrors can be a nice addition to the nursery – just be sure they aren't hanging near the cot or changing table, or anywhere an older baby can climb to dislodge them.

You can also add some colour with your choice of flooring. It should be comfortable, easy to clean and slip-resistant. Wood or laminate are good choices, and you might consider rubber and bamboo. Sadly, flooring isn't mess-resistant, but as long as books and toys don't cause you to stumble, your baby won't mind a muddle.

Parents**Ask...**

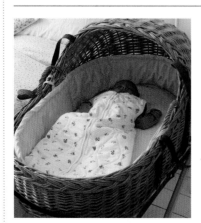

Moses baskets are good for the first couple of months – they are very portable, and small enough to feel cosy.

Will I need a nightlight for my baby?

Nightlights can be useful for toddlers who are afraid of the dark but babies don't need them. That's because children don't experience night-time anxiety until they are two or three years old, when they're capable of imagining scary things lurking in the dark. In the meantime, your baby will sleep better in a dark room.

Should we buy a breathing monitor?

A breathing monitor makes a sound to alert you if your baby stops breathing. The DH says that normal, healthy babies do not need one and that there is no evidence to show that they prevent cot deaths. If at all possible, your baby should sleep in the same room as you for the first six months. This will help you to keep a closer eye on any changes in your baby's breathing during the night.

Are baby sleeping bags a good idea?

The great thing about baby sleeping bags is that your baby can't kick them off. If you use one, the Foundation for the Study of Infant Deaths recommends using one without a hood and making sure that it is the right size around the neck so your baby won't slip down inside the bag. It also advises that you should never use a sleeping bag with a quilt or duvet, as this will make your baby far too hot.

Seating and storage

A comfortable chair will be your back's best friend, so invest time in finding one that suits you. You may love the idea of your grandmother's rocking chair, but consider how you will position your baby for feeding and whether it can accommodate both of you. Don't underestimate how much you will come to rely on a sturdy seat at the end of a long day: the last thing you'll want is one that puts you in an awkward, hunched or twisted position. Some mums couldn't live without a glider chair – a soothing but expensive option – while others are content with the simplest bench. You might even be able to incorporate a seat into an existing space, creating built-in storage.

Storage is such a simple concept, yet so hard for exhausted parents to put into practice. Luckily, there are business empires built on getting organised – just do a quick search online. Try not to be overwhelmed by the options when a few simple baskets, stackable boxes or shelves could be all you need to minimise the nursery mess.

Convenience is key, but storage can also be designed so it complements the décor. Give baskets the flourish of a ribbon so that they match the curtains or paint wooden boxes to go with the skirting board. Keep nappy supplies on a shelf near the changing table or in a decorative hanging pocket on a peg. You can even display your favourite baby hats or outfits on wall hooks.

Dad's Diary

Getting the nursery ready
"We started preparing the baby's nursery this week. When I say we, I mean Emma has chosen the colour scheme, the furniture, the curtains – the tasteful selection of soft toys. I'm doing all the hard work: all the painting and varnishing (Emma's staying out of the way to be on the safe side), putting up the cot and the wardrobe (do babies really need wardrobes? Surely their clothes are too small?), fixing the shelves, hanging the blackout blind, lugging the rocking chair up the stairs. Phew! When I've finished, all Emma will have to do is arrange the soft furnishings in a decorative manner."

Sharing with a sibling

It is recommended that a baby sleeps in the same room as his parents for the first six months of life. This helps reduce the risk of cot death and is also convenient because babies tend to wake several times a night for feeding in the early part of their lives.

After that time, if your baby and toddler both sleep well, it is fine for them to share a room. Problems only arise if they wake frequently and prevent each other from falling back to sleep, although many babies and children aren't bothered by their siblings crying. Also, bedtimes can vary with differing age groups and could potentially cause disturbances. Do make sure, though, that an unchecked toddler is not able to "feed" any unsuitable toys through the bars of the cot, as these could be a hazard to your baby. Being together at night-time may enhance your children's relationship and could be a source of comfort and security to them while they are both young. As they grow, sharing a bedroom will teach important lessons about boundaries and sharing.

Once your new baby is sleeping well it can be comforting for him and his older sibling to share a bedroom.

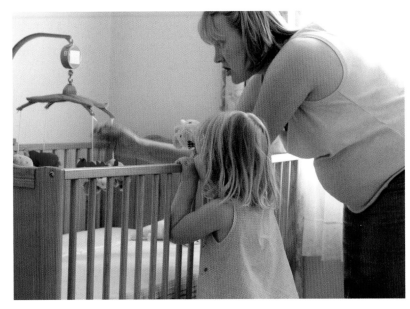

Getting ready for pregnancy

Staying safe and healthy

Your pregnancy diary

Birth and beyond

Essential baby buys

A stroll around a baby equipment shop can be a bewildering and overwhelming experience for parents-to-be. Does your baby really need so much stuff? The truth is that he probably doesn't. Try to stick to the basics – you can always pick up other things you need after he's born.

Clothing for your newborn

When you are buying for your newborn, it's helpful to know what is actually useful – and what you can do without. Here are the essentials:

● Cotton vests/body suits with envelope necks and poppers underneath: you need three or four.

● Babygros/sleepsuits/all-in-ones: at least three or four and/or nighties with drawstrings at the bottom – very useful for night-time nappy changing.

● A soft hat or bonnet to wear outside, for a winter baby, or a wide-brimmed sunhat for a summer baby.

● A soft blanket or two to wrap and cuddle your baby in.

● An all-in-one warm suit (with poppers between the legs) is also useful for a winter baby. He can wear it over a sleepsuit and it's handy for outdoors.

● A cardigan or two to provide an extra layer. Cardigans are better than jumpers because small babies tend not to like having clothes pulled over their heads.

Practicalities

Make sure everything is machine-washable! And where possible, 100 per cent cotton so that it's gentle on your baby's skin. Fleecy polyester jackets and blankets can make your baby too hot and irritate his skin. Also, wash all clothing before use in non-biological washing powder, to avoid irritation.

Some warmer clothes are a must for a winter baby. For going out, opt for an all-in-one suit with a cosy hood.

You'll need several little vests with envelope necks since new babies don't like having clothing pulled over their faces.

Cellular cotton blankets double up as bedding or to wrap your baby in for a cuddle. A couple of soft hats are useful, too.

Bedding and equipment

Although you can now get baby sleeping bags for newborn babies (see p.104), most parents start off with cotton sheets and cotton cellular blankets.

You will need about four sheets and two or three blankets to start with. Sheets are usually either traditional woven cotton, brushed flannelette, stretch cotton terry or cotton jersey. Stretch fitted sheets are useful as they are less likely to come untucked, and are quick and easy to put on and take off.

If your baby's bedroom is very cold, you can use acrylic cellular blankets, which wash well. If you buy traditional

Other key equipment

As well as a Moses basket or a cot and mattress (see pp.102–103) there are a number of other essential items that you need to have ready:

- A baby bath or a newborn bath support that you can put in your own bath (you could use a washing-up bowl to begin with).
- Nappies (disposable or reusable) – as newborn babies need their nappies changed eight to 10 times a day, buy enough disposable nappies to keep you going for at least the first few days or so. If you are planning to use cloth nappies,

- If you have a car, you will need a rear-facing car seat (see p.109).
- If you are planning to bottle feed, you will need bottles, teats, bottle brushes and a sterilisation method (see p.108).
- If you are planning to breastfeed, you will need nursing bras and breast pads.
- Baby wipes or cotton wool, nappy cream and nappy sacks, for (plenty of!) nappy changing.
- A changing mat, or changing unit.
- Top-and-tail bowl – this has separate compartments for cooled, boiled water to clean your baby's face and bottom with cotton wool in the early months.

> "If you are going to **use cloth nappies** have at least **one packet of disposables** handy too."

wool blankets, check to see that they can be machine-washed. Polyester fleece blankets are available, too, and are useful in the pram on a cold day.

Duvets and pillows aren't recommended for your baby until he is a year old because they can restrict his movement and may make him too hot.

it's a good idea to have at least one packet of disposables handy too. For cloth nappies, you may also need nappy liners and waterproof wraps, and a bucket with a lid to store dirty nappies.

- A buggy that has a padded seat and a lie-flat position so it is suitable for a newborn (see p.109).

It also has a smaller compartment that holds the soap.

- A couple of small towels and some mild baby bath.
- Changing bag – essential for holding clean nappies, wipes, baby cream, nappy sacks, muslins and a change of clothes on outings.

A rear-facing car seat is essential for a new baby. You must make sure it is properly installed and fits your car perfectly.

A baby bath is useful, although you could start with a washing-up bowl. A changing mat or changing unit is a must-have.

You'll definitely need a changing bag with lots of pockets to hold all your baby's supplies when you go on outings.

Getting ready for pregnancy

Staying safe and healthy

Your pregnancy diary

Birth and beyond

If you intend to breastfeed, you will need a nursing bra and breast pads, and a breast pump will be useful for expressing milk.

A steriliser is essential for bottle-feeding equipment, and will come in handy if you use a breast pump to express your milk.

In the first few months, your baby will appreciate small brightly coloured soft toys, such as rattles, and soft books with a mirror.

Baby goes green

The greenest choice is not to buy much baby equipment at all and borrow where possible. But here are some unusual green buys:

- A natural cot mattress made from coir with an organic cotton cover. It's more expensive than a traditional mattress but lasts longer.
- Hooded bamboo baby towels: they are extra-absorbent.

Sometimes you don't have to buy anything – or very little! Try the following:

- Join a toy library.
- Have baby in the bath with you.
- Raid the larder for olive oil – great for dry skin and baby massage.
- A sling or front carrier (you won't need a car seat if you're walking everywhere), and a borrowed pram.
- Washable breast pads and a couple of breastfeeding bras (organic cotton if possible).
- Second-hand or borrowed baby clothes. If you want to buy new, choose organic Fairtrade cotton.
- Choose long-lasting toys that can be passed down to the next generation.

Feeding

All you really need in order to breastfeed are your baby and your breasts. For bottle-feeding mums, though, there are some products and accessories that will make life easier.

- **Breast pumps** If you're going to be expressing at work and want to make your pumping time as short as possible, get an electric pump that is reliable, quiet and fast. If you only plan to express once or twice a week, a hand pump will probably do just as well.
- **Nursing bras** A good nursing bra needs to be comfortable and adjustable, should give good support and must be easy to get in and out of. It's worth being fitted for one after you have reached 36 weeks of pregnancy.
- **Feeding bottles** If you're planning to bottle feed, basic bottles are inexpensive and available in wide-neck or standard. Each bottle generally comes with a teat and a lid.

Anti-colic bottles claim to reduce the amount of air a baby takes in while feeding, which is thought to be a possible cause of colic. If your baby is unsettled after feeds and suffers with wind, it might be worth investing in one of these systems, but they don't work for all babies. Steriliser bottles are handy as they can be microwave sterilised without needing any other equipment.

- **Sterilisers** You have a choice of four ways to sterilise your baby's feeding equipment to kill the germs that cause tummy upsets: boiling, cold water sterilising, steam sterilising and microwave sterilising. For boiling, you just need a pan with a lid. Cold water sterilising is also cheap and convenient, and involves soaking everything in a special non-toxic sterilising solution.

Electric steam sterilisers hold up to six bottles at a time and sterilise in under 10 minutes, while microwave steam sterilisers fit inside your microwave and use water to create steam when heated up.

- **Teats** These come in various "flow" sizes, in different types of material – latex or silicone – and in different shapes, including standard and "natural", which mimic the shape of a nipple. Generally, you should start with slow flow for newborn babies.

Entertaining your baby

When it comes to entertaining baby, you'll find that, in her first months, she will most appreciate things she can look at and listen to. She might enjoy:

● **Mobiles** Look for mobiles with high-contrast colours and patterns as well as those that play music. For safety's sake, keep the mobile out of baby's reach.

● **Mirrors** Although she won't realise it's herself she's seeing at this stage, your baby will find her own reflection fascinating. By three months, she may begin smiling at it. Look for a mirror you can hang near a changing table.

● **Soft books with high-contrast patterns** There are plenty of these on sale. Lie down next to her so she can watch you as you read aloud to her.

● **Sock and wrist rattles** Attach a soft rattle to your baby's wrist or ankle. That way she can experiment with sounds she makes herself.

● **Wind chimes** Hang a set of these in a place where she can watch them move and listen to the sound.

● **Black, white and red toys** These high-contrast toys and playmats will help your child pick out the differences in shapes and patterns.

Taking your baby out

You may be the sort who likes to have the coolest pram on the block. Perhaps you need a car seat for long journeys. Maybe you fancy keeping your baby cuddled up next to you in a sling. Whatever your needs, there's a baby-carrying system that will be just right for you and your baby.

● **Prams** Few parents buy traditional old prams any more, but you can buy "pram-style" pushchairs that are suitable for newborns. They also have modern features, such as swivel wheels, and they fold up so that they can (just about) go in and out of the car boot.

● **Pushchairs or buggies** There are two main types: umbrella-folding and flat-folding. Flat-folding models are usually suitable for newborn babies (but their seats must go completely flat and the seat should be padded).

Umbrella-folding pushchairs fold up into an umbrella shape. These folding buggies are convenient, but are usually only suitable for babies from three or six months onwards.

● **Travel systems** A travel system is a type of pushchair that is compatible with a rear-facing car seat and, usually, with a carrycot. Both will "click" in and out of the pushchair frame.

● **Car seats** Choosing the right car seat for your child's age and weight is very important. A newborn baby should always be put in a rear-facing car seat. You must also make completely sure that the car seat is properly installed. It should be held tightly by the seatbelt with very little sideways movement. Some child seats work better in some models of car than others, so you should try before you buy.

● **Slings** These let you keep your baby close to you, but still have your hands free for other activities. Small babies often like the feel of being carried about in a sling or carrier, and will often happily go to sleep in them.

Laid-back mum

If you want to be able to get up and go without faffing around with a buggy, then try a sling.

"With my first baby I found using a buggy really cumbersome so I ended up mostly using a sling. It was dead easy. It was really just a long piece of stretchy fabric but it was very comfortable to wear. And my baby loved it – and often went straight off to sleep in it, too.

Sometimes I would use the sling around the house when I wanted to get on with something and needed my hands free, but it was absolutely brilliant when we were out and about. It was a really nice feeling to be able to go where I wanted without worrying about how I was going to get there. I'm pregnant again now and I know that having a sling is going to help me look after the new baby and my toddler at the same time. Sounds silly but I can't wait to start using it again."

A sling is a convenient way of taking your baby out and about, and many babies just love the closeness a sling gives.

Getting ready for pregnancy

Staying safe and healthy

Your pregnancy diary

Birth and beyond

Your pregnancy diary

A week-by-week guide

The first trimester

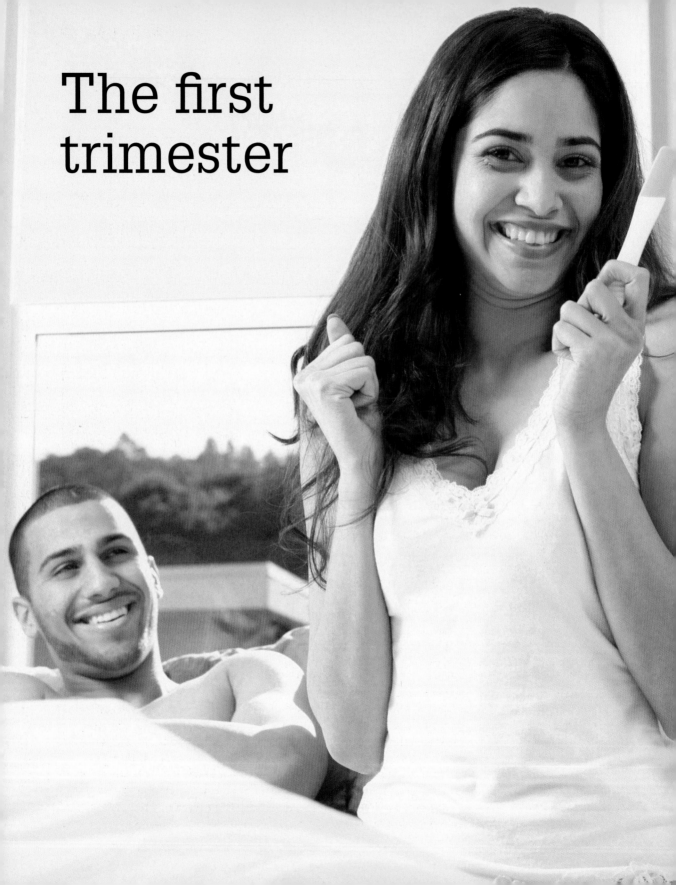

All change

There are many changes to get used to in the first trimester, so take things one step at a time. Remember to eat well, rest when your body tells you to, and remind yourself that women have been growing babies for thousands of years, so your body knows what it should be doing.

The start of the journey

The first trimester (or three months) lasts to the end of week 13. This is the trimester when you may be experiencing some of the most unpleasant pregnancy symptoms, such as nausea and fatigue. It's an emotional time, too, as you flit between excitement and joy, and anxiety and uncertainty. Try to enjoy these early weeks as much as you can. You're at the start of an incredible journey.

From cell to tiny human

During the first trimester, your baby develops from a microscopic single cell to a fully formed tiny human being with all the major organs in place and ready to grow. At 12 weeks, your baby will have grown to around 5.5 centimetres (2¼ inches) long from crown to rump (about the size of a lime) and will weigh around 14 grams (½ ounce). She'll even have toothbuds and finger nails. Her heart will start beating during week six, and will beat 150 times a minute – roughly twice the rate of an adult heart.

You'll experience a lot of physical changes too. Your uterus will expand to accommodate your growing baby. Before pregnancy it was the size of a clenched fist; by six weeks it will be as big as a grapefruit. You may experience some aching in your lower abdomen as your muscles and ligaments stretch to support it. You'll find you need to urinate more often too, as your uterus presses on your bladder. Your breasts may feel sore and they may grow large enough for you to need a bigger bra by the end of this trimester. By seven weeks, you'll have 10 per cent more blood than you did before you were pregnant (by the end of your pregnancy, you'll have 40 to 45 per cent more blood running through your veins and arteries to meet the demands of your full-term baby).

Once you know you are pregnant, make an appointment to arrange antenatal care. It's usual to be seen for a booking appointment at around eight to 10 weeks. This allows time to arrange any first trimester screening tests. You'll be offered your first scan when you're 10 to 14 weeks pregnant to confirm your dates. This scan will also tell you if you're carrying more than one baby. If you've decided to have a nuchal translucency (NT) scan (see p.137) to screen for Down's syndrome, it needs to be carried out at 11 to 14 weeks. Sometimes an early scan is needed, for example, if you are feeling pain or are bleeding, or if you've had a miscarriage in the past.

Once you know you're pregnant, take the opportunity to learn from your friends about their experiences of pregnancy.

Laid-back mum

Staying relaxed about falling pregnant can help you keep calm when your test's positive.

"I'd been on the pill for five years, but a couple of months ago, my partner and I decided I should come off it and we'd let nature take its course. I've just done a pregnancy test and I'm delighted that it's positive. I thought I'd feel a bit panicked when it actually happened, and I certainly didn't expect to fall pregnant so quickly, but I think because we've been so relaxed about the whole thing, I still feel perfectly calm. I'm just ridiculously happy now!"

Getting ready for pregnancy

Staying safe and healthy

Your pregnancy diary

Birth and beyond

▼ Your body at **03** Weeks

03 Weeks

❋ A momentous meeting has taken place inside you – a single sperm has broken into and fertilised your egg.

❋ You probably don't know you're pregnant yet, but you may see a little spotting by the end of this week.

While you're waiting for your period a huge amount of activity is going on in your body. Your fertilised egg is busy implanting itself in your uterus and your hormone levels are going crazy.

I think I may be pregnant

A momentous meeting has taken place inside you – a single sperm has broken through the tough outer membrane of your egg and fertilised it, triggering conception. Several days later, the fertilised egg has burrowed into the lining of your uterus and has started to grow. A baby is in the making! You probably don't know you're pregnant yet, but you may notice a little spotting by the end of this week. This so-called "implantation bleeding" may be caused by the egg burrowing into the blood-rich uterine lining (a process that began six days after fertilisation), but no one knows for sure. In any case, the spotting is very light and only a minority of pregnant women experience it at all.

Hormonal changes

What's going on in your uterus now? A lot. Your baby-in-the-making is just a tiny ball, or blastocyst (see pp.34–5), consisting of several hundred cells that are multiplying wildly. Once the blastocyst takes up residence in your uterus it is called an embryo (see pp.34–5). The part of the embryo that will develop into the placenta starts producing the pregnancy hormone human chorionic gonadotrophin (hCG), which tells your ovaries to stop releasing eggs and triggers increased production of oestrogen and progesterone. These keep your uterus from shedding its lining – together with its tiny passenger – and stimulate placental growth. The hormone that turns a pregnancy test positive is hCG; by the end of this week, you may be able to take a pregnancy test and get a positive result. (If your test is negative and you still haven't got your period in two or three days, then try again.)

While all this is going on, amniotic fluid is beginning to collect around your multiplying ball of cells in the cavity that will eventually become the amniotic sac. This fluid will cushion your baby during the weeks and months ahead.

Right now, your little embryo is receiving oxygen and nutrients (and discarding waste products) through a primitive circulation system made up of microscopic tunnels. These connect your developing baby to the blood vessels in your uterine wall. By the end of next week, the placenta will be well enough developed to take over this task.

 Your baby at **03** Weeks

Amazing things are happening, perhaps even before you know you're pregnant.

❋ This week, a rush of activity occurs. In the 12 to 24 hours after you ovulate and an egg is swept into a fallopian tube, that egg can be fertilised if one of 300 million sperm (an average ejaculation) manages to swim all the way to the fallopian tube – from the vagina through the uterus – to penetrate it.

Pregnant again?

Many of us find that second and subsequent pregnancies pass in a flash and suddenly the birth is approaching, without you having gone through any of the emotional preparation or made any of the practical arrangements that you did first time.

It's different

You will probably find that your bump starts to show much earlier than last time, and that you feel the new baby moving several weeks before you did with your first. For a lot of women, nausea and vomiting aren't as bad in the second pregnancy, but this isn't universal. Symptoms you had during your first pregnancy, such as varicose veins and piles, may well recur, but you'll know better how to manage them.

If you had a medical problem in your first pregnancy, such as gestational diabetes (see p.229) or obstetric cholestasis (see pp.230–31), it may recur in your second. If you had pre-eclampsia (see p.233) in a first pregnancy, you have about a one-in-five chance of it recurring. However, you now know the kind of diet you need to have, the medication you should take, and the specialists you have to see, so both you and your doctors can manage the condition much more effectively.

Recurring worries

You may find yourself worrying about problems you had during your first pregnancy or labour. Perhaps you pushed these bad experiences to the back of your mind once they were over, but now they're resurfacing because you're pregnant again. Don't struggle along without talking to someone. Ask for a chat with your midwife or doctor,

or talk to a friend or antenatal teacher. Or arrange to get a copy of your maternity notes from your previous pregnancy and read through them. National guidelines advise that healthy women should have seven antenatal appointments during their second pregnancy, while first-timers have 10. You may feel that you're not receiving the same level of attention as you did before, but this is because second pregnancies are generally straightforward. If there is anything worrying you, give your midwife a ring.

Shared experiences

Perhaps you are pregnant with your second child at the same time as other friends. You can share experiences with them, sympathise with each other over

If you're pregnant for the second time, take every opportunity to spend time with your first child before your new baby arrives.

pregnancy symptoms and snatch a quick cup of coffee while your toddlers play together! If there is a big gap between your pregnancies, perhaps contact your local National Childbirth Trust (NCT) branch; they run "refresher" courses for women expecting their second or subsequent babies.

Getting ready for pregnancy

Staying safe and healthy

Your pregnancy diary

Birth and beyond

Parents**Ask...**

I've had some light bleeding. Is that a period or something else?

It's impossible to say for sure at this stage. If your period is usually right on schedule and you are now late, you may well be pregnant. On the other hand, it's not uncommon for women to get their period a few days late sometimes.

It's thought that implantation (when the embryo attaches itself to the lining of the uterus) can sometimes cause spotting. However, one small study in the United States found that nine per cent of women had at least one day of bleeding during their early pregnancy, and this was more likely to happen when a woman's period was due than around implantation.

If you have other symptoms, such as a one-sided pain low down in your tummy, see your midwife or doctor immediately; it might be an ectopic pregnancy (when the embryo has implanted in the fallopian tube rather than in the uterus; see pp.44–5). Bleeding with abdominal pain may also be a sign of an impending miscarriage, but that certainly isn't true in every case.

Finally, it's possible that the blood you saw may have nothing to do with pregnancy. Your cervix could be inflamed and bleed easily, especially after cervical smears, internal examinations or sex. Or you may have an infection. Either way, it's always important to report any bleeding between periods or after sex to your doctor.

▼ Your body at **04** Weeks

04 Weeks

❄ You may not feel pregnant yet, but your body is already going through enormous changes.

❄ Feeling queasy yet? If not, brace yourself – nausea and vomiting (morning sickness) can strike any time.

If finding out you're pregnant brings mixed feelings, listen to those feelings and talk them through. Remember, you have another eight months or so to get used to the idea of becoming a mum.

Feelings of anticipation

The two layers of the embryo form organs and tissue

Excitement, joy, anticipation – all of these emotions run high once you find out you're pregnant. But pregnancy brings out the worrier in us, too. And for good reason: you're growing a life inside of you. It's natural to fret about what you eat, drink, think, feel and do because you don't want anything to hurt your baby. You may also worry about how this new person will change your life and personal relationships.

Pregnancy can be a stressful and overwhelming time. You may be overjoyed at the thought of having a baby one day, and then the next day start wondering what you've got yourself into. You may be worried about whether you'll be a good mum, whether the baby will be healthy, and how the cost of having a child will affect your family's future finances. And you may worry about how your relationship with your partner and your other children will be affected – whether you'll still be able to give them the attention they need. As

unsettling as this is (especially if you pride yourself on being in control), try to remind yourself that this kind of emotional upheaval is normal at this stage. Mood swings are thought to be caused partly by fluctuating hormones (see p.71 and p.76). They tend to be most pronounced in the first 12 weeks of pregnancy. They should gradually diminish as you sort things out and as your body adapts to its new role.

To help with mood swings if you're feeling low, try these suggestions:

● **Talk it over** Air your worries about the future with your partner or understanding friends. Just putting your concerns into words often helps dispel them or helps you find solutions.

● **Do something that makes you feel good** This might mean carving out some special time for you and your partner. Or it might mean taking some time alone for yourself: curl up for a nap, go for a walk, have a massage, or see a film with a friend.

● **Take care of yourself** Get plenty of sleep, eat well, exercise, and try to have some fun. If you still find anxiety creeping in, try taking a pregnancy yoga class, practising meditation or other relaxation techniques.

▼ Your baby at **04** Weeks

Your ball of cells is now, officially, called an embryo (see p.34) and it's changing fast.

❄ The embryo is now divided into two layers that will form your baby's organs and tissues. It is attached to the developing placenta by a stalk that will form part of the umbilical cord. It also starts changing from a disc to an upside-down pear shape with a line – the primitive streak – down the centre.

My cluster of cells

This week marks the beginning of the embryonic period, when the blastocyst has implanted and become an embryo. From now until 10 weeks, all of your baby's organs will begin to develop and some will even begin to function. As a result, this is the stage when he'll be most vulnerable to anything that might interfere with his development.

He is now the size of a poppy seed and consists of two layers: the epiblast and the hypoblast. All his organs and body parts develop from these.

The primitive placenta is also made up of two layers at this point. Its cells are busy tunnelling into the lining of your uterus, creating spaces for your blood to flow so that the developed placenta will be able to provide nutrients and oxygen to your growing baby when it starts to function at the end of this week.

Also present now are the amniotic sac, which will house your baby, the amniotic fluid, which will cushion him as he grows, and the yolk sac, which produces your baby's red blood cells and helps deliver nutrients to him until the placenta has developed and is ready to take over this duty.

If you're taking any medications – prescription or over-the-counter – ask now whether it's safe to keep taking them. And be sure to alert your doctor to any other issues of concern.

The next six weeks are critical to your baby's development. The rudimentary versions of the placenta and umbilical cord, which deliver nourishment and oxygen to your baby, are already functioning. Through the placenta, your baby is exposed to what you take into your body, so make sure it's good for both of you.

Eleven days after fertilisation the inner cells of the embryo start developing into two layers – the epiblast and the hypoblast.

If you haven't already tried a home pregnancy test, taking one now will confirm your pregnancy. Once you get confirmation, you can call your doctor and make an appointment. Good consistent antenatal care is one of the best ways to ensure that you and your baby are healthy throughout pregnancy.

Dad's **Diary**

From pharmacy to father

" 'Can I help you?' the pharmacist enquires. I blush bright red. 'Condoms?' she second guesses. 'Actually, I need a pregnancy test.'

'Oh! Any preference for the type?'

The wee-on-a-stick type? The words form in my mind, but somehow I resist saying them. I shake my head. I don't have a preferred pregnancy-testing method.

The pharmacist passes me a box with a reassuring warm smile. 'This one should be fine.' I hurriedly exit the shop, feeling like some naughty schoolboy. But at nearly 40 years old, I am anything but.

Now back at home with Jo, I supervise a controlled test under strict laboratory conditions; we have to do it properly.

'Two minutes.' I begin a countdown as if commentating on a space-shuttle launch. My stopwatch bleeps. It's the moment of truth. We stare at each other in silence for a moment before I flip the test over. 'Well?' Jo begs.

Through the gaps in my fingers I am staring at the test window. I'm staring at the very faint blue line which is starting to appear. I can hear Jo's voice somewhere in the distance, but I daren't take my eyes off that line. Come on! You can do it! I will it on as if we have just fast-forwarded nine months to the birth.

'Yes!' At last I can afford to look up at Jo. 'Yes. I'm going to be a Dad!' "

If you've decided to start a family, the joy of discovering you're pregnant is one that you'll want to share with your partner.

▼ Your body at **05** Weeks

05 Weeks

✱ Pregnancy symptoms continue or start this week. Most women notice nausea, fatigue and sore breasts.

✱ Hormonal changes this week will start to expand your kidneys, making you need to urinate more often.

You're thrilled to be pregnant, but not so thrilled by the effect it has on your party-animal lifestyle. But remember, giving up the booze, cigarettes and recreational drugs is the best way to protect your baby.

Time to kick those bad habits

We all have our vices, but while you're pregnant it pays to put the partying on hold – at least for a while!

I'm a smoker...

Even if you haven't managed to stop smoking in the past, you can do it this time. About 30 per cent of all pregnant women who smoke manage to give up. Different people take different approaches to giving up smoking.

Most successful quitters set a "giving-up date" and make it public by telling friends, family and colleagues. Once you've established the "when",

bite to eat; others go for a walk. Find something to distract your mind for a few minutes. Giving up smoking can be much easier if you don't try to do it by yourself. Support from friends and family can increase your chances of success. Ask the people close to you for help.

I take drugs

Giving up any drug is never easy when you are addicted, even when you are pregnant. Although it may take courage, it is always better to let your maternity care providers know if you are taking a particular drug. Then they will be able to

▼ Your baby at **05** Weeks

You may not look pregnant yet, but plenty of changes are happening inside you.

✱ At this early stage you may not even have had any pregnancy symptoms but your baby is growing rapidly. The embryo still looks more like a tadpole than a human, but by the end of this week the tiny S-shaped heart may have begun to beat and the eyes and ears will have started to develop.

"Binge drinking **is dangerous** for your **developing baby**."

it's time to think about the "how". Ask yourself if you're ready to go cold turkey or if you'd prefer to use nicotine replacement therapy (NRT). You'll need to plan ahead for cravings too. These last only two or three minutes on average so your plan can be a simple one. Some people chew gum or grab a

make sure you and your baby receive the specific help and care you need. Remember: you won't be the first mum-to-be in this position that they've ever met, and they will do what they can to help. By asking for help you will be demonstrating your willingness to put your baby's health first. If you take just

Now that you are pregnant you can still enjoy a night out with your girlfriends at a bar or restaurant, but go easy on the alcohol.

Systemised mum

Writing a pregnancy diary can have practical uses as well as being part of your family history.

"I haven't written a diary since I was a teenager, but as soon as I discovered I was pregnant, I really wanted to make a record of all the weird and wonderful things that are happening to me. Whenever I ask my mum about when she was pregnant with me, she can never quite remember. I don't want to forget a thing – and I'd like my baby to be able to read my pregnancy journal one day, too. I make a note of changes to my body, how I'm feeling, all my anxieties. It's great to get things off my chest, even though no one else reads it. It's also quite practical. I note down what I've eaten so I can keep track of my calorie intake and make sure I'm getting all the right nutrients."

recreational drugs occasionally or at the weekends, these will still harm your baby, so now is the time to stop.

I like a drink or two

Binge drinking or getting drunk during pregnancy is dangerous for your developing baby. Binge drinking is drinking five or more units of alcohol on one occasion. Alcohol is a toxin. When you drink, it rapidly reaches your baby through your bloodstream and across the placenta. Too much alcohol can cause permanent damage to a developing baby. The damage can lead to a range of problems called fetal alcohol spectrum disorders (FASD). It can also cause problems during pregnancy, such as miscarriage and premature birth. The Department of Health (DH) recommends that you give up drinking before getting pregnant, and FASD experts suggest not drinking at all during pregnancy. Other experts are less sure whether drinking at moderate levels is dangerous or not. According to the Royal College of Obstetricians and Gynaecologists, there is no proof of harm from drinking within the limit of no more than one to two units of alcohol, no more than once or twice a week during pregnancy. If you did drink, don't worry too much. Thousands of women have a drink or two before they know they are pregnant, or conceived around the time of a binge-drinking session, and their babies have been fine.

Recreational drugs and pregnancy

Recreational drugs can be harmful to you and your baby during pregnancy. Here's an idea of how they affect you:
● **Marijuana** Several studies have associated regular use of marijuana during pregnancy with fetal growth retardation and low birthweight.
● **LSD** One study showed that the pure form of LSD did not cause any fetal abnormalities or an increased risk of miscarriage. However, there have been reports of congenital abnormalities in the babies of women who use LSD and other drugs. As we do not know exactly what effect these drugs have on unborn babies, it's wise to avoid them.
● **Cocaine** This drug can cause serious problems. If used in the early months, it can increase the risk of miscarriage. Used later, it could trigger premature labour. It may also cause the placenta to separate from the wall of the uterus before labour begins.
● **Ecstasy and amphetamines** These substances have been linked to birth defects, mainly of the limbs and heart.
● **Heroin** This can cause growth restriction, premature delivery – around half of the babies who are born to heroin-addicted mothers are born early – and stillbirth.

Diet in the first trimester

If you live on cheese sandwiches and coffee, it's time to spruce up your diet. Not only will this help you cope with early pregnancy symptoms like fatigue and nausea, but it will ensure that you and your baby get all the vital nutrients you need while you're pregnant.

The perfect pregnancy diet

You may not have much of an appetite at the moment, especially if you're suffering from nausea and vomiting. On the other hand, you may be packing away more food than you ever dreamed possible. However you find that pregnancy is affecting your appetite, it's important to try to eat healthily when you can. A healthy diet will make you feel better, and give your baby all the nutrients she needs to develop.

Small regular meals, and frequent (non-caffeinated) drinks, can combat any nausea or tiredness. Contrary to popular belief, you don't need any extra calories in your first two trimesters, so you definitely should not feel that you have to try to eat for two.

Fruit and veg

Government guidelines suggest eating five portions of fruit and vegetables a day as part of a healthy diet, and this is particularly important during pregnancy. If you're not a fan of fruit and vegetables make a start by eating more of those you do like. Add sliced bananas or apple to your breakfast cereal, grate carrots onto your lunch time roll, drink a lunch time glass of pure fruit juice (this counts as one portion) or have two different vegetables with your main meal instead of your usual one.

Folic acid is a particularly important nutrient during the first trimester (see opposite). Overcooking destroys folates, so try to eat your vegetables lightly steamed, microwaved or raw.

And finally, eat when you are hungry. As long as you are eating fresh, wholesome foods and gaining weight at the appropriate rate, relax!

Five portions of fruit or vegetables (*above*) should be a regular part of your diet. A handful of grapes or two handfuls of cherries or berry fruits make up a portion. **Milk and dairy products (*left*)** such as cheese and yogurt are sources of calcium.

If you're suffering from nausea and sickness in the early months of your pregnancy, eating small, regular meals will be better than infrequent, large ones. You'll probably feel better if you eat lightly cooked food. Stir-fries are better than fry-ups.

Essential vitamins and minerals

In some circumstances it can be difficult to get all the nutrients you need through diet alone – if you are suffering badly with nausea and vomiting, for example. In this case, your doctor or midwife may advise you to take a vitamin and mineral supplement especially designed for pregnant women.

There are no hard-and-fast rules as to what has to be in a multivitamin in order for it to be called an antenatal supplement, but a good supplement generally contains more folic acid, iron and calcium than a general multivitamin. It also mustn't contain the retinol form of vitamin A, which can be harmful to your growing baby.

Folic acid

Folic acid is a B vitamin, which is found in a number of foods, including leafy greens, black-eyed beans, chickpeas, broccoli, asparagus, peas, brown rice and fortified cereals, wheatgerm and papaya. The body does not store much folic acid, so doctors recommend that you take a daily supplement containing 400 micrograms (mcg) of folic acid during the first 12 weeks of pregnancy, and ideally for at least three months before trying to conceive. This can reduce your risk of having a baby with a neural tube defect, such as spina bifida.

Fact: Riboflavin, found in milk, eggs, and mushrooms, not only promotes good vision and healthy skin in you – it is also essential for your baby's bone, muscle, and nerve development.

Iron

Iron is needed to make the extra blood required to support your growing baby. Your body makes so much extra blood when you're pregnant that you need about 30 to 60 milligrams (mg) of iron every day – that's 15 to 45mg more than the recommended daily allowance of 15mg. Good sources of iron in your diet include lean red meat, fortified bread and cereals, dark green leafy vegetables (such as curly kale and watercress), beans and lentils, and dried fruits such as figs. Although liver is a good source of iron, if you're pregnant you should avoid eating it because a build-up in your body can harm your unborn baby.

Calcium

A woman needs twice as much calcium when she's pregnant: 1,500mg a day. It is found in milk products, dark green leafy vegetables, tofu, and tinned salmon and sardines (you should eat the bones).

Other nutrients

Besides folic acid, iron and calcium, a good antenatal supplement should also contain vitamin C, vitamin D, B vitamins, such as B6 and B12, potassium, zinc and vitamin E. Once you have found the right supplement, never take more than the recommended daily intake (usually one multivitamin a day). Taking megadoses of certain vitamins can be harmful to you and your baby.

Strict vegetarians and women suffering from conditions such as diabetes, epilepsy, gestational diabetes or anaemia, should talk with their doctor or midwife about any special supplements they might need.

If your diet doesn't give you all the nutrients you need, you may need to take a multivitamin supplement for pregnancy.

 Green mum

A vegetarian diet during pregnancy can provide all the nutrients you need.

"Now that I know I'm pregnant, I've been eating lots of pulses, nuts, seeds and soya products just to make sure I'm getting enough protein. And I know that iron and calcium are two nutrients that are particularly important during pregnancy. I've read up about it and discovered that the iron's important for the extra blood I'll need, and the calcium will protect my bones. As a vegetarian I've had to adapt slightly to make sure I'm getting enough in my diet. For iron I've been eating more wholemeal bread, pulses, fortified cereals and green vegetables, and for calcium I've been having plenty of cheese and milk, although one of my pregnant vegetarian friends who doesn't eat dairy products has been taking a calcium supplement."

Nuts are a good source of protein and many contain calcium, too.

Getting ready for pregnancy

Staying safe and healthy

Your pregnancy diary

Birth and beyond

▼ Your body at **06** Weeks

06 Weeks

❋ Sore breasts and frequent trips to the loo may start to disturb your sleep about now.

❋ It's common to feel tired or even exhausted as your body becomes used to changing hormone levels.

As soon as you know you're pregnant, visit your doctor. She can confirm your pregnancy, answer any questions you may have and book your first midwife appointment. She may also suggest a few health checks.

Your first visit to the doctor

A large head and developing organs can now be seen

It's best to contact your doctor's surgery as soon as you know you're pregnant. Your doctor will be happy to meet you in early pregnancy to start to plan your antenatal care. You may be asked to bring a urine sample to confirm your pregnancy, although many doctors are happy to accept home test results.

At the first appointment, your doctor will calculate how many weeks pregnant you are based on the first day of your last period, so if you haven't already made a note of it, try to remember what day it was. From this, she'll also be able to estimate your due date. She'll check your blood pressure, weight and height, and examine your abdomen. It's unlikely that you'll have a vaginal examination, unless you have any bleeding or abdominal pain.

You may be asked about any medical problems you've had in the past, and about problems in previous pregnancies, such as miscarriage or high blood pressure. If you have a pre-existing medical condition, such as epilepsy or diabetes, that may affect your pregnancy, she'll be able to organise the appropriate antenatal care for you, and advise you on how to manage your condition now that you're pregnant.

She may discuss what you can do to keep yourself and the baby healthy. She'll advise you to take folic acid (see p.49) and possibly vitamin D supplements. If you smoke, she'll outline the health risks to your unborn baby (see p.17) and will be able to offer advice or refer you to organisations that can help you quit. She'll also ask how much

▼ Your baby at **06** Weeks

At this stage, your baby has reached about the size of a small bean.

❋ If you could see inside yourself at the end of this week, you'd see that your baby has a large head with dark spots where the eyes are beginning to form, and tiny ears just appearing. The liver, lungs, stomach and pancreas are starting to develop and his blood-circulation system continues to become more sophisticated.

Your doctor will calculate your due date, answer any questions you may have and arrange your booking appointment.

alcohol you drink (see p.119) and may ask you if you take any recreational or prescription drugs.

If you have any questions for your doctor, make a note of them before you go. It's a good time to air any early worries you may have, whether it's about workplace safety, pre-booked travel plans, or a hereditary illness that you are concerned may affect your baby. After this appointment, your doctor will arrange your booking appointment with your midwife (see pp.128–9).

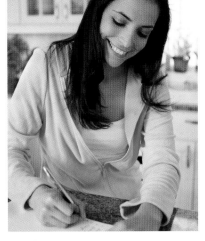

Making a list of questions that you'd like to ask your doctor can help you to focus during your antenatal appointment.

Healthcare professionals

Confused about who will care for you while you're pregnant and after the birth? Here are the main players.

● **Midwife** Almost always female, midwives provide care to women during pregnancy, labour, birth, and after your baby is born – usually for the first 10 days, although this can be extended to 28 days if you have particular needs.
● **Doctor** You may see your family doctor for all or some of your antenatal checks. Even if you have midwife-led care, you'll still be able to consult your doctor if you have any health problems while you're pregnant, whether these are related to the pregnancy or not.
● **Obstetrician** This is a doctor or surgeon who specialises in pregnancy, childbirth and the immediate postnatal period. If you have a medical or obstetric history that's in any way out-of-the-ordinary, you may be put under the care of a hospital obstetrician, in which case you'll see a doctor as well as a midwife at your antenatal checks.

Systemised mum

If you never shop without a list, you're sure to have a list ready for that first antenatal appointment.

"I'm so excited about being pregnant but, as this will be my first baby, I don't want to forget to ask the doctor anything important. I've prepared a list of questions for when I get to see her at my first antenatal appointment. Here they are:
● Is there anything special I can do to make sure I stay healthy?
● Do I need to take any supplements?
● Which foods should I avoid?
● Which screening tests can I have?
● When will I have my first scan?
● Do I have any other options for giving birth apart from my local hospital (for example, at home)?
● When do I need to book antenatal classes, to be sure of getting a place?
● What exercise can I do, and are there any pregnancy exercise classes I can join?
● Which over-the-counter and prescription drugs should I stop taking now I'm pregnant?"

The role of the amniotic sac

The amniotic sac is the bag of fluid inside your uterus that contains your baby. It's made up of two membranes called the amnion and the chorion. The amniotic sac is filled with amniotic fluid (also known as "the waters"), which helps to cushion your baby from bumps and injury, as well as providing him with fluids that he can breathe and swallow. This clear, slightly yellow fluid maintains a constant temperature for your baby and provides a barrier against infection.

The amniotic sac begins to form and fill with fluid within just a day or two of conception. The amount of fluid in the sac will increase gradually until around week 38, when it will reduce slightly until your baby is born.

The membranes which make up the sac occasionally rupture as labour begins, but they usually remain intact until the end of the first stage of labour. The membranes may also be broken by a midwife or doctor to induce or to speed up labour.

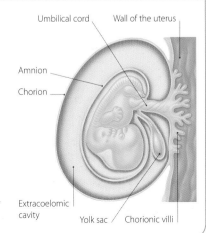

Umbilical cord
Wall of the uterus
Amnion
Chorion
Extracoelomic cavity
Yolk sac
Chorionic villi

FIRST TRIMESTER	SECOND TRIMESTER	THIRD TRIMESTER

Your body at **07** Weeks

07 Weeks

✳ Your uterus has doubled in size in just two months but you're unlikely to look pregnant yet.

✳ Emotions run high in the early weeks so you're bound to feel fragile or irritated occasionally.

If you are one of the unlucky mums-to-be who is suffering from nausea and vomiting, be gentle on yourself, accept all offers of help and see if any of our tried-and-tested tips work for you.

Nausea and vomiting

The small tail of the embryo will soon disappear

No one knows why the first sign of pregnancy for many mums-to-be is an early morning dash to the bathroom. With around eight out of 10 pregnant women feeling sick, and half of them actually vomiting, many women spend the early weeks of pregnancy feeling awful rather than "blooming".

How badly affected you may be varies widely from woman to woman. You may get the odd bout of mild queasiness when you first wake, or you may endure weeks or even months of feeling or actually being sick.

Pregnancy sickness used to be known as "morning sickness" but this name is misleading. It may be worse in the morning, but most sufferers get it throughout the day and into the evening. It can take over your life for a time. If you get it badly you may find yourself unable to work, to care for your toddler or other children, to cook, shop or run your home.

The cause is unknown, but nausea and vomiting are thought to be connected to the effects of the hormone hCG. Although it won't help your nausea, feeling sick is actually a good sign as it means that your pregnancy-hormone levels are high enough. Other hormones, such as oestrogen and the thyroid hormone thyroxine, are also thought to play a part.

Nausea and vomiting usually start at around five or six weeks of pregnancy but most women find that it improves by 14 weeks. Some have it until 16 weeks, whereas others experience varying degrees of it for the whole nine months. Luckily, this is unusual, and there may be support available.

The most severe form of pregnancy sickness is called hyperemesis gravidarum (literally "excessive vomiting in pregnancy"). If you are vomiting frequently, are unable to eat and drink without vomiting, or are losing weight, then you are probably suffering from hyperemesis. This can affect your health and that of your baby, so talk to your doctor or midwife about it as soon as you can. There are certain treatments that can help you at home, or you may need to go to hospital.

Your baby at **07** Weeks

Your baby's growing fast now. She's doubled her size since last week.

✳ In theory, your baby is still an embryo because she has the remains of a small tail, which will disappear in the next few weeks. Her heart and brain are becoming more complicated, her eyelid folds are forming, and her nostrils may be visible. Her arm buds are starting to look more like arms and curve slightly over her heart.

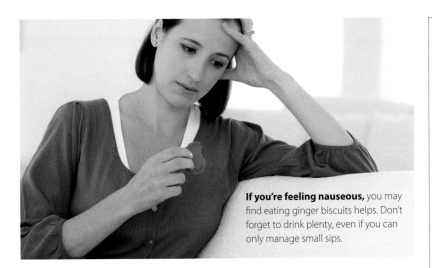

If you're feeling nauseous, you may find eating ginger biscuits helps. Don't forget to drink plenty, even if you can only manage small sips.

It is a good idea to tell your partner, family and friends how you're feeling, and what you need, as they may be struggling to know how to help you. You may also have to tell people at work about your pregnancy (and about your nausea and vomiting) earlier than you were planning, so you can get the support you need.

Try not to get overtired and to minimise stress. If necessary, take time off work. Eat little and often, and try to see which foods suit you and which make you worse. Rich, fatty, highly spiced foods are often the culprits. Most importantly, keep well hydrated, sipping iced water, lemon squash, barley water or whatever you can manage.

Safe remedies for nausea and vomiting

If pregnancy sickness is making your life a misery, hopefully one of the remedies below will help.

Ginger Steep grated root ginger in boiled water, leave to cool and sip it throughout the day.

Acupressure You could try wearing wristbands that stimulate an acupuncture point (the Pericardium 6, or PC6, point), which can relieve sickness. Try putting the bands on first thing in the morning before you even get out of bed. During the day, if you experience a wave of nausea, press on the button (one wrist and then the other) about 20 to 30 times at one-second intervals.

Mint Sip peppermint or spearmint tea. Sugar-free chewing gum or peppermint sweets may also help.

Fetal development

Big news this week. Hands and feet are just starting to emerge from developing arms and legs – although they look more like paddles at this point than the tiny, pudgy extremities you're daydreaming about holding and tickling. Technically, your baby is still considered an embryo and has something of a small tail, which is an extension of her tailbone. The tail will disappear within a few weeks, but that's the only thing that is getting smaller. Your baby has doubled in size since last week and now measures 1.25cm (½in) long – about the size of a blueberry. Developing muscles mean she's also becoming a jumping bean, moving in fits and starts.

Your baby now has eyelid folds partially covering her eyes, which already have some colour, and tiny veins are visible beneath parchment-thin skin. Right now, the teeth and palate are forming, and the ears continue to develop.

Both hemispheres of her brain are growing, too, and her liver is making red blood cells. This continues until her bone marrow forms and takes over this role. She also has an appendix and a pancreas, which will eventually produce insulin to aid in digestion. A loop in her growing intestines is bulging into her umbilical cord, which now has distinct blood vessels to carry oxygen and nutrients to and from her tiny body.

Identifiable hands and arms are starting to develop in this six- to seven-week embryo, although the hands look a bit like paddles.

Getting ready for pregnancy

Staying safe and healthy

Your pregnancy diary

Birth and beyond

▼ Your body at **08** Weeks

08 Weeks

✳ Although you're unlikely to have gained much weight, parts of you, like your breasts, are certainly growing.

✳ As your uterus grows, you may feel cramps in your lower abdomen as your ligaments stretch.

It's time to think about your antenatal care. If things are straightforward, you'll probably have most appointments with a midwife at your local clinic. If complications develop, you'll see an obstetrician.

Planning your antenatal care

Your options for antenatal care vary according to the area in which you live. You're likely to be offered some variation on the following:

● **Shared care** This means you are looked after by your doctor and community midwife, seeing each alternately.

● **Midwife-only care** If you have this, you'll see one of the team of community midwives – not necessarily the same one – at each antenatal visit.

● **One-to-one care** With this type of care, you'll be seen by the same midwife for almost all of your antenatal visits, although you'll also meet at least one other midwife during the course of your pregnancy. Your main midwife or her back-up will also help you give birth to your baby.

● **Consultant care** This means you'll be under the care of a named hospital consultant – an obstetrician (a specialist in pregnant women) – and you will see her or a member of her staff at some or perhaps all of your antenatal visits.

Another option is to have private antenatal care with an independent midwife. In this case, your antenatal checks can be done entirely at home, and you can either have a home birth or go to hospital with your independent midwife. Expect to pay around £2,500 plus for this service.

Guidelines commissioned by the National Institute for Health and Clinical Excellence (NICE) say that women with an uncomplicated pregnancy are best looked after by midwives and doctors. There should be no need to involve an obstetrician.

First and subsequent checks
It's increasingly common for the first appointment, known as the booking appointment, to be done at your home. After that, you're likely to have your checks at your local doctor's surgery or health clinic. You'll only have all of your checks at the hospital if you need consultant care. It's now common in many parts of the country for pregnant women to go right through their 40 weeks without seeing an obstetrician at all. However, if there's any problem, however small, your midwife will refer you immediately to an obstetrician.

Now officially a fetus

▼ Your baby at **08** Weeks

Congratulations – your embryo is now called a fetus, which means "offspring".

✳ He now measures approximately 1.6cm/½in. His embryonic tail is gone, and all his organs, muscles, and nerves are beginning to function. His hands now bend at the wrist, and his feet begin to lose their webbed appearance. Eyelids are beginning to cover his eyes and taste buds start to form on his tongue.

Going to the hospital

Many women go to hospital at least once during their pregnancy, and that is usually for an ultrasound scan. NICE recommends that women are offered a dating scan (see p.136) between 10 and 13 weeks and an anomaly scan (see pp.156–7) between 18 and 20 weeks.

All scans and tests are optional. Your midwife or doctor should be able to tell you exactly what is involved in each and will leave it up to you to decide if you want it. Don't go along with something because it seems like "the thing to do". Make sure you know exactly what's being checked for, and how and when you'll be given the results.

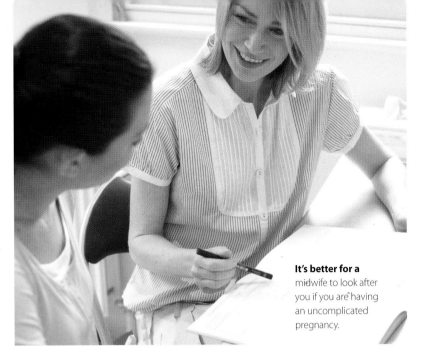

It's better for a midwife to look after you if you are having an uncomplicated pregnancy.

Single mum

Planning your antenatal care can help you feel in control of your pregnancy.

"Despite the fact that I've progressed from feeling nauseous to actually being sick, I'm starting to feel positive about my pregnancy. I was a little nervous about my first appointment with the doctor. I was worried he might be judgemental about me being single and pregnant, but he wasn't at all. He explained what antenatal care is available where I live, when I'll have my scans, and what will happen at my booking appointment. It all feels very real now and I feel much more confident now that I know I'll have total control over what happens in the next seven months.

So, I've stopped worrying so much about how I'll cope alone, and how I'll manage financially, and I've started worrying about all the usual things that bother pregnant mums – and that actually feels quite good!"

Private screening tests

Despite government recommendations that all women should have access to the same screening tests on the NHS, there is still great variation in what is available. Some hospitals can offer women the recommended scans and tests, while others are short of funds and resources, so it is difficult for them to do so.

If your local hospital does not offer the scans or tests you would like, you may decide to pay for one privately. Here is a round-up of what's available privately:

● Nuchal translucency (NT) scans between 11 and 14 weeks of pregnancy, with or without an assessment of the nasal bone. If this bone is absent, small or poorly formed, it may be an indication of Down's syndrome.

● The combined test – a NT scan, plus a blood test for hCG (see p.37) and for Pregnancy-Associated Plasma Protein A (PAPP-A) between 11 and 14 weeks of pregnancy

● The integrated test – the combined test at 11 to 14 weeks of pregnancy (NT scan and a blood test for hCG and PAPP-A)

with a further blood test for alpha-feto-protein (AFP), unconjugated estriol (uE3) and inhibin A at 15 to 20 weeks.

The combined test and the integrated test are the most accurate screening tests that are available privately. They cost between £110 and £200 depending on where you have the tests. There are around 90 test centres in the UK.

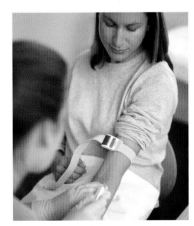

A shortage of funds in your area may mean you can't have the tests you want. If that's the case you can choose to pay.

FIRST TRIMESTER	SECOND TRIMESTER	THIRD TRIMESTER

▼ Your body at **09** Weeks

09 Weeks

❋ By now you'll find that hormonal fluctuations are really making your emotions yo-yo.

❋ At this stage, pregnancy hormones in your body may be causing some painful headaches.

You'll have your first antenatal appointment before 12 weeks of pregnancy so that your doctor or midwife can book you in for early scans and tests if necessary. Here's what to expect.

Your first antenatal visit

Your first official check-up in pregnancy is known as your booking appointment. For this, you're most likely to see your community midwife and it may be done at home. After that, you can opt to have all your appointments with the community midwives, or shared with your doctor. If you have a serious health condition or other complication, you will also see a consultant obstetrician from time to time. Be prepared for lots of questions and form filling! Here are some of the things the midwife may ask:

- **Date of last period** This allows your midwife to calculate your due date. You should also be offered a dating scan to get a more accurate idea of how pregnant you are.
- **Miscarriages, abortions and births** Your "obstetric history" could have a bearing on this pregnancy and birth, in case you need extra treatment.
- **Family history of disease/genetic conditions** Screening is now available for known genetic conditions, such as cystic fibrosis.

Your baby at **09** Weeks

Your baby weighs under 10g/½oz – but she is poised for growth.

❋ All of her body parts are now present and correct, including arms, legs, eyes, genitals and other organs. Her eyelids are fused and won't open until 27 weeks. Her wrists are more developed, her ankles have formed, and her fingers and toes are clearly visible. Her arms can even bend at the elbows now.

Understanding your notes

Mystified by the shorthand on your notes? Here's what all those abbreviations mean:

Length of pregnancy 8+3 (8 weeks and three days pregnant)

Blood pressure 120/70 (the lower figure should not be higher than 90)

Urine PGO – contains Protein, Glucose or anything else (Other); NAD – no abnormalities detected

Height of uterus The number of centimetres corresponds to the number of weeks you have been pregnant.

Position of your baby (see p.197)
Cephalic (or ceph) – head-down
Br – bottom down or breech

Heartbeat or activity FHH: fetal heart heard; FHNH: fetal heart not heard; FMF: fetal movements felt; FMNF: fetal movements not felt

● **Your lifestyle** Your midwife will ask how much alcohol you drink and whether you smoke. She'll also have information for you on diet and exercise in pregnancy.

● **Where to have your baby** You will be told about your options so you've got plenty of time to think about them.

Your midwife will also want to carry out some tests.

● **Blood tests** She will take at least a couple of test tubes of blood for analysis.

● **Screening tests** Your midwife may also ask if you want a blood test to screen for your baby's risk of Down's syndrome and spina bifida.

● **Urine check** She will check for protein in your urine (an early sign of pre-eclampsia; see p.233) and urinary tract infections (see p.228).

● **Blood pressure check** The result will be used as a "baseline average" for future checks.

● **Ultrasound scan** If your midwife is based at the local hospital, your first antenatal appointment may be combined with a dating scan (see p.136).

● **Measuring your weight and height** Your midwife will record your weight at the first appointment, but won't keep close tabs on it unless you start to put on a large amount.

Telling everyone you're pregnant

When you tell people you're pregnant is entirely up to you. Many mums-to-be wait until they're at least 13 weeks pregnant and the risk of miscarriage drops. Some wait until they've had their first scan, while others, particularly first-time parents, can't wait to share their news with everyone.

Keeping your baby news a secret is understandable in the first trimester, particularly if you've had a miscarriage in the past. But if your pregnancy ends and no one knows, it can be hard to cope with your loss on your own.

If you have children already, their age may help you decide when and how to tell them. If you have an older child, you'll probably want to tell her at around the same time as you tell other family members. Once she knows, she'll want to share the news.

A toddler won't really understand that you're having a baby until you start to show – or even until you have your baby. You'll need to let your employer know about your pregnancy by the 15th week before the week that your baby is due to arrive (see p.64).

It's best to tell your older child your news when you tell the rest of the family.

Getting ready for pregnancy

Staying safe and healthy

Your pregnancy diary

Birth and beyond

Sleep in early pregnancy

If you can't remember when you last had a good night's sleep, don't despair. In early pregnancy, high levels of pregnancy hormones can leave you feeling shattered during the day and tossing and turning at night. But this should pass once you enter your second trimester.

Exhaustion in the early days is normal. Listen to your body and get as much rest as you can for your sake and your baby's.

Bedtime ritual for a good night's sleep

If you're suffering from disrupted sleep now that you're pregnant, try some or all of these useful tips:
● Cut down on caffeinated drinks, such as tea and coffee, and avoid them completely during the afternoon and evening.
● Keep your bedroom cool.
● Use your bed for sleep and sex only.
● If your chores aren't done by suppertime, leave them for tomorrow.
● Finish exercising at least three or four hours before you go to bed.
● Regulate your body clock by going to bed at the same time every night.

Tired all the time

At this stage you'll probably be feeling very sleepy during the day. This is caused by raised levels of progesterone in your body. Although this hormone makes you drowsy, it can also disrupt your sleep at night. Sadly, there's no real way around this problem other than to rest when you can, even if you can't actually sleep.

Your newly tender breasts may make it hard for you to find a comfortable sleeping position as well, especially if you normally sleep on your stomach. Your first trimester is the perfect time to get used to sleeping on your left side. This improves the flow of blood and nutrients to your baby, and helps your kidneys to get rid of waste and fluids.

Another sleep stealer is your growing uterus, which puts pressure on your bladder and sends you scrambling for the loo seemingly endlessly. You may find that it helps if you drink plenty of fluids during the day, but cut down in the late afternoon or evening.

If you feel caught in a vicious circle of wakefulness at night and exhaustion during the day, you're not alone. More than half of all pregnant women take at least one nap during weekdays, while 60 per cent take at least one weekend nap. You should expect this first three months to be the most tiring time of your pregnancy, so remember to listen to your body when it's telling you to slow down or rest.

Parents**Ask...**

Am I too tired? Could I be anaemic?
Fatigue is a common sign of anaemia (see p.229) – but it's also experienced by many pregnant women who are not anaemic. Breathlessness, headaches, tinnitus and palpitations are other symptoms of anaemia, along with unusual food cravings. Your eyelids, nail beds and tongue may also look paler than usual.

How will I know if I'm anaemic?
The routine blood tests that you will have at the antenatal clinic will check whether your haemoglobin levels are satisfactory or not. It's normal for the levels to drop a little during pregnancy because there's far more fluid in your blood to dilute the red blood cells. Only if your levels drop very low indeed will your doctor prescribe iron tablets for you.

In your dreams...

First your husband sleeps with your best friend. Then you sleep with an old boyfriend from your school days. Now you're trying to make a quick getaway – but from what? As you travel down the motorway, you have a nagging feeling that you've forgotten something. Suddenly you remember: you've left your baby at the gym!

Have you lost your mind? No – not your waking mind, anyway. During pregnancy, your dreams have more twists and turns than ever before. It's all down to your surging hormones, perhaps entwined with mixed feelings about your changing shape, and maybe the added ingredients of anxiety and excitement about becoming a mother.

Another reason why your dreams may have changed in style is that you are more likely to interrupt a dream-filled cycle of REM sleep by frequent waking during the night to go to the loo, ease a leg cramp, or move to a more comfortable position.

Some common images

Although it's impossible to predict what dreams you may have, there are some images that can often appear at certain stages of pregnancy. It's common to dream about birth and motherhood, sex, tall buildings, and water.

You could record your dreams and what you think they mean in a journal. Share your weird and wonderful tales with your partner, and don't forget to ask him what expectant father's dreams he's having. As a dad-to-be, his feelings of excitement, anticipation, anxiety, and worry may open a floodgate of dreams, too. Sharing your dreams and feelings throughout your pregnancy will help you both feel loved and needed.

Working mum

Usually on top of things at work? Now finding you can hardly keep your eyes open? It's just normal.

"I'm 10 weeks pregnant and the worst pregnancy symptom I'm suffering right now is the tiredness. I can barely stay awake while I'm at work sometimes. This week, I've been going back to the car at lunchtimes for a 20-minute cat nap to recharge my batteries. I feel a bit better afterwards, but it's been very difficult to concentrate. The hardest time is mid-afternoon – I could literally fall asleep at my desk around that time. None of my colleagues know that I'm pregnant, and my workload hasn't changed, so I guess I just have to plough on as best I can. When I finally manage to get home, I'm usually asleep in front of the TV by 7.30pm."

Raised levels of progesterone can disrupt your night-time sleep and make you crave a daytime nap. You're not alone!

Getting ready for pregnancy

Staying safe and healthy

Your pregnancy diary

Birth and beyond

FIRST TRIMESTER	SECOND TRIMESTER	THIRD TRIMESTER

▼ Your body at **10** Weeks

10 Weeks

✳ Your uterus is now about the size of a grapefruit – almost big enough to fill your pelvis.

✳ Strange dreams are common during pregnancy and could also contribute to disrupted nights.

It's natural to be concerned about twinges in your tummy when you are pregnant. They're common and usually nothing to worry about. You do need to be on the look out for certain warning signs, though.

Aches and pains in the early weeks

The fetus swallows and starts to have taste buds

Pains in the stomach are fairly common in early pregnancy and, on their own, are rarely a sign of a serious problem. Carrying a baby puts a lot of pressure on muscles, veins, ligaments, and the rest of your insides, so it's not surprising that you feel some discomfort, especially around your midriff.

This may be because the veins of your pelvis are congested. Or you may be tense: some people feel nervous about having sex during pregnancy. This can occur any time during pregnancy. Although you needn't avoid sex during a normal pregnancy, you may want to take it soft and slow. A gentle post-orgasm back rub may help soothe the pain. However, if you experience cramping along with spotting, heavy bleeding, fever, chills, vaginal discharge, continuous tenderness and pain, or if the cramps don't subside after several minutes, call your doctor.

Pregnancy cramps

Some common causes of cramps in early pregnancy include:

● **Ligament stretching** You might experience mild cramps on one or both sides of your abdomen. This is caused by the ligaments stretching so that they can support your growing uterus. It might occur from early through to late pregnancy. To help alleviate this, try sitting down, or lie down and put your feet up. Resting comfortably when you get any pain will usually alleviate it.

● **Orgasm** You may find that you get cramps during and after orgasm, sometimes combined with a backache.

Could it be more serious?

Some of the ailments that cause cramps during the first trimester are ectopic pregnancy (see pp.44–5) and early miscarriage (see pp.42–3). If your symptoms match those of either of these conditions, you should call your doctor immediately. If you think you may be having an early miscarriage, lie or sit down with your feet up, and relax as much as you possibly can.

If your cramping is accompanied by heavy bleeding, call 999 or go to the accident and emergency department of your nearest hospital.

▼ Your baby at **10** Weeks

Another three weeks, and your baby will have doubled his size.

✳ He is now swallowing and kicking, and all his major organs are fully developed. The external sex organs are just starting to show and, in a few weeks' time, they will be developed enough to reveal if you're going to be mum to a boy or a girl. More minute details are appearing too, such as fingernails and peach-fuzz hair.

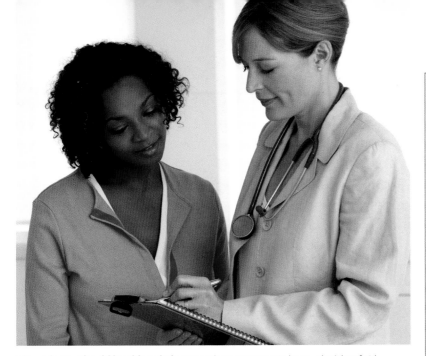

Your doctor should be able to help you with any queries you have – don't be afraid to ask, even if you think they're silly. You may be able to get a double appointment.

Getting the best out of your family doctor

When you are pregnant you may find yourself visiting your general practitioner or family doctor more frequently. Family doctors are "generalists", which means they know a little about each body system. Some will have more experience in some fields than others. Female doctors often specialise in women's health problems.

It's a good idea to contact your doctor's surgery as soon as you know you are pregnant. You can call your midwife or doctor's surgery any time if you have a pregnancy symptom that is worrying you, or if you just "don't feel right" – it's better to be safe than sorry.

Because of the number of appointments needed each day, the maximum amount of time a family doctor can allocate for each appointment is about 10 minutes.

If it were more than this, the waiting time to see a doctor would be too long. This means that it's vital to make the most of each consultation. Here are some tips that can help:

- If you've got more than one problem that you need to discuss with your doctor, write down an "agenda" and either give it to your doctor at the start of the consultation or tell your doctor what is on your list so that the most important items are discussed first.
- If you really feel that your problems cannot be dealt with in 10 minutes, ask the receptionist if it is possible to get a double appointment. Doctors can occasionally do this for a patient.
- If you have a recurring or long-term problem, try to see a doctor who is familiar with you and your condition. She then won't have to waste time

catching up with what has happened before and can use the appointment time more effectively.

Sometimes your problem can be easily dealt with by another member of the practice team. If you have a pregnancy-related problem, your midwife can usually help. Practice nurses can often deal with blood tests, holiday vaccinations and health check-ups for conditions such as asthma, diabetes and epilepsy.

Some doctors' surgeries have nurse practitioners. These are nurses who have undergone extra training that allows them to be able to deal with more straightforward complaints, such as cystitis (urinary tract infection), skin complaints or sore throats. Nurse practitioners are also allowed to write you a prescription.

Systemised mum

It's good to know you can always contact your doctor or midwife if you have a worrying symptom.

"I've been poring through pregnancy books and I'm really aware of every single ache and pain, hoping that it's nothing serious. I know it's early days, though, and I'm sure that once I've had my first scan I'll calm down a bit!

I've been getting odd twinges in my lower tummy. I know it can be a symptom of something perfectly normal like ligament stretching. But I also know that sometimes it can be something more serious like a urine infection or an ectopic pregnancy.

My style is to err on the side of caution. If I'm really worried, I know I can ring my doctor or midwife who can rule out anything serious and put my mind at rest."

| FIRST TRIMESTER | SECOND TRIMESTER | THIRD TRIMESTER |

▼ Your body at **11** Weeks

11 Weeks

❋ Leg cramps and heartburn may be annoying you during the day and keeping you up at night.

❋ A dark vertical line of pigmentation, called the linea nigra, may appear on your belly.

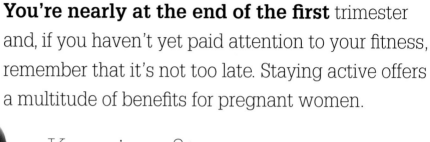

You're nearly at the end of the first trimester and, if you haven't yet paid attention to your fitness, remember that it's not too late. Staying active offers a multitude of benefits for pregnant women.

Keeping fit

Giving birth is akin to running a marathon – it requires stamina, determination, and focus. Keeping physically active during the months of your pregnancy is good preparation for the hard work of labour.

The Royal College of Obstetricians and Gynaecologists says that weight-bearing exercise throughout pregnancy can reduce the length of labour and decrease delivery complications. Weight-bearing exercise can mean simply using the weight of your body when you exercise, for instance when you walk briskly, jog, or dance. Or it can involve weight training, using free weights or a machine. If you already do weight-bearing exercise you may well be able to continue now you're pregnant, but check with your doctor first. If you are new to exercise, ask your doctor what's safe for you. If you join an exercise class, always tell the teacher that you are pregnant.

Other reasons for keeping fit

You may not have a bump yet, but you'll soon reach the stage where your body's not the svelte thing it used to be.

Although you know it's for a good cause, watching the scale creep its way up to numbers you've never seen before can be disheartening. Staying active can make you feel less frumpy. It can also help you shed weight faster postnatally. What is more, some research has shown that babies of women who exercised during pregnancy may do better in labour than those of the non-exercisers.

And if that weren't enough, exercise also strengthens your cardiovascular system so you don't tire as easily – a real plus now that you're pregnant. It also helps you to cope with stress and can give you a better night's sleep. Read pp.56–7 to learn more about the types of exercise that are suitable during pregnancy and about how to exercise safely. What are you waiting for?

Tips: Pelvic floor exercises help to prevent stress incontinence in later life and help ensure that your sex life is as good after your baby is born as it was before; they are often called "sexercises".

 Your baby at **11** Weeks

Your 4-cm/1½-in baby now has all her parts, from tooth buds to toenails.

❋ She is now really busy kicking and stretching; her movements are so fluid that, if you could watch them, you would think it was a sort of water ballet. Her fingers and toes have fully separated, too. Now her main task is to grow larger and stronger until she can survive on her own outside your uterus.

The benefits of Pilates

The tummy and pelvic floor muscles (see below) are known in Pilates as the "stable core". Pregnancy can weaken these muscles, leading to poor posture and back pain. Pilates exercises are useful for pregnant women as many of them strengthen the core muscles. Some exercises are performed in a hands-and-knees position, which lessens the weight on your back and pelvis. The Wall Slide strengthens your core muscles and also improves the mobility of your hips, so it is a sound pregnancy investment.

Press your back against a wall, feet hip-distance apart. Raise your arms as you bend your knees and slide gently down the wall. Go as far as you can, then slide back up.

Active mum

When you've always exercised, it can be a shock to realise you may need to try a gentler routine.

"I'm a bit of a gym bunny. Before I fell pregnant I'd go at least five times a week after work. I did weight training, an aerobics class, spinning. You name it – I'd give it a try.

During that first trimester, though, I started feeling so unbelievably tired. There was no way I could keep it up because after work all I wanted to do was go home and crawl into bed.

I felt so guilty for abandoning my fitness regime and started to panic about just how much weight I was going to put on. I spoke to my midwife about it, and she said that while the routine I did at the gym might be a bit too much for me now, there was no need to give up on exercise altogether. So now I've started a gentle routine that includes swimming, yoga and lots of walking. I feel just great and ready for the months ahead!"

Your pelvic floor

Your pelvic floor muscles form a broad sling between your legs from the pubic bone in front to the base of your spine at the back. Being pregnant can place a lot of stress on those muscles. They can become weak and stretched from as early as 12 weeks, increasing your risk of stress incontinence (urine leaks when you laugh, cough, sneeze or exercise) after you have given birth. To strengthen these important muscles, try this exercise:
● Place one hand at the top of your bump and the other on one of your shoulders. Breathe normally for four or five breaths.
● You should find that the hand on your tummy moves up and down more than the hand on your shoulder. If this is not happening, try to stop your shoulders moving, but don't try to make

your tummy move – this should happen completely naturally.
● Once you have mastered this, gently pull up and in "down below" as you breathe out.
● Then try to hold a contraction for a few seconds while you breathe in and out as normal.
● You may feel your lower tummy muscles tightening – this is not a problem. If you are tightening the muscles above your belly button you are trying too hard!
● When you've done all this, go back to the beginning and start again.

You should aim to be able to hold a pelvic floor contraction for 10 seconds while breathing normally. If you lose your breathing control, stop and start again. Try to repeat the exercise at least eight times, three times a day.

Pelvic floor muscle | Vagina

Your pelvic floor muscles are like a sling or hammock running from front to back. During pregnancy they stretch, which can cause stress incontinence.

Scans at 10 to 14 weeks

Around now, you'll probably be looking forward to your first scan. It's an amazing moment in your pregnancy, and one to share with your partner or a friend. Bear in mind, though, that scans occasionally pick up problems – speak to your midwife if you are worried.

The dating scan

All pregnant women should now be offered a dating scan at between 10 and 14 weeks of pregnancy. If you have an irregular cycle or if you've been taking the contraceptive pill, working out your due date from your last menstrual period (LMP) isn't very accurate. Ultrasound scans are more accurate; if the scan date differs from your period dates, the scan date will be used.

As the due date given by a scan is usually later than a period date, scan dating reduces the number of inductions of labour for "overdue" babies. A dating scan is also recommended before you have a nuchal translucency (NT) scan (see opposite); having an accurate due date makes that test more reliable.

The scan is done at the maternity unit and they usually ask you to come with a full bladder. The sonographer puts some gel on your tummy and moves a small hand-held transducer over your skin to get views of the baby.

You'll be given a report, which tells you exactly how many weeks pregnant you are. And of course, the scan will also show if you're expecting twins, triplets or more. It's a good idea to keep your report with your maternity notes.

Chorionic villus sampling (CVS)

Chorionic villi are tiny projections on the placenta that reveal the chromosomal make-up of your baby. CVS involves extracting a fragment of chorionic villi to detect chromosomal abnormalities such as Down's syndrome. You will be able to discuss the pros and cons before you decide to have the test. It can be done using one of the following methods:

● **Transabdominal CVS** You may be given a local anaesthetic before a needle is inserted through your abdomen into your uterus to the placenta.

● **Transvaginal CVS** Your doctor inserts fine forceps or a small tube through your vagina and cervix into the uterus. You might have to wait two to three weeks for the results of the CVS.

Transabdominal procedure

Transvaginal procedure

The nuchal fold (red) of this fetus is narrow and clear. With a more opaque fold, the baby is at higher risk of having Down's syndrome.

At the age of 12 weeks, an ultrasound scan clearly shows the profile and part of the body of the fetus (left).

Getting ready for pregnancy

Staying safe and healthy

Your pregnancy diary

Birth and beyond

The nuchal translucency scan

A nuchal translucency (NT) scan assesses whether your baby is likely to have Down's syndrome. Nuchal translucency refers to the collection of fluid under the skin at the back of your baby's neck. All babies have some of this fluid, but many babies with Down's syndrome have an increased amount.

What the results can tell you

The NT scan can't tell for certain if your baby is affected, but it can help you decide whether or not to proceed to having a diagnostic test, such as CVS (see opposite) or amniocentesis (see p.147). The NT scan must be performed between 11 weeks and 13 weeks and 6 days of pregnancy. It is usually done through your tummy, but occasionally a vaginal scan, which will give better views, is required.

To date your pregnancy accurately, the sonographer measures your baby from the top of his head to the bottom of his spine. She then measures the width of the nuchal translucency. An NT measurement of up to 2 millimetres (mm) is normal at about 11 weeks, and up to 2.8mm is normal by 13 weeks and 6 days. An increased NT doesn't definitely mean there's a problem. However, as the NT increases, so does the risk of Down's and other chromosomal abnormalities.

Your scan measurements will be combined with your age to generate your own individual risk for this pregnancy. This may be higher or lower than your background risk (the average risk that applies to all women of your age). You'll be given the results straight after your scan.

Most women given a high risk (a one-in-150 chance, or less) of having a baby with Down's syndrome will go on to have a normal baby. Even with a risk as high as one in five, your baby has four chances out of five of NOT having Down's syndrome. The only way to know for certain if your baby has Down's syndrome or another chromosomal abnormality is to have a CVS test or amniocentesis.

The decision to have invasive tests can be very difficult, but you don't have to decide in a hurry. Sometimes, a screening test suggests that a normal baby has a high risk of having Down's. This is called a false positive. Combining an NT scan with a blood test (called the combined test) gives a more accurate result. At the moment, the NT scan is offered routinely in some NHS antenatal clinics. Few hospitals offer the combined test so you may like to consider having this done privately (see p.127).

75% of babies with Down's syndrome are picked up by an nuchal translucency scan and another five per cent of women are given a false positive. This means that one in 20 women are wrongly given a high risk.

▼ Your body at **12** Weeks

12 Weeks

�֍ With luck your nausea will be on the wane and you'll soon be feeling more energetic.

�֍ This is roughly the stage when your raging hormones should start calming down.

If you're over 35 you may be wondering how your age will affect your pregnancy. The good news is that the vast majority of pregnancies for women in this age group are uneventful and lead to healthy babies.

Concerns of older mums

Organs grow quickly and eyes move closer

Overall, the risks faced by women over 35 during pregnancy tend to be exaggerated. Many recent studies have shown that, in healthy women, the risks of delaying pregnancy are low, even though being over 35 is associated with an increased risk of certain complications. It appears that it's not just your age that matters: the state of your health before you conceive matters, too. There is evidence that older women are more likely to develop diabetes, high blood pressure or placenta praevia during pregnancy. But both mother and baby usually still do well. And, although the risks of stillbirth are higher for older women, the rates are still very, very low.

Modern maternity units are able to take older women's complications in their stride. By working with your maternity-care team and, for example, by controlling your diet if you are diabetic, you can help reduce the risks for yourself and your baby. An increased rate of induced labour, forceps delivery and caesarean has been found for women over 35 in the UK, although the exact reasons for this are not clear. It may be that obstetricians are more likely to intervene in older women's deliveries.

Genetic defects

The odds of having a baby with a genetic defect such as Down's syndrome increase as you get older. For example, figures from the NHS for 2007 show that if you are aged 20 to 30, the risk of having a baby with Down's syndrome is just one in 1,500. If you are 35 to 40 years of age, that rises to a risk of one in 270 and, if you are aged over 45, it rises still more to one in 50. If you're almost, or over, 40 you should strongly consider genetic testing (see pp.222–3) because the risk of genetic problems increases significantly. And since genetic abnormalities are the most common reason for miscarriage, the risk of miscarriage also increases with age.

Whatever your age, if you're considering pregnancy, see your doctor for a preconception check-up (see p.16). The doctor will take a detailed medical and family history for both you and your partner to identify conditions that might affect the health of you or your baby.

▼ Your baby at **12** Weeks

Now your baby's tissues and organs begin to grow and mature rapidly.

✷ Starting with your baby's face, his eyes, which began to form on the sides of his head, have moved closer together, and his ears are now almost in their normal position. His intestines, which started out as a large swelling in the umbilical cord, will begin moving into his abdominal cavity about now.

How the placenta works

The placenta develops in the lining of the uterus. It is fully formed, with two arteries and a vein, and functioning by about 10 weeks after fertilisation.

Your baby's blood flows into the placenta through the arteries. Oxygen and food from your blood are carried into the baby's blood in the placenta. The baby's blood returns through the vein, taking waste products and carbon dioxide back to the placenta for disposal. Although the circulation of your blood and your baby's blood come close, there is no direct connection.

Another of the placenta's functions is to produce hormones, such as oestrogen and progesterone. These help your baby to grow and develop and cause many of your body's changes during pregnancy.

The placenta also protects your baby from infections and harmful substances. What is more, its large surface area, plus the amount of blood flowing through it, provides the perfect mechanism for dispersing heat and helping control your baby's body temperature.

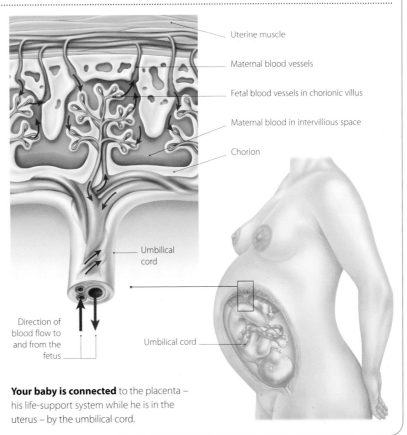

Uterine muscle

Maternal blood vessels

Fetal blood vessels in chorionic villus

Maternal blood in intervillious space

Chorion

Umbilical cord

Direction of blood flow to and from the fetus

Umbilical cord

Your baby is connected to the placenta – his life-support system while he is in the uterus – by the umbilical cord.

Fetal development

The most dramatic development this week: reflexes. Your baby's fingers will soon begin to open and close, his toes will curl, his eye muscles will clench, and his mouth will start to make sucking movements. In fact, if you prod your abdomen, your baby will squirm in response, even though you won't be able to feel it.

His intestines, which have grown so fast that they now protrude into the umbilical cord, will begin to move into their proper place in his abdominal cavity at about this time. His kidneys are developing, too: they begin excreting urine into his bladder.

Meanwhile, nerve cells are multiplying rapidly, and in your baby's brain, synapses – where two nerve cells connect – are forming furiously. His face looks unquestionably human: his eyes are now at the front of his head, and his ears are almost where they should be. From crown to rump, your baby-to-be is just over 5.5cm (2¼in) long (about the size of a lime) and he weighs 14g (½oz).

Now your doctor or midwife can feel the top of your uterus (the fundus) low in your abdomen, just above your pubic bone. You may already be wearing maternity clothes, especially if this isn't your first pregnancy, but if you're still small and not yet ready for maternity clothes, you've no doubt noticed that your waist is thickening and that you're more comfortable in loose, less restrictive clothing. You may now find that, once the feeling of sickness has passed, your appetite returns.

| FIRST TRIMESTER | SECOND TRIMESTER | THIRD TRIMESTER |

Your body at **13** Weeks

13 Weeks

❋ If you are lucky, you may find that your sex drive is making a comeback this week.

❋ Your breasts may have already started making colostrum, the first milk that nourishes your baby.

You're almost in the second trimester now and you may soon find your energy levels returning to normal. Use your newfound energy to take some exercise, but don't forget to get some rest, too.

Feeling better now?

By the end of your first trimester, you will hopefully be over the worst of any nausea and vomiting. Once the nausea has passed, you may even feel ravenous. By 16 weeks you may have gained as much as 4.5 kilograms (kg)/10 pounds (lb) and by week 22 you'll be putting on about 225g (8oz) a week. You may also notice that you have sudden cravings for weird and wonderful foods. So go ahead and satisfy your heightened sense of taste and smell! Now is not the time to be worrying about your weight. Eat healthily, especially if you're hungry, but don't deprive yourself – remember that gradual weight gain is a positive sign of a healthy pregnancy. So why not arrange to meet a friend for a good chat over a leisurely lunch?

Exercise and rest
Take advantage of your revived energy levels to strengthen and prepare your body for the physical demands of labour, birth, and motherhood that lie ahead. Yoga (see p.59) and Pilates (see p.57) exercises can help relieve aches and pains in your back and pelvis and, towards the end of pregnancy, can

even help to position your baby ready for delivery. Regular, gentle exercise also makes it easier to get your body back in shape once the baby's born. You'll find useful tips on exercising on pp.56–7 and on p.134.

Although you'll soon be feeling livelier, make sure you set aside a few quiet hours to relax. Your physical and emotional wellbeing are important right now, so put your feet up – or better still, have a cat nap – whenever you get the chance. If your feet are sore and swollen, have a long, luxurious soak in the bath and massage them afterwards with your favourite moisturising lotion or foot balm.

A key moment
One of the most exciting moments of the second trimester is feeling your baby move. In a first pregnancy, most women notice this "quickening" some time between 16 and 20 weeks. You may feel these first wiggles as a flutter low down in your tummy.

Around this time you will also be offered an anomaly scan – an antenatal test to screen for any possible birth defects (see pp.156–7).

▼ Your baby at **13** Weeks

Amazingly, although your baby is still really tiny, she already has fingerprints.

❋ Your baby is now nearly 7 to 8 cm/2¾ to 3¼in long and weighs nearly 23g/¾oz. When you poke your stomach, she may start rooting (searching for a nipple). If you're having a girl, she now has approximately 2 million eggs in her ovaries, although she will have only half this number by the time she's born.

That loving feeling

As the tiredness of early pregnancy lifts, you may feel your libido return, which is sure to please your partner. In fact, some women find that their libido is at a high in the second trimester but, with any stage of pregnancy, there is a wide variety in how women feel and how sexually active couples are.

Meanwhile, for your partner, your pregnant physique is a constant reminder of his virility – he may well find your blossoming breasts and soft curves irresistible. Why not celebrate your sensuality with some new, sexy lingerie? Or plan a romantic evening

with your partner – at the theatre, cinema, a favourite restaurant, or somewhere else where you can appreciate each other's company before you become Mum and Dad! If you can't afford to go out, get your partner to cook an intimate dinner for two, or turn your bedroom into a romantic hideaway, with candles and soft music. Turn off your phones and hide anything that reminds you of work.

Going shopping

Last but by no means least, there's shopping. Although at 13 weeks many women "make do" with their existing wardrobe, soon it will be worth buying some maternity clothes. As your breasts expand with extra milk ducts, you'll need to make sure you're regularly fitted for a good maternity bra (see p.92).

If your feet tend to swell it might be wise to invest in a pair of shoes a size bigger than normal. Switch to flat styles as you begin to carry more weight. Your growing bump alters your centre of gravity – which makes balancing on high heels even trickier than usual.

As well as being functional, maternity bras come in all sorts of shapes and colours – you can find some very attractive designs.

Parents**Ask**...

Now I'm at 13 weeks, is my risk of miscarriage over?

About 15 per cent of known pregnancies end in miscarriage. About 98 per cent of women who miscarry do so in the first 13 weeks, but occasionally a woman will miscarry much later.

What causes miscarriage?

Probably at least half of all miscarriages in the first trimester of pregnancy are the result of chromosomal abnormalities that prevent the baby from developing normally. Later miscarriages – after 20 weeks – may be the result of an infection or an abnormality of the uterus or placenta, or a weak cervix that is not strong enough to keep the womb tightly closed until the baby is ready to be born.

Is it true that some tests can cause miscarriage?

Unfortunately, two of the tests used to detect abnormalities in babies – amniocentesis (see p.147) and CVS (see p.136) – can make you miscarry. Amniocentesis results in miscarriage for around one per cent of women. CVS may cause miscarriage in between one and two per cent. Discuss the risks and how you feel about them with your midwife.

Getting ready for pregnancy

Staying safe and healthy

Your pregnancy diary

Birth and beyond

Twins and more

If you're carrying twins or more, chances are you'll already have had a scan and you'll be coming to terms with your amazing news.

During the rest of your pregnancy, you'll have more antenatal appointments and ultrasound scans than you would in a single pregnancy. In a singleton pregnancy, you would normally have an appointment every four weeks until week 32. If you're expecting twins, your appointments will be more frequent. And because a multiple pregnancy is considered higher risk, you'll probably be referred to a consultant obstetrician for your antenatal care. This means that you'll have regular appointments at the hospital, and also see your midwife at a health centre, doctor's surgery or at home. You'll also have scans more frequently in the last trimester to check the growth and position of your babies and placentas.

The second
trimester

The time of your life

The second trimester is an exciting time. With nausea and vomiting and miscarriage worries behind them, most women feel full of beans and excited about their growing bump. Why not treat yourself to a few new clothes and maybe even a romantic pre-baby break?

Making the most of it

Most women find the second three months the easiest stage of pregnancy. They can sleep sounder and their bump isn't too big to impede their movements. Make the most of these middle months to enjoy low-impact exercise (see p.57) and maybe arrange a last-minute holiday too, while you can still move about easily – and before you need to worry about the possibility of baby arriving early. You may also notice a distinct improvement in your libido as the nausea and tiredness recede and your energy levels rise!

At this stage of your pregnancy you'll probably be feeling at your best and looking forward to the arrival of your new baby.

Your growing bump

At the start of the second trimester your uterus may be big enough to show the world that you're expecting, but your baby is still tiny – only about the size of half a banana.

Over the next few weeks she will sprout hair – not only on her head and brows but all over her body – in the form of ultrafine hair called lanugo. Some of her muscles are starting to work, too – she will soon be grasping, frowning, grimacing and sucking her thumb.

From 17 weeks her eyes will start to look forwards instead of to the sides and the rubbery cartilage that will eventually become her skeleton is about to start hardening into bone. By 18 weeks she can both feel and hear. Admittedly, all she can hear at the moment is your heartbeat and the sound of your digestive system, but soon she will be able to detect noise outside the womb and identify your voice.

After you reach the halfway stage of pregnancy your baby will start to gain weight rapidly. By 21 weeks she could measure about 27cm (10½in) from crown to heel. Her eyebrows and eyelids are fully developed and fingernails now cover her fingertips. She is really starting to look like a miniature newborn.

At 24 weeks your baby becomes "viable" – meaning that if she were born prematurely now, she might survive, with special care. At 26 weeks, her eyes begin to open and, towards the end of the seventh month, her response to sound grows more consistent. As you approach the final stage of pregnancy – your third trimester – your baby is really starting to grow and fill the available space in your uterus.

 Active mum

Most women experience a massive improvement in the way they feel in the second trimester.

"The first trimester was an absolute nightmare for me, what with all that nausea and vomiting, plus the exhaustion. I genuinely don't think I've ever felt so rough in my whole life. The good news is that, once I entered the second trimester, everything got heaps better. I stopped feeling nauseous, the overwhelming fatigue vanished, and I could get back into an exercise routine. I try to swim or go for a walk every day. I'm definitely rocking the pregnancy glow now!"

Getting ready for pregnancy

Staying safe and healthy

Your pregnancy diary

Birth and beyond

▼ Your body at **14** Weeks

14 Weeks

❋ Some women find that nausea drags on. If you're still being very sick, consult your doctor or midwife.

❋ You may notice that your hair is now more lustrous – becoming thicker and fuller.

Your baby is beginning to look like a real person now, and is practising different facial expressions. Meanwhile, your uterus is starting to show above your pelvis – a reassuring sign that your baby is growing.

How your baby's growing

You've reached 14 weeks and your baby is stretching out and starting to look like a real little human. He's about the size of a lemon and has nearly doubled his weight in just the last week. His body's growing faster than his head right now, and his head sits upon a neck that's starting to look more like a real neck. By the end of this week, his arms will have grown so that they're more in proportion to the rest of his body. His legs still have some lengthening to do, though.

Your baby's skin is extremely sensitive now, and he's starting to develop an ultra-fine, downy covering of hair all over his body known as lanugo. It usually disappears before birth. Although his eyebrows are beginning to grow and the hair on top of his head is sprouting, this hair may change in both texture and colour once he is born. He now has sockets in his gumline ready for 20 little teeth to form, and he even has tiny vocal cords, although he won't actually make any sounds until he's born. Thanks to impulses from his brain, your baby's facial muscles are getting a really good workout as his tiny features form one

expression after another. He can squint, frown and grimace. Although you can't feel his tiny punches and kicks yet, your little boxer's hands and feet measure about 1.25cm (½in) long and are quite flexible and active. Tiny fingernails are starting to grow. He can grasp, too, and if you have an ultrasound scan, you may catch him sucking his thumb.

Your baby's organs

Crucially, your baby's liver starts making bile this week – a sign that it's doing its job properly – and his spleen starts helping in the production of red blood cells. His intestines have moved into his abdominal cavity from the umbilical cord, and the muscles in his digestive tract are already contracting. His kidneys are producing urine, which he releases (pees) into the amniotic fluid around him – a process that he'll keep up until birth.

And last but not least, your baby's genitals are starting to take on male or female characteristics. This won't be visible on scans just yet. You'll have to wait until your mid-pregnancy scan to know if it's a boy or a girl.

▼ Your baby at **14** Weeks

This week, your baby's parchment-thin skin is starting to cover itself with lanugo.

❋ This will disappear by the time he is born unless he's born prematurely. He can now grasp, squint, frown, and grimace. He may even be able to suck his thumb. His movements probably correspond to the development of impulses in the brain. Crown to rump, he's now about 8cm/3¼in long and weighs 43g/1½oz.

How your body's changing

The top of your uterus is peeking above your pubic bone now, which may be enough to push your tummy out a tad. Starting to show can be quite a thrill, giving you and your partner visible evidence of the baby you've been waiting for. Take some time to plan, daydream, and enjoy this amazing time. It's normal to worry a bit now and then, but try to focus on taking care of yourself and your baby.

Birth is still months away, but your breasts may have already started making colostrum, the first milk that's designed for your baby immediately after birth. Even if your breasts are small or you have inverted nipples, you should still be able to breastfeed if you want to.

Pregnancy is a challenge for your immune system so you may find that you have more coughs and colds than usual.

Your immune system is slightly impaired when you're pregnant so you may have noticed that you've had a few more coughs and colds recently than you normally would. Although they are annoying and tiring, these sniffles won't harm your baby.

ParentsAsk...

Why are my hands and feet always warm?

It is quite common to feel warmer than normal when you are pregnant, and many women say they find that their hands and feet become particularly hot. This is probably due to the hormonal changes that occur during pregnancy and to an increase in blood supply to the skin. Do not despair. There are measures you can take. It might help if you:

● Fill a footspa or small tub with cool water and soak your feet.

● Buy a mini battery-operated fan and carry it with you everywhere.

● Wear clothing and shoes that are made of natural fibres, which allow the skin to breathe.

● Run your hands and wrists under a cold tap to cool your pulse points, and use a cool wet flannel on your forehead and the back of your neck – this should help to cool you down quickly.

Getting ready for pregnancy

Staying safe and healthy

Your pregnancy diary

Birth and beyond

Dad's **Diary**

So Dad, your life is about to be turned upside down by the latest addition to your family. But how up to date on baby information are you? Take our quick quiz to see how much you know, and what you still need to learn about life as a dad. Then turn to p.320 for the correct answers.

1 How long should you let your newborn cry at night before picking him up?
(a) Less than one minute
(b) Five to ten minutes
(c) Ten to 15 minutes
(d) Until he stops.

2 How many times a day does the average newborn eat?
(a) Three meals a day
(b) Every four hours
(c) Eight to ten times
(d) On the hour every hour.

3 What's the standard advice on how long after childbirth you should wait until you and your partner can have sex again?
(a) One week
(b) Six weeks
(c) Until your partner says so
(d) Until her doctor gives the green light.

4 What's the number one never-leave-home-without-it item you should bring for an afternoon at the park with your 6-month-old?
(a) Your mobile phone
(b) A muslin or other soft cloth

(c) The video camera
(d) A nappy.

5 What should you always bring your partner whenever she is busy breastfeeding baby?
(a) A glass of water
(b) A magazine
(c) Her favourite beer
(d) The TV remote.

6 What's the recommended position for a sleeping baby?
(a) On his tummy
(b) On his side
(c) On his back
(d) In his car seat.

▼ Your body at **15** Weeks

15 Weeks

❋ You may feel your baby's first wiggles as a flutter low down in your tummy.

❋ Your immune system is slightly impaired so you may suffer from coughs and colds more easily.

You may have discovered that you're a sensitive soul now you're pregnant. We're not just talking about crying over soppy films either. Your skin can be more easily irritated than usual, so take extra care with it.

Skin changes

Minor skin problems during pregnancy are common and most won't cause any harm. However, talk to your doctor if your skin is inflamed or blistered, or if you have a rash, irritation or itchiness that lasts more than a couple of days.

Chafing

As you put on weight, chafing can take place between your thighs or under your breasts, resulting in red, moist skin. Your skin may then become inflamed and blistered and you may notice an odour. This is a condition known as intertrigo.

Keep the affected area as dry as possible and try to keep your skin cool by wearing cotton clothes and avoiding wearing tights. See your doctor, as intertrigo may cause thrush (see p.238).

Sensitive, irritated skin

Skin tends to become more sensitive during pregnancy, not only because of the higher levels of hormones in your body, but because the skin has become more stretched and delicate. Soaps and detergents may suddenly cause irritation, or conditions such as eczema may become worse.

Try to identify what could be causing the irritation – could it be your washing powder or a perfume that you use? Choose loose, cotton clothes and keep your body well moisturised. Long soaks in a warm bath will dry out your skin, so keep these to a minimum.

Rashes and itchiness

It's pretty common for rashes and itchiness to come and go during pregnancy, without any obvious cause. Dabbing on calamine lotion should help to reduce any itching.

Intense itching all over – particularly at night and on the palms of your hands and the soles of your feet – can be a sign of a rare pregnancy-related liver disorder called obstetric cholestasis (see pp.230–31). As with any itching, report it to your doctor if it doesn't go away within days.

75–90% of pregnant women will be affected by stretch marks, but they will fade closer to your own skin colour after your baby is born.

▼ Your baby at **15** Weeks

Her legs are now growing longer than her arms and her fingernails are fully formed.

❋ You may not know it, but your tiny tenant frequently gets hiccups now. Babies don't make any sound, though, because their trachea is filled with fluid rather than air. Your baby now weighs around 70g/2½oz and measures nearly 11cm/4½in long. All her joints and limbs are now able to move.

Amniocentesis test

Amniocentesis is a diagnostic test that involves taking a sample of amniotic fluid from your uterus to see whether your baby has any serious abnormalities. It is usually used to detect chromosomal disorders in your baby, such as Down's syndrome (see pp.214–15).

Amniocentesis is usually performed in the second trimester, from 15 weeks of pregnancy. Your doctor will insert a long, thin, hollow needle through your abdominal wall and extract some of the fluid around your baby. You may not get the results until two to three weeks after you have the procedure.

Sadly, it's estimated that about one in 100 women miscarries as a direct result of amniocentesis. If you're uncertain whether or not to have an amniocentesis, or if you're very anxious about the procedure, talk through your concerns with your midwife.

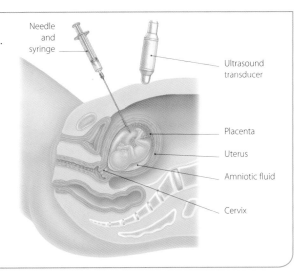

Needle and syringe — Ultrasound transducer — Placenta — Uterus — Amniotic fluid — Cervix

Antenatal care in the second trimester

Your next routine antenatal appointment is due at around 16 weeks, but you may have a blood test before 16 weeks if you're having screening tests for Down's syndrome. Here are the various tests you can expect during the second trimester:

- **14 to 20 weeks** If you are having the quadruple test to check for Down's syndrome (see pp.214–15), you'll have a single blood test between 15 and 20 weeks (ideally at about 15 to 16 weeks). If you are having the integrated test (see p.127) you will have your second blood test at around this time, again ideally at about 15 to 16 weeks.
- **16 weeks** At this appointment your midwife will discuss with you the blood and urine test results from your booking visit. If your iron levels are low, she may recommend that you take an iron supplement (see p.149).

She'll also check your blood pressure and, as before, test your urine for traces of protein, which can be a sign of pre-eclampsia. As with all your antenatal appointments, this is a good opportunity to ask questions and raise any issues that may be worrying you. You may also want to chat through your birth choices and ask about antenatal classes in your area.

- **18 to 20 weeks** If you've decided to have an anomaly scan (see pp.156–7), this should take place at 18 to 20 weeks. If they find that your placenta is blocking the entrance to your cervix, you will be booked in for another scan at 34 to 36 weeks to make sure the placenta has moved out of the way, which it usually does.
- **25 weeks (first pregnancy only)** As usual at your appointments, your midwife will check your blood pressure and test your urine for protein. She'll also measure the distance from your pubic bone to the top of your bump with a tape measure to check that your baby is growing well.

Systemised mum

Noticing your baby move for the first time is very special. You're sure to want to record it.

"I felt my baby kick for the first time when I was 19 weeks pregnant. I was at work, in a meeting. At first, I wasn't sure if I'd imagined it or if it was my stomach rumbling because I was hungry. Then a few minutes later it happened again, and it was different to anything I'd felt before – like butterfly wings flapping. I was so excited and wanted to share it with my colleagues. They all gathered round to try and feel it, but it was so gentle they couldn't.

As soon as I could, I rang my partner to tell him and he was excited too. In fact, he sat all evening with his hand on my stomach, hoping to feel the movements. It took a week or so before they were really strong enough for that, though. The next day I wrote about it in my pregnancy diary. I don't want to forget a thing."

Getting ready for pregnancy

Staying safe and healthy

Your pregnancy diary

Birth and beyond

Diet in the second trimester

Your baby grows rapidly during this trimester and your appetite may start to grow too. Try not to snack on junk food. Instead, prepare healthy snacks like raw veg and hummus for when the munchies strike. And take care to eat a diet that gives you all the necessary nutrients.

Healthy essentials

You should now be getting some of your energy back. On the other hand, you may find that you are suddenly more susceptible to coughs and colds and to minor infections.

Antioxidants
Fresh fruit and vegetables are rich in antioxidants, which can help you fight off infections, so try to get plenty of fruit and veg into your diet. (At least five portions a day is the recommended intake anyway, whether you are pregnant or not.) Some experts believe that a diet rich in antioxidants may also help prevent pre-eclampsia.

Omega 3 essential fatty acids
These are important in pregnancy for your baby's brain, eye and vision development. Oily fish, such as mackerel, herrings and sardines, are good sources. If you're a vegetarian, try linseed or flax seed oil instead. The Food Standards Agency (FSA) recommends that you should eat no more than two portions of oily fish a week. This is because oily fish can contain environmental pollutants that may affect the development of your unborn baby (see p.53). However, oily fish is still a good source of omega 3 fats and is rich in other nutrients.

Four healthy pregnancy snacks

Now that you're in the second trimester, hopefully you should feel that you are getting some of your energy back – and your appetite, if you suffered from nausea and vomiting. However busy your life is, make the time to eat well. Try these healthy snacks to help satisfy those hunger pangs.

Cranberry and soft cheese wrap with watercress
Mix some dried cranberries and cream cheese together. Spread over a tortilla wrap and arrange some watercress on top. Roll up and serve with cherry tomatoes or a green salad with balsamic dressing, and a glass of cranberry juice.

Papaya smoothie
Take half a small, ripe papaya, and remove all the seeds and skin. Chop roughly and place in a blender. Add 200ml (7fl oz) chilled apple and mango juice, and blend together until smooth.

Melon with blueberries and yogurt
Mix some cubes of cantaloupe melon with a handful of fresh blackberries or blueberries. Serve with a spoonful of Greek yogurt and a drizzle of honey.

Hummus with pitta bread
Drain a 400g (14oz) tin of chickpeas and whizz them in a food processor together with 15g (1 tbsp) tahini, the juice of half

a lemon and a clove of garlic. Drizzle in 15ml (1 tbsp) olive oil and a little water to make the mixture creamy. Serve with fingers of pitta bread.

Get your infection-fighting antioxidants by eating plenty of fresh fruit and vegetables. It's believed they can help prevent pre-eclampsia, too.

Vitamin A

Our bodies need vitamin A for vision, the skin, and to stay healthy in pregnancy. Vitamin A comes in two forms – retinol and betacarotene. Both are needed, but too much retinol can harm a developing baby by causing birth defects. Liver and liver products are very high in the retinol form of vitamin A and should be avoided when you are pregnant. Other foods, such as egg yolk, butter or margarine and milk, also have retinol in them, but at levels that are safe. Good sources of betacarotene are carrots, sweet potatoes, papaya, oranges, and green vegetables, especially broccoli, watercress, spinach and spring greens.

ParentsAsk...

I've just been told I've got gestational diabetes. What is it and what can I do about it?

This is diabetes that develops for the first time during pregnancy (see p.229). You can usually manage it by changing your diet and taking regular exercise. Your midwife or the specialist at the diabetic clinic will advise you on how to control your blood sugar levels by cutting down on sugary foods and drinks. You will be helped to look at your eating patterns, and advised to choose a balanced diet of wholegrain carbohydrates, lean proteins and healthy fats.

You will also be asked to monitor your blood sugar levels to check whether the changes you've made are making a difference – your doctor or diabetes specialist will show you how to do this. You should be offered extra ultrasound scans every four weeks from 28 to 36 weeks of pregnancy to see how your baby is growing and how much amniotic fluid you have.

Getting your iron

Before you conceived, you needed about 15mg of iron a day. That's quite a lot and many of us probably don't actually get the recommended daily amount. During pregnancy, you need extra iron to help keep you and your baby healthy – it helps your blood to transport oxygen around your body.

If you don't have enough iron to fuel haemoglobin production (to make red blood cells) for both you and your baby, you may develop iron-deficiency anaemia (see p.229). This is the most common type of anaemia in pregnancy. A surprisingly high proportion of women – about one in five – develop iron-deficiency anaemia when they are pregnant, so it is something that you need to be on your guard about.

As with most vitamins and minerals, food is the best source of iron. You shouldn't need iron supplements if you take care to have a diet that's rich in iron. This means eating lots of dark green leafy vegetables, wholemeal bread, iron-fortified cereals, lean red meat, dried fruit and pulses. Vitamin C helps your body absorb the iron in your diet. Try drinking plenty of orange juice or eating fruit or vegetables that are rich in vitamin C when you have an iron-rich meal. Tea and coffee make it difficult for your body to absorb iron, so it's best not to drink them at mealtimes. If you do have to take iron supplements, the drawback is that they have some unpleasant side effects. They can cause constipation and other tummy upsets, such as nausea, diarrhoea and tummy ache. Increasing the fibre in your diet can help prevent constipation, and taking the tablets with a meal can help the other side effects.

If the side effects become a serious problem, ask your doctor to prescribe you another brand or to reduce the dose. Taking less is probably better than not taking any at all.

▼ Your body at **16** Weeks

16 Weeks

❊ Your uterus has expanded so much that the ligaments in your abdomen are stretching to make room.

❊ You've probably gained at least 2.2kg (5lb) by now, and maybe as much as 4.5kg (10lb).

The effect of pregnancy hormones and your extra weight can lead to back problems. Help keep backache at bay by watching your posture, ditching the high heels and getting some regular exercise.

Protecting your back

The muscles of your back, lower abdomen and pelvic floor help to move and stabilise the joints of your back and pelvis. As your uterus and baby grow, it can become more difficult for the muscles to do this, which can give you back pain.

Tips for avoiding back pain

● **Avoid heavy lifting** If you have to lift or carry anything, hold it close to your body, bend your knees rather than your back and try not to twist. If you have a toddler, see if they can climb onto a chair or sofa before you pick them up.

● **Exercise regularly** You can reduce the risk of developing back pain if you exercise regularly. See pp.57, 134 and 184–5 for advice on the best forms of exercise during pregnancy.

● **Wear shoes that are comfortable for you** Some women will only be comfortable in flat shoes, but other women need a bit of a heel to take the pressure off their back.

● **Improve your posture** When standing, imagine that someone is making you taller by pulling a string attached to the top and back of your head. Tightening your pelvic floor muscles (see p.135) and your tummy muscles will help to support your back in this posture.

● **Try pelvic tilting** Stand with your back against a wall, feet a few centimetres away from the wall, and knees slightly bent. Put one hand in the hollow of your back and tilt your pelvis backwards so that your back squashes your hand. Now tilt your pelvis the other way to take the pressure off your hand. Continue to tilt forwards and backwards in a rhythmical fashion. (See also Back exercises for pregnancy, opposite.)

● **Get into a good sitting posture** When sitting, ensure that your back is well supported. Try placing a small towel rolled into a sausage shape in the hollow of your back.

● **Kneeling on your hands and knees** This reduces pressure on your back from your baby. Round your back up into a hump shape (tucking your tailbone under you), then gently arch your back in the opposite direction so you stick your bottom out (humping and hollowing). Repeating this in a rocking motion helps relieve back or pelvic pain.

▼ Your baby at **16** Weeks

Your baby has now grown to about the size of a large avocado.

❊ He weighs approximately 100g/3½oz and, in the next three weeks, he will double his weight and add quite a bit to his length. In or out of the uterus, babies are playful creatures. Yours may already have discovered his first toy – the umbilical cord – which he'll enjoy pulling and grabbing.

Planning a break

If you're having a final fling with your partner before settling down to the delights of family holidays, opt for comfort over adventure as well as good standards of hygiene and medical care. Choose shortish flights (north to south rather than east to west to minimise jet lag) and look for a place with a pleasant rather than baking temperature.

Make sure you have the following packed in your hand-luggage:

● **Your passport if travelling abroad** It sounds obvious, but double-check if you're suffering from pregnancy-related forgetfulness! If you are flying within the United Kingdom you will need photo ID. Don't forget your driving licence if you're planning to drive on holiday.

● **A letter from your doctor or midwife** If you are flying in late pregnancy, this must give your due date and confirm that you are fit to fly. Most airlines won't let you fly after 32 weeks.

● **Your maternity notes** If you do have a pregnancy-related problem while you're away, the local midwife or doctor can see your notes and can also fill in details of any treatment you have.

● **Any prescribed medication** If you are travelling abroad, it's wise to carry a note from your doctor explaining what the medication is and why you need it.

● **Copies of your travel insurance** It's also worth writing the helpline number on several postcards and keeping them in different places.

● **Details of how to contact a local doctor or hospital** In the UK, NHS Direct can put you in touch with local services. If you are going abroad, some research on the internet may be useful before you go.

Back exercises for pregnancy

Kneeling pelvic tilt
Done on all fours, this strengthens the abdominal muscles and eases back pain.
● Get down on your hands and knees, arms shoulder-width apart and knees hip-width apart, keeping your arms straight but not locking the elbows.
● As you breathe in, tighten your abdominal muscles, tuck your buttocks under and round your back.

● Relax your back into a neutral position as you breathe out.
● Repeat these movements, following the rhythm of your breath as you do so.

Tailor or cobbler pose
This yoga position helps open your pelvis and loosen your hip joints in preparation for birth. It can also improve your posture and ease tension in your lower back.

● Sit up straight against a wall with the soles of your feet touching each other (sit on a folded towel if that's more comfortable for you).
● Gently press your knees down and away from each other, but make sure you don't force them.
● Remain in this position for as long as you feel comfortable. Release, take a few breaths, then repeat.

Get down on all fours to do your pelvic tilts. Follow the rhythm of your breath by breathing in and tightening your abs. On the out breath, relax your abs and return your back to a neutral position.

Sit in tailor or cobbler pose to open your hip joints and prepare them for the birth ahead. Gently press your knees down without forcing them. Hold as long as it's comfortable, then relax and repeat.

Getting ready for pregnancy

Staying safe and healthy

Your pregnancy diary

Birth and beyond

FIRST TRIMESTER	SECOND TRIMESTER	THIRD TRIMESTER

 Your body at **17** Weeks

17 Weeks

❋ If you are a first-time mum, you may well start to feel your baby's movements around now.

❋ You may be gaining weight rapidly at this point as your baby grows, even if you're not eating much.

Pregnancy is mostly seen as a woman's thing. Few women believe that their partner really understands what's involved. But dads-to-be can participate. You'll also need to think about antenatal classes soon.

How dads can get involved

Dads – you can't be pregnant, but you can be an active observer. Let your partner know you're enjoying seeing her pregnant body. Take pictures to record her growing bump. Give her a back massage. Feel the baby kick. If you read the week-by-week pregnancy diary in this book, you'll know just what's happening, and what needs doing.

Be there

Try to make it to some of your partner's many antenatal appointments. And don't miss the chance to get a glimpse of your baby during a scan. If your partner has an amniocentesis or other procedure, make sure you're there. And, of course, attend antenatal classes, and work through the breathing and relaxation exercises together.

As your partner tries to improve her diet, give up alcohol and drink more fluids, you can support her by sharing these lifestyle changes. Eliminate from the house and shopping trolley any bad-for-baby foods that might tempt her. Cut down or cut out alcohol yourself. Don't smoke. Treat yourselves to some healthy pastimes too – a walk in the park, a swim, or even surprise her with a stay at a spa with treatments for pregnant women.

Love her changing body

Your partner may feel unattractive now she's pregnant, so do your very best to compliment her on how lovely she looks, and tell her what you love about her pregnant body. Meanwhile, you may also find that, what with hormone changes, back pain and nausea, your sex life takes a back seat for a while.

Your partner may also be pretty demanding. Go with it. She's doing most of the hard work. The least you can do is sort the food shopping, send her flowers and indulge her demands for cottage cheese and strawberry jam sandwiches.

75% of dads-to-be experience pregnancy

"sympathy symptoms". Strange as it may sound, some men start to feel pregnant while their partner's expecting – even to the point of exhibiting similar symptoms.

 Your baby at **17** Weeks

With a bit of luck, your midwife may be able to hear your baby's heartbeat now.

❋ There's almost nothing more exciting than knowing your baby's heartbeat can be heard. She is now nearly 13cm/5in long and weighs approximately 140g/5oz. Her skeleton is mostly rubbery cartilage, which will harden later. A protective substance called myelin slowly begins to wrap around her spinal cord.

Attending antenatal classes gives you the opportunity to practise positions for labour and birth as well as the breathing exercises. It's also a social occasion.

Antenatal classes

Antenatal classes may come in various forms, but all have the same aim – to help prepare you for labour, birth and early parenthood. Those run by midwives or at your local hospital are free, but you may have to pay for other types, such as NCT classes and The Active Birth Centre or aquanatal exercise classes. You may find it helpful to go to more than one type of class. Just remember when attending classes other than those run by your hospital or health centre to check that the teacher has been properly trained.

Antenatal classes not only help you focus on your pregnancy and forthcoming labour and birth, but they are also a great place to meet other parents-to-be. The content of the classes will vary from place to place, but classes on offer could include:

● Early pregnancy classes that cover topics such as: looking after yourself, including suggestions about eating well and the appropriate exercise for pregnancy; emotional and physical changes you might experience during pregnancy; giving up smoking and preparing for labour and birth.

● Women-only classes, which are a good option if your partner is male and you don't want to take him to an antenatal class, or if your birth partner is female. Sometimes a fathers' session is offered during the course as well.

● Couples' classes, which are usually for first-time parents and help both partners get involved in the preparations for labour and birth.

● Refresher classes, which are aimed at women who already have children. You may find it useful to see what's changed since you were first pregnant. Childcare facilities may be offered during the class. Most antenatal classes respond to what you want to know, but this is especially true of refresher classes.

● Tamba, the twins and multiple birth association, offers multiple birth antenatal classes.

 Systemised mum

Antenatal classes prepare you well for your baby's birth and are great for involving your partner.

"When I found out I was pregnant, I couldn't wait to start my antenatal classes. I hate feeling out of control and knew that they would teach me what to expect and how to make pregnancy and birth as enjoyable and healthy as possible. As soon as I could, I booked myself and my husband into a couples' class. I thought it would be a great way to make the whole thing seem more real for my partner, too."

FIRST TRIMESTER	SECOND TRIMESTER	THIRD TRIMESTER

Your body at **18** Weeks

18 Weeks

�֍ Bigger, more comfortable clothes are a must now. You may even need bigger shoes as your feet swell.

✖ Nose bleeds are common as your increased blood supply puts pressure on the delicate veins of your nose.

With your bump growing rapidly it's probably obvious that you're pregnant. Strangers may smile at you or even start a conversation. You need to be prepared for well-meaning but unwanted advice.

Time for rapid growth

A boy's genitals are visible; a girl's are in place

Your baby at **18** Weeks

Your baby's chest moves up and down, but he's taking in amniotic fluid, not air.

✖ The amniotic fluid protects him as he grows inside the amniotic sac. He is now about 12cm/4¾in long from crown to rump and weighs about 190g/6¾oz. If you're having a girl, the vagina, uterus (womb), and fallopian tubes are already in place. If it's a boy, the genitals are distinct and recognisable.

Your baby is now about 12cm (4¾in) long and he weighs almost 190g (6¾oz). He's busy flexing his arms and legs – movements that you'll start noticing more and more in the weeks ahead. His blood vessels are visible through his thin skin, and his ears are now in their final position, although they're still standing out from his head a bit.

A protective covering of myelin is beginning to form around his spinal cord and nerves, a process that will continue for a year after he's born. If you're having a girl, her uterus and fallopian tubes are formed and in place. If you're having a boy, his genitals are noticeable now, but he may hide them from you during an ultrasound! His chest moves up and down to mimic breathing but he's not taking in air, only amniotic fluid.

Because your baby's growing so rapidly, an increase in your appetite is pretty common about now. Make it count by choosing meals and snacks that are nutrient-rich instead of empty calories. Bigger, more comfortable clothes are a must now as your appetite and waistline grow.

Your cardiovascular system is undergoing dramatic changes, and during this trimester your blood pressure will probably be lower than usual. Don't spring up too fast from lying or sitting or you might feel a little dizzy.

From now on, it's best to lie on your side – or tilted to one side. If you're flat on your back, your uterus can compress a major vein, which can decrease the blood return to your heart and your baby. Try a pillow behind you or under your hip or upper leg for comfort.

Mid-pregnancy ultrasound

This scan is often done sometime in the second trimester (usually between 18 and 22 weeks) to assess fetal growth and development, screen for certain birth defects, check the placenta and umbilical cord and determine whether the gestational age is accurate. During this scan, you might see your baby kick, flex, reach, roll, or even suck his thumb. Bring your partner along, and whether or not he's able to accompany you, make sure you ask for printouts of the baby in various poses.

Feeling baby's first movements

Pregnant women usually feel the first movements of their fetus around 16 to 20 weeks, although this can vary from woman to woman. At first, the movements feel like a gentle fluttering, and it can often be mistaken for "wind". As your baby grows, these sensations change so that you start to feel thumping or kicking movements which become stronger as your pregnancy progresses. First-time mums often feel movements later than mums who have been pregnant before as they are not exactly sure what to expect. Women who are very active may also miss the subtle feelings of early movement.

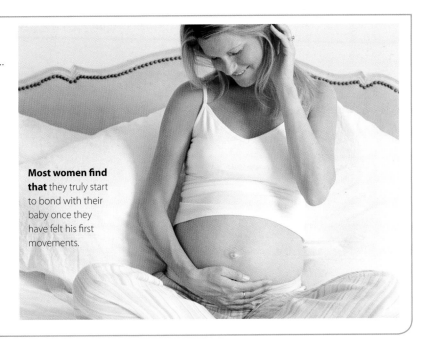

Most women find that they truly start to bond with their baby once they have felt his first movements.

Dealing with unwanted or unhelpful advice

Now that you're pregnant, you'll probably find you're given lots of advice by friends and relatives – and even complete strangers – especially once you start showing. Some of it will be helpful: "try sleeping with a pillow under your legs" or "make up lots of freezer meals before the baby arrives". And some of it not so helpful: "sleep while you can now – you'll get no sleep when the baby's born!" or "you look small for seven months – are you sure your dates are right?"

Dealing with unwanted advice and tactless comments can be tricky – especially when you're battling with pregnancy hormones. Remember, most people offer you advice with the best of intentions and, in the case of friends and family, it's because they care for you.

It's a good idea to have some stock responses prepared for those moments when you're given unsolicited – or even questionable – advice. Politely thank the giver for their concern and tell them you'll think about their suggestion, or that you'll ask your midwife or doctor when you go for your next appointment. If Granny tells you to stock up on stout to help you to breastfeed successfully, it might be worth updating her on current alcohol guidelines.

When people give you unasked-for advice, or advice that makes you worry, try not to get cross or upset. It's really not worth it. If you're having a particular problem with a friend's or relative's intrusive comments, and you don't feel able to confront them, ask someone to mediate for you.

Working mum

You may have to compromise on the shoe front, but you can still look smart and be comfortable.

"I finally caved in and bought some new work shoes. All my work shoes have really high heels, but I've had some lower-back pain lately. I'm told the ligaments in your back soften during pregnancy and I don't want to cause any lasting damage. So I bought a couple of pairs of ballet pumps. They're very comfortable and quite smart. I'm sure they'll be great as I get bigger. I'll still wear my killer heels – but only for special occasions."

Wearing flat shoes can help prevent lower-back pain.

Screening at the halfway stage

You'll probably have your detailed anomaly scan around this time. It's an exciting moment in your pregnancy and one you'll want to share with your partner. Occasionally, problems do get picked up, but chances are your baby will be absolutely fine.

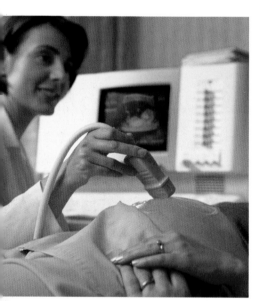

Anomaly scan

Most women are offered a detailed scan at about 20 weeks to check that their baby is developing normally. This is usually called the anomaly scan. It is carried out in order to look for any abnormalities in your baby's development and growth, and to check the position of the placenta.

Seeing your baby on a screen is an exciting and emotional time. Most hospitals welcome your partner and

> **Partners are usually** welcome when you have a scan and you can normally watch what's happening in your uterus on a screen.

your other children to share the experience with you. Many couples want to know the sex of their baby and get some photos. It's important to remember, though, that this scan's main purpose is to look for abnormalities.

You are usually allowed to watch the scan as it is being performed. If you haven't already had a scan, the sonographer will check that there is only one baby and will confirm your due date. She will point out your baby's heartbeat, face and hands before looking at him in detail. The scan normally takes about 15 to 20 minutes.

ParentsAsk...

Will I be able to find out the sex of my baby at the anomaly scan?

By 20 weeks, when the anomaly scan is normally done, your baby's sex is often clearly visible, but not all hospitals will tell you so you need to check with your midwife to find out what the policy is at your particular hospital. You can often buy pictures of your baby from the scan. These will probably be on thermal paper, which is heat sensitive, so don't laminate them. If you want copies, it's best to scan them into a computer or photocopy them.

What happens next if they find a problem at the anomaly scan?

If your sonographer suspects a problem, you will be told straightaway and you should be given an appointment for a repeat scan with a fetal medicine specialist within 72 hours. If a heart problem is suspected, you'll be invited for a detailed heart scan (a fetal echo).

What support will we have if something's seriously wrong?

If you are one of the few unlucky ones and a scan reveals a serious problem, you should be

given plenty of support to guide you through all the options. Although such serious problems are rare, some families are faced with the most difficult decision of all – whether to end the pregnancy. Other problems may mean that a baby needs surgery or treatment after birth, or even surgery while it is still in the uterus. There will be a whole range of people to support you through any painful times, including midwives, obstetricians, paediatricians, physiotherapists and the hospital chaplain.

Sometimes the sonographer sees or suspects a problem. About 15 per cent of scans will be done again for one reason or another, but most problems that need repeat scanning do not prove to be serious.

Abnormalities

About half of all major abnormalities can be picked up during an anomaly scan. These include:

- **Major limb abnormalities (missing or very short limbs)** Around 90 per cent of these are picked up by the scan.
- **Diaphragmatic hernia (hole in the muscle separating chest and abdomen)** Around 60 per cent of these cases are picked up by the scan.

- **Spina bifida (open spinal cord)** Around 90 per cent of these cases are picked up by the scan.
- **Major kidney problems (missing or abnormal kidneys)** Around 85 per cent of these are picked up by the scan.
- **Hydrocephalus (excess fluid within the brain)** Around 60 per cent of cases are picked up by the scan.
- **Down's syndrome** Around 40 per cent of these cases are picked up by the scan. Babies with Down's sometimes have heart or bowel problems that are visible.
- **Major heart problems (such as defects of the chambers, valves or vessels)** Around 25 per cent of these are picked up by the scan.

Some problems, including heart defects and bowel obstructions, may not be visible until later on in pregnancy. Your regular antenatal checks usually pick up any signs of problems that develop later. Sometimes the notes of the scan describe the placenta as "low-lying". Usually this means it is in the lower third of the uterus but it is almost certain that it will move up out of the way as pregnancy progresses. If a scan reveals a low-lying placenta, you will be given an extra scan later in pregnancy to check that it has moved up.

If you have a history of going into labour too early, or of late miscarriage, you may also have a scan to measure the length of your cervix.

Anomaly scan checks and measurements

Head The shape and size of the head are usually checked first.

Legs and feet These will be checked in case there are any abnormalities.

The heart The four chambers of the fetal heart can be clearly seen and checked.

Spine The vertebrae will be counted and checked to make sure they are aligned.

The sonographer will check the various parts of your baby's body that show how well he is growing.

- The head is usually examined first, to check its shape and internal structures.
- The spine is checked to make sure that all the vertebrae are aligned and that the skin properly covers the spine at the back.
- The baby's abdominal wall is also checked to make sure it covers all the internal organs.
- The heart is looked at to check its size and shape.
- The stomach should be visible below the heart.
- The sonographer will check that your baby has two kidneys, and that urine flows freely into the bladder.
- The arms and legs will be checked in case of abnormalities.
- Your baby's hands and feet will be examined.
- The placenta, umbilical cord and amniotic fluid will all be checked.

Your body at **19** Weeks

19 Weeks

✳ Your uterus has grown well into your abdomen – the top of it probably reaches your belly button.

✳ You may ache in your lower abdomen as muscles and ligaments stretch to support your bump.

Congratulations – you're at the halfway mark!

You may be suffering from some aches and pains in your back and lower abdomen now. There's no need to worry. Most of these pains are perfectly normal.

Aches and pains

It's common to get aches and pains in your lower abdomen during this stage of pregnancy. Aching (as opposed to cramping) is usually caused by the stretching of the muscles and ligaments supporting your uterus. You'll probably feel it most when you're getting up from a bed or chair, when you cough or when you get out of the bath.

Sitting comfortably with your feet up should alleviate your symptoms. These symptoms are perfectly normal and give you an excuse to get off your feet – and even be waited on! However, don't hesitate to call your midwife or doctor any time abdominal aching is accompanied by severe pain or cramping, bleeding, fever, chills or a feeling of faintness.

Backache is also common during pregnancy (see p.150). Pain at the back of the pelvis is known as pelvic pain (see p.231). The pain is often one-sided and may be concentrated in the buttock area. It is often confused with, or misdiagnosed as, sciatica.

If you have pain on or around the front of your pubic bone, you may be suffering from symphysis pubis dysfunction (SPD; p.231). It's sometimes common to feel a grinding or clicking in your pubic area and the pain may travel down the inside of the thighs or between your legs. The pain is usually made worse by separating your legs, walking, going up or down stairs, or moving around in bed.

Hip pain is also common. It can be particularly problematic in bed, and can make sleeping difficult. Sleeping on your side with your legs bent and a pillow between your knees may help. If any of these conditions are a problem, talk to your doctor or midwife. Alternatively, your doctor can refer you to a physiotherapist who will be able to help differentiate between these conditions.

"Sitting with **your feet up** will help **alleviate your symptoms**."

▼ Your baby at **19** Weeks

At this stage of your pregnancy your baby's five senses are starting to develop.

✳ The nerve cells serving each of her senses – taste, smell, hearing, seeing and touch – are now developing in their specialised areas of her brain. She now measures around 15cm/6in, and weighs about 240g/8½oz.. If you are carrying a girl baby, she now has roughly six million eggs in her ovaries.

What's happening to your breasts?

By now you have no doubt noticed the huge changes taking place in your bra cups: larger breasts and darkened nipples and areolas (the circles of skin surrounding your nipples). You may also have noticed the appearance of tiny bumps around your areolas. These are called the glands of Montgomery. They produce an oily substance that cleanses, lubricates and protects the nipples from infection during breastfeeding.

Perhaps even more remarkable than this visible transformation are the extensive changes taking place on the inside. Your breasts are made up of supportive tissue, milk glands and protective fat. Amid the fat cells and glandular tissue is an intricate network of channels or canals called milk ducts.

Pregnancy hormones make the milk ducts increase in number and size. Each one branches off into smaller canals near the chest wall called ductules. At the end of each ductule is a cluster of small, grapelike sacs called alveoli. A cluster of alveoli is called a lobule; a cluster of lobules is called a lobe. Each breast contains 15 to 20 lobes.

Milk is produced inside the alveoli, which are surrounded by tiny muscles that squeeze the milk out into the ductules. These ductules converge and lead to bigger ducts that end at your nipple. Your milk-duct system becomes fully developed sometime during your second trimester. This means that you can breastfeed your baby even if she's born prematurely.

You'll begin full-scale milk production within 24 to 48 hours of giving birth. The oestrogen and progesterone levels in your body start to drop. The hormone prolactin then signals your body to make lots of milk to nourish your baby.

Working mum

Finding a comfortable pair of maternity tights can prove to be an unexpected challenge.

"It's taken me ages to find a pair of maternity tights that I like. None of them look particularly sexy before you put your clothes on top of them (my other half laughed his head off when he saw me try the first pair on), but then tights never do look that great!

Some are more comfortable than others – and the prices range from cheap and cheerful to pretty pricey. It's much more comfortable to wear tights with a high cotton content – the last thing you need is hot, sweaty legs when you're pregnant. I may invest in a more expensive pair when my bump gets bigger – some of them have built-in support around the bump, which sounds like a good idea."

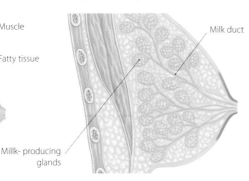

Muscle

Fatty tissue

Millk- producing glands

Milk duct

Before pregnancy your breasts consist of fatty tissue on top of a layer of muscle.

During pregnancy milk-producing glands are stimulated. Ducts take milk to the nipple.

Parents**Talk...**

"I was really worried when doing nothing more energetic than getting out of bed or up from a chair made the lower part of my stomach ache. I called my midwife and she reassured me that it's nothing to worry about, as long as it's not a severe pain or cramp. She said it's just my muscles stretching as my baby grows."
Fritha, 27, first-time mum

"Whenever I start to feel uncomfortable, if possible I'll sit down and put my feet up. After a few minutes, I usually find that the aching eases or stops altogether. I must admit that I do sometimes milk the situation though. My partner has brought me many a cup of tea while I've been exaggeratedly sighing in my chair."
Dee, 33, pregnant for the second time

Getting ready for pregnancy

Staying safe and healthy

Your pregnancy diary

Birth and beyond

FIRST TRIMESTER	SECOND TRIMESTER	THIRD TRIMESTER

 Your body at **20** Weeks

20 Weeks

❋ Some breathlessness is normal and may get a little worse as your uterus pushes up against your lungs.

❋ You can probably feel your baby move around now. Those flutters are one of the joys of pregnancy.

You may be feeling a little heavy now, especially if you're carrying twins. It's not just the weight of your baby that's the problem, but your uterus becoming increasingly muscular as it starts preparing for birth.

Pregnant with twins

When you are expecting twins, you might suffer more from some of the usual symptoms of pregnancy. Anaemia (see p.229) is more common with twins, for example, and can make you feel very tired. You are also likely to gain more weight than mothers expecting one baby. As in any pregnancy, try to eat a healthy, balanced diet and also to ensure that you gain enough weight to help your babies to grow well.

Later on in pregnancy there is more strain on your muscles because you are carrying extra weight, so back pain (see p.150) might be a problem. Another problem is breathlessness (see opposite); having two babies pushing up against your diaphragm can make it worse.

Extra care

You should be offered extra scans to see how your babies are positioned in the uterus, how well they are growing, and whether any complications are developing. Regular blood pressure and urine tests are especially important, too, as you have a higher-than-usual risk of developing gestational hypertension (see pp.229–30), pre-eclampsia (see

Fact : If it were possible, more than two-thirds of mums-to-be said they would choose to have twins. They love the idea – you only have to be pregnant once to have a big family straight away.

p.233), or gestational diabetes (see p.229). Bed rest is not often recommended these days, just because you're pregnant with twins. However, you will still need extra rest. If you have older children, arrange more childcare if you can. And snatch daytime naps whenever possible.

If you are at work, think about taking maternity leave early. This makes sense because carrying twins is hard work and premature birth happens in about half of twin pregnancies. One of the most important lessons to learn when you have twins is to ask for help. If people offer to lend a hand, let them; if not, ask them. You could also contact a multiple-birth support group for advice and that is a good way to make friends who also have twins. Ask your midwife for details.

▼ Your baby at **20** Weeks

This week your baby will be swallowing more of the amniotic fluid.

❋ Any excess water will move into his large bowel. He now measures about 16.5cm/6½in from crown to rump. A whitish coat of a slick, fatty substance called vernix caseosa is beginning to cover him. This helps to protect his skin during its long immersion in the amniotic fluid. It also helps to ease delivery.

Breathlessness

About seven out of 10 pregnant women feel breathless at some point. It can start in the first or second trimester, and is probably due to your respiratory system adapting to the effects of pregnancy hormones. In addition, your ribcage moves up and outwards. This gives you a greater lung capacity and helps your body to process oxygen and carbon dioxide more efficiently.

Later on, as your uterus pushes your diaphragm towards your lungs, you'll probably have some breathlessness too, especially if you're expecting twins or carrying your baby high.

Most women in their first pregnancy find that their baby engages, or drops down into the pelvis, from around 36 weeks (see p.205). You may well find that this helps to relieve the breathlessness. In later pregnancies your baby may not engage until the very end. If you've still got a while to go, try doing some light exercise. If you are unfit, you are more likely to feel breathless, which is why a gentle workout can help.

Although breathlessness is normal during pregnancy you should always call your midwife or doctor if you notice other alarming symptoms, such as chest pain, palpitations or a racing pulse. Breathlessness can also be a sign of anaemia (see p.229). Ask your midwife to check for this with a blood test if it hasn't been done recently.

There is no need to worry about your baby. You may fear that you're depriving him of oxygen, but rest assured that he is getting what he needs.

"Rest assured that **your baby** is getting the **oxygen he needs**."

Diaphragm is pushed towards the lungs

Ribcage moves up and out to make extra space for your lungs

Expanding uterus pushes the diaphragm up

You'll probably be feeling breathless whichever way up your baby is now (most turn head down in readiness for birth). That's because your expanding uterus squeezes your other organs up, especially your diaphragm and ribcage.

ParentsAsk...

I'm having twins. Will I be able to have a normal delivery?
Many women carrying twins are able to have a vaginal birth, although around six out of 10 twin births are by caesarean section. Talk to your doctor and midwife about the policy in your local hospital and chat through your options. It may depend in part on the position your babies are in when you go into labour. If your first twin is in a head-down position and the placenta isn't in the way of the cervix, a vaginal birth is often possible. Also, ask your doctor about the amount of experience she has of delivering twins vaginally.

Getting ready for pregnancy

Staying safe and healthy

Your pregnancy diary

Birth and beyond

Sleep in the second trimester

By now your body will be adjusting to the huge hormonal and physical changes of pregnancy, and you can sleep more peacefully as a result – barring a few minor sleep disturbances, such as leg cramps, weird dreams and a stuffy nose, of course!

Dad's **Diary**

Sharing a bed

"Sally's sleep has really improved now we've passed the first trimester. She isn't running to the loo so often, or waking up early feeling sick. It's a shame I can't say the same for myself. While she's happily knocking out the zeds, I'm putting up with all manner of nocturnal nuisances. She's usually a peaceful sleeper, but lately, sleeping next to Sally has been like sleeping next to a pneumatic drill. It's lucky she's not so big that I can't move her onto her side to stop the snoring. And she's fidgety too. Even when she's sound asleep her legs are on the move, kicking out and twitching."

You may be sleeping better now but disturbing your partner with your snoring.

Sleeping in comfort

Chances are that you're sleeping better now than you have in months. That's because the influx of progesterone that started when you became pregnant has tapered down to a steady drizzle. So

"You won't be **scurrying to the bathroom** as often as **before**."

although your hormone levels are still rising, it's happening more slowly now, and you'll probably be feeling less tired than you did during the early months.

The other good news is that your baby is now positioned above your bladder, rather than next to it, so you won't be scurrying for the bathroom as often as you have been.

Bear in mind, though, that the quality of your sleep, as well as the amount of time you spend asleep, still won't be as good as it was before you were pregnant and you may at times be affected by snoring and congestion, leg cramps (see opposite) and vivid dreams.

You are more likely to snore because the increase in progesterone can make your nasal passages swell slightly, causing congestion. Try sleeping on your side rather than your back, or try

wearing a nasal strip to keep your nostrils wide open (these are available at most pharmacists). If you are having problems getting comfortable, you can use pillows to support both your tummy and your back in bed. Tucking a pillow between your legs supports your lower back and may make sleeping on your side more comfortable. You can also get pillows that are made especially for pregnancy, although you may need to scour the classified ads in baby magazines or surf the net to find them.

Bizarre dreamworld

If you are having strange dreams, which may or may not include pregnancy and baby-related images, it may be that your sleep and dream patterns are being affected by your hormones, your changing shape and mixed feelings of anxiety and excitement about becoming a mum. All you can do is try to enjoy your new technicolour dreamworld. You could also record your dreams and what you think they mean in a journal.

Leg cramps and other night-time miseries

Your leg muscles are now bearing your increasing weight and can sometimes seize up during the night in protest. Too little calcium and potassium circulating in your blood can also cause spasms, as can your expanding uterus pressing on the nerves leading to your legs.

To prevent night-time cramps, eat a banana or drink a glass of milk before bed for a quick calcium and potassium boost. Rotate your ankles and wiggle your toes whenever you can. Try stretching your calf muscles several times before you go to bed.

If you do get a cramp, straighten your leg, heel first, and gently flex your ankles and toes. You can also relax the cramp by massaging the muscle or warming it with a hot-water bottle. Walking around for a few minutes may help, too.

Your sleep may also be disturbed by restless legs – crawling, creeping, or tingling sensations inside your foot and calf. Nearly all sufferers report an overpowering urge to move their legs. No one knows exactly what causes restless legs, but it may be inherited.

Drugs are available for the problem but none are safe during pregnancy. Try keeping a journal of what you eat and drink, what you do, and your emotions. After a few weeks, you may be able to tell if diet, stress or even environmental factors are causing your symptoms.

If you get a leg cramp at night, straighten and stretch your leg, then flex your ankles.

How exercise can help you sleep

Regular exercise during pregnancy makes you healthier, both physically and mentally, and it can help you to sleep more soundly, too – provided you do the right amount at the right time of day.

For a start, exercise helps you work off any excess energy, and will tire you enough to lull you into a deeper, more restful slumber. Gently stretching your muscles helps ward off sleep-disturbing aches and pains, such as leg cramps.

On the other hand, if you exercise shortly before you go to bed, you may feel revved up instead of ready to wind down. Some experts say that working up a sweat too close to bedtime can interfere with your natural sleep cycle and rob you of restorative deep sleep. So it's important to set aside the late afternoon or early evening for exercise and give yourself at least four hours to unwind before you hit the sack.

Natural sleep remedies

If you're having trouble getting to sleep now you're pregnant, try some tried-and-tested natural remedies.

Herbal remedies A hop pillow may help if you wish to use herbal remedies, but avoid drinking hop teas unless prescribed by a qualified medical herbalist.

Aromatherapy Lavender, chamomile or ylang ylang essential oils may help when used for a massage, but use occasionally and only two to three drops in 10ml (two teaspoons) of a base oil such as almond oil.

Flower remedies Remedies containing a mixture of flower essences are specifically designed to ease general stress and tension and may help you to sleep.

Homeopathy Homeopathic remedies can help but are best prescribed by a professional homeopath according to your precise symptoms. If your mind refuses to "shut off", try one 30c tablet of the homeopathic remedy coffea under your tongue before retiring or if you wake in the night. Aconite is useful if you have vivid dreams and are restless, waking at the slightest sound.

The occasional aromatherapy massage with lavender oil can help with sleeplessness.

Your body at **21** Weeks

21 Weeks

✳ It's hard to be graceful when you're pregnant. Don't be surprised if you find you're more clumsy now.

✳ You're carrying more weight, your centre of gravity has changed and all your joints are loosening up.

By now you should be feeling your baby moving regularly – often when you are trying to rest! Those kicks and nudges will help you and your partner to bond with the little person growing inside you.

Your baby's movements

If this is your first pregnancy you will probably first be aware of your baby's movements at around 18 to 20 weeks. For subsequent pregnancies, when you are already familiar with the tell-tale signs, you will probably first feel her movements a bit earlier, at around 15 to 18 weeks.

After the initial vague stirrings, which some women say feel like a butterfly's wings flapping, your baby's movements become stronger and more regular. Later, you will start to feel thumping or kicking movements, though not all the time because she sometimes just wants to rest.

While you are busy you will probably be less aware of the movements your baby is making. It's more likely you'll start to notice them when you sit down and relax. Every baby has his or her own individual pattern of waking and sleeping. By late pregnancy you will probably have become tuned into your baby's particular pattern of movements. This is what you might expect as your baby grows.

● **From 20 to 24 weeks** As the weeks go by, you'll notice how your baby's activity will gradually increase. From now onwards, over the next 10 weeks, your baby will be having a busy period while she floats in the amniotic fluid, with lots of kicking and somersaults.

● **From 24 to 28 weeks** Baby hiccups are common at this time but start earlier in pregnancy. This explains the jerking movements you may feel. The amniotic sac now contains up to 750ml (1¼ pints) of fluid. This helps your baby to move about freely. At around this time, you may notice her jump at sudden noises.

● **At 29 weeks** At this stage in your pregnancy, your baby will begin to make smaller, more definite movements. She is starting to get more cramped inside your uterus.

● **At 32 weeks** Your baby's movements will reach a peak of activity and, from now on, you will notice an increase in the frequency and type of movements as your baby gets bigger and stronger.

● **From around 36 weeks** Your baby may take up her final (usually head-down) position at about this time, particularly if this is your first pregnancy. That is because, in a first pregnancy, the

---

▼ Your baby at **21** Weeks

From now on, watch what you say as your baby can probably hear you!

✳ Now you can communicate with her by talking, singing or reading aloud. Studies even suggest a newborn will suck more vigorously when feeding if you read aloud from a book that you've read aloud from during pregnancy. Your baby now measures about 27cm/10½in and has proper eyebrows, eyelids and fingernails.

As your pregnancy progresses your baby's movements get stronger and your partner should be able to feel them, too.

muscles of your uterus and abdomen are still firm and will help to keep her in place. The main movements you are likely to feel now are jabs from her arms and legs, and possibly a few painful kicks to your ribs.

If this isn't your first pregnancy, your abdominal muscles are likely to be weaker. This gives your baby the chance to keep changing her position and she could continue to do so even right up to your due date.

● **From 36 to 40 weeks** Now you are in the last weeks of your pregnancy and your baby will be getting larger and her roll-over movements will become less frequent. If she's sucking her thumb and "loses" it, you may feel quick, darting movements. This is her head turning from side-to-side while she tries to find her thumb again.

Working mum

Feeling your baby kick can have its embarrassing moments, but it's a great bonding experience.

"My baby's definitely not a night owl. She's moving around and kicking a lot now, but only during the day. She even tickles me at work, which makes me laugh for no apparent reason. Very amusing for my colleagues! Feeling her inside me is wonderful. I feel like I'm bonding with her already."

During the last two weeks of your pregnancy, the movements are likely to slow down and your baby's growth rate will decline slightly. This is all completely normal and nothing to worry about.

Avoiding excess weight gain

If you are worried about how much weight you are putting on, keep a food diary for a few days. This will quickly show you how balanced your diet is. If you're eating plenty of fruit and vegetables, lots of multigrain foods and some good proteins and dairy products, then there is less need to worry than if you find you are filling up on chips and chocolate. If you are eating well but still piling on the pounds, then it's time to see a dietician who has experience of working with pregnant women. She will help you to find out how to make the best of your nutrient intake without loading up on calories.

Your best strategy is to eat healthily and incorporate regular exercise into your daily life. Evidence has shown that exercise in addition to a healthy diet during pregnancy results in less weight gain than eating a healthy diet alone. The researchers also found that the women who exercised reduced their risk of giving birth to a large baby.

If you're a relative newcomer to exercise, though, you should start with low-impact exercise such as walking, swimming or low-impact aerobics (see p.57). And never begin a new exercise regime without first discussing with your doctor or midwife what is safe.

Parents**Ask...**

It's my second pregnancy and I'm a bit big. Is this OK?
Women expecting second or subsequent babies are sometimes slightly large for dates. This may be because their muscles have been weakened by a previous pregnancy. Everything is probably quite normal.

Why are my ankles swollen?
This is called oedema (see p.238) and it's quite common. Your growing uterus makes blood pool, which forces water down into the tissues of your feet and ankles. Just raise your feet whenever possible. Although your swollen ankles will probably add to your feelings of ungainliness, oedema is temporary and will pass soon after you give birth.

"Keeping a food diary **will show** if your diet is **well balanced**."

Getting ready for pregnancy

Staying safe and healthy

Your pregnancy diary

Birth and beyond

Your body at **22** Weeks

22 Weeks

✳ At this point, you'll probably notice a steady gain in weight – about 225g (½lb) each week.

✳ You may notice increased vaginal discharge. It's due to increased blood flow in that part of the body.

Have you found yourself longing for cocktail sausages with ice cream, or salivating over cheese and chocolate? Don't worry – lots of women have weird food cravings in pregnancy.

Cravings in pregnancy

 Your baby at **22** Weeks

Now the baby inside you is beginning to look like a miniature newborn.

✳ This is a very exciting time because your baby is now looking recognisably like a baby. His lips are becoming more distinct and his eyes have developed; though the irises haven't got their colour yet, his eyebrows and eyelids are in place. His pancreas, which is essential for hormone production, is developing steadily and the first signs of teeth are there now, showing beneath his gum line. If you could see inside your womb, you would be able to spot the fine hair (lanugo) now covering his body.

Don't be surprised if you find you have a craving to eat something particular during pregnancy. This kind of yearning is an undeniable part of carrying a baby for many women, and not all of these cravings can be neatly catalogued – or stomached. You may find yourself yearning for pickles wrapped in cheese, or mayonnaise spooned straight from the jar – or even seeking out a good helping of pure steak fat!

Some pregnant women develop strong cravings for non-food items such as dirt, ashes, clay, chalk, coal, ice, laundry starch, baking soda, soap, toothpaste, paint chips, plaster, wax, hair, coffee grounds, and even cigarette butts. This phenomenon is called pica, which is Latin for magpie – a bird that will eat almost anything.

The causes

No one knows what causes these cravings, but a combination of biochemical, psychological, and cultural factors may be at work. In some studies, these bizarre cravings have been linked to an iron deficiency – even though none of the craved items contain a significant amount of iron. Some women who have iron-deficiency anaemia crave

ice until the deficiency is cured. And pica is sometimes listed as a symptom of iron-deficiency anaemia.

If you crave non-food items, it doesn't necessarily mean you have any sort of deficiency, and it definitely doesn't mean you should consume them! In fact, eating non-food substances can interfere with your body's ability to absorb nutrients and may even cause a deficiency. And while eating ice is not likely to be harmful (except possibly to your teeth!), eating dirt and most of the other items mentioned can lead to illness, such as lead poisoning or bowel blockage, which could have very serious consequences.

Get some advice

If you're having strong cravings for any non-food items, it's a good idea to talk to your doctor or midwife. While this kind of craving does occur in healthy pregnant women, it's worth getting yourself checked for any underlying physical or psychological problem. You may also be able to curb unhealthy cravings by eating breakfast every day (just some fruit could do), getting plenty of exercise and making sure you have a wide ranging and healthy diet.

Planning ahead for working parenthood

If you have a job you enjoy, finding dependable childcare means you can return to work after the birth.

All parents work, of course, and staying at home with a demanding baby or toddler is equally, if not more, taxing than going back to your old job. There are new skills to be learned, but there is no one around to train you. Added to that, there is no recognition of the hard work done and no pay cheque at the end of the month. It's not all about money, of course, but dropping one person's income is something that many couples find difficult to afford.

Deciding to return to work means balancing your time between work and family, and you will need to develop a raft of new skills. One of the most valuable is the ability to plan and juggle your time so that you meet different demands. You will also need to develop strong organisational skills.

Solid and dependable childcare arrangements are a must if you want to enjoy your new life to the full. Be prepared to devote plenty of time to choosing the right option for you, as you are handing over a huge responsibility to someone when you employ them to care for your baby. You have to be confident that you are leaving your little one in the hands of a skilled and caring professional. You don't want to be fretting about your baby's well-being while you're trying to work.

If you have a job that you find satisfying and your child is entrusted to capable hands, you can have a very rewarding life as a working parent. Work can give you a challenge, an income and the pleasure of adult company during part of the day. Then, you can return home and really enjoy spending time with your child.

 ## Working mum

It can be hard to know when – and how – to tell your work colleagues you're pregnant.

"It's so much easier now that my work colleagues know I'm pregnant. I don't need to hold in my stomach any more! I was quite nervous before I told them, so I told the colleagues I work with most closely first. It didn't take long for the news to travel after that. I've had lots of congratulations – everyone seems to be really happy for me. It created a bit of a buzz in the office for the morning. A couple of my workmates even said that they suspected I might be pregnant – I guess I wasn't that good at hiding my nausea and tiredness after all!"

 ## Green mum

Urinary tract infections (UTIs) are common in pregnancy, but there are ways of avoiding them.

"Over the years, since I had my last baby, I've learnt quite a few natural methods for warding off UTIs. I think they're better than taking pills and medicines and they seem to have worked, as I haven't had a UTI during my pregnancy so far. By this stage last time around, I'd already had a couple and I was really fed up.

Firstly, when I go to the loo, I always take care to wipe myself front to back and empty my bladder completely. And I always make sure I go to the loo soon after having sex, too.

Then, whenever I have a shower, I wash carefully between my legs with an organic body wash. And of course it helps to always wear cotton knickers and change my underwear and tights every day. And I also drink a couple of glasses of cranberry juice a day. As well as being full of antioxidants and vitamin C, they say it helps flush out the bacteria which cause UTIs."

Many women find that drinking a glass or two of cranberry juice daily helps to treat UTIs.

Getting ready for pregnancy

Staying safe and healthy

Your pregnancy diary

Birth and beyond

Your body at **23** Weeks

23 Weeks

✻ You may notice some bleeding when you brush your teeth – it's a common pregnancy complaint.

✻ Your belly button, once an "innie", may now stick out. Don't worry. It'll revert soon after you give birth.

Are you a blooming mum-to-be, or just feeling blooming awful? Remind yourself why pregnancy makes you beautiful. And if you're still struggling to choose a name for your baby, we have a few tips.

You're blooming pregnant!

Even though you're probably overjoyed by the new life that's been growing inside you for the last 23 weeks, there may be days when you can't wait for the whole thing to be over. As your breasts grow, your abdomen swells and your waistline disappears, you may long to have your old shape back – or even to remember what it was! While you're revelling in being pregnant, you may not be revelling in looking pregnant.

The second trimester of pregnancy is usually when women are looking – as well as feeling – at their best. Read on for a reminder of some of the beauty bonuses of pregnancy.

● **You will probably have that celebrated "glow"** You may notice that your skin looks brighter than usual. Hormones are partly responsible, but an increase in blood volume brings more blood to the skin, which helps to give it that radiant look.

● **Fast-growing fingernails** Around the fourth month, your nails may start to grow faster than usual. Pregnancy hormones get the credit for this, but also the blame, as fingernails may become softer or more brittle.

● **A fabulous head of hair** Many women find that pregnancy brings out the best in their hair. You might start to notice your hair has more volume.

● **Bigger breasts** It's common to go up a cup size or two during your pregnancy, so by now you may have a new cleavage to show off!

● **A very happy mate** Believe it or not, your partner may be crazy about your new physique. Men tend to see the sensuality in blossoming breasts and soft curves. The sight of your pregnant form is a constant reminder of his virility too, and we all know how important that is to him!

Whether or not you're blossoming and blooming, it is worth trying out these two look-good strategies:

● **Emphasise the positive** If your legs are gorgeous, flaunt them by wearing a short dress. Toned upper arms like a supermodel's? Show them off with a sleeveless top. Proud of your new, improved cleavage? Don't be shy – highlight it with a scoop- or V-neck top.

● **Spoil yourself occasionally** Treat yourself to a pedicure, a manicure, a new lipstick or some lacy underwear.

 Your baby at **23** Weeks

Her hearing's well established now so she's getting used to all sorts of sounds.

✻ She can make out a distorted version of your voice, the beating of your heart and your stomach rumblings. Loud noises that she has often heard in the uterus – a dog's bark, the vacuum cleaner – probably won't bother her when she is born. She now weighs a little more than 500g/1lb and measures about 29cm/11½in.

Anything you do that's just for you will make you feel more glam. Meanwhile, don't forget to exercise. It'll make you feel better about the way you look, keep your energy levels up and help you bounce back after the birth.

And here's a little perk that no one told you about: pregnant women often bring out the kindness in people. People fall over themselves to hold doors open for you. They give up seats on trains and buses. Enjoy it while it lasts!

45–50% more blood will be running through your veins and arteries

by the time you get to the end of your pregnancy. This is all part of the way your body adapts during pregnancy to meet the demands of your baby.

Dad's **Diary**

Getting to grips with being a stay-at-home dad

"Our childcare plans were turned upside-down when I was made redundant. My partner was just three months pregnant, and our little girl was almost three. After months of job-hunting (and our baby's birth just weeks away) we started to think seriously about me staying at home with the children. Laura earns more than I did anyway, and had planned to go back part-time after the birth. Her company has happily agreed to her returning full time, so she'll be the main breadwinner. Now we've made the decision, I'm not worried about staying at home – I'm not hugely career minded and I don't have a problem with not being the primary earner. I'm happy at the thought of being able to spend more time with my children."

Many fathers relish the thought of being a stay-at-home dad.

Choosing a name

If you've already started thinking about baby names, you'll know that naming your baby is one of the best bits about being pregnant. But it's a big responsibility too. After all, your baby

will have the name you choose for life. Here are a few things to consider before you make your choice:

● **Sound and compatibility** How your baby's name sounds when it is said aloud is one of the most essential things to think about. Is it melodious? Harsh? Does it go well with your surname? Often, longer first names work better with shorter surnames, and vice versa.

● **Uniqueness** An unusual name has the advantage of making the bearer stand out from the crowd. On the other hand, a name that no one has heard of and can't pronounce can draw unwanted attention.

Choose what you will call your baby with careful consideration. Remember, she'll be stuck with your choice for life.

● **Relatives and friends** Many parents choose to name their babies after a grandparent, other relative, or close friend. This option can provide you with a good pool of names to consider.

● **Ancestry and heritage** Your child's heritage is an essential part of who she is, and you may want her name to reflect that heritage.

● **Meaning** No one is likely to treat your daughter Ingrid differently because her name means "hero's daughter", but the derivation of your baby's name is something you may want to think about.

● **Initials and nicknames** People, especially children, can be cruel when it comes to nicknames, so try to anticipate any potentially embarrassing ones that your little one may be given if you choose something unfortunate.

Getting ready for pregnancy

Staying safe and healthy

Your pregnancy diary

Birth and beyond

Your body at **24** Weeks

24 Weeks

✲ By now, you probably have a definite "pregnant" shape and the linea nigra down your abdomen.

✲ You may notice faint red streaks – striae or stretch marks – on your tummy, hips, buttocks and breasts.

If you're feeling hot, heavy and fed up, it's time to spoil yourself with a few treats. Don't feel guilty if you have the urge to splash out on a bit of pampering and de-stressing now and again.

Go on, treat yourself

You're a few weeks beyond the halfway point in your pregnancy but the end probably still feels a long way off. You can be excused if you sometimes feel a little down, but if ever there was a time to pamper yourself, then pregnancy is it. Banish the blues by trying some of our indulgent ideas.

● **Give yourself a home spa** Make your bathroom a tranquil space: dim the lights and add scented candles and a relaxing CD. Have some fluffy bath towels handy – keep them on a warm radiator or heated towel rail for added comfort. Then get the facemasks, bubbles and nail polish out and enjoy.

● **Get a great haircut** Book yourself in for a consultation and cut with a really good stylist. He'll be able to help you find a lower-maintenance style that will see you right through pregnancy and into those first few weeks of living with a baby. While you're there, ask about nourishing salon products. Pregnant women often find their hair is much glossier, so now is the time to make the most of that shine.

● **Go out on a date** Spend a romantic evening with your partner this week, at the theatre, cinema, a favourite restaurant, or somewhere else where you can appreciate each other's company. If you already have children, ask a favourite grandparent or friend to do the babysitting.

● **Ditch the lenses** The shape of your eyeballs can change during pregnancy due to fluid retention, or you may even be suffering from dry eyes. If you wear contact lenses and they're becoming uncomfortable, think about investing in a chic pair of glasses instead. Some designer frames can look very stylish and sexy. Glasses could be a good investment for your early days of motherhood too, when you might not have time to fiddle about with your contact lenses – especially in the early hours of the morning.

● **Buy even more shoes!** If your feet are swollen, it might be wise to invest in a pair of shoes a size bigger than normal. Opting for something practical and comfortable doesn't mean sacrificing style – flat shoes can be just as pretty as their high-heeled counterparts and look great with the right outfits.

▼ Your baby at **24** Weeks

If your baby arrives from now onwards, he may survive, with special care.

✲ This is the week when your baby becomes "viable", which means that if he's born prematurely, he could be OK with special care. His skin is thin and fragile but his body is filling out and taking up more room in your uterus. Taste buds are now forming and, believe it or not, your baby may already have a sweet tooth.

Looking at childcare options

It is important to start thinking about childcare early on, and certainly once you're into your second trimester of pregnancy, because the best childcare choices are often snapped up very quickly. The first thing to do is to look at all the options that are available in your

Finding suitable childcare takes time. Make sure you start researching your options as early as possible.

area. You can do this by talking to other parents and parents-to-be or by contacting ChildcareLink or the Children's Information Service in your area. You'll find the numbers in your local phone book.

If you are looking for a nanny, it may be hard to find someone who is prepared to commit themselves to a job before handing in their notice to their current employer (usually a month beforehand). However, you can start a general search for nanny agencies, begin to see people and build up a picture of quality and availability.

If you are looking at childminders, you may find that the same principles apply. Many childminders are unwilling to commit themselves too far in advance. You may be asked to pay a fee to keep a place available.

When you start looking, don't expect to find someone immediately – in fact, it's a good idea to see a number of different people and places before making any decision, so you get an idea of the variety in quality, price and style.

If your first choice is oversubscribed or out of your reach financially, don't despair, but be prepared to compromise. and consider alternatives. The only thing you should not compromise on is your certainty that your child will be looked after by caring, qualified people.

Premature labour

A premature birth is when a baby arrives before 37 complete weeks of pregnancy. It's difficult for doctors to predict which women will go into labour prematurely, but there is evidence that certain bacteria in your urine make premature labour more likely. It is now recommended that all women have their urine tested for bacteria early in pregnancy.

Other risk factors include smoking, using recreational drugs, expecting twins or more, and previous premature births. If your waters break or you start contractions before 37 weeks, contact your midwife, doctor or hospital immediately.

Most premature babies do well nowadays, but you can minimise your risk of having a premature labour.

Parents**Talk...**

"I'm about halfway through my pregnancy and my skin is really itchy. It's especially bad on my tummy, and my midwife says that's because the skin is stretching there as my bump grows, which I guess makes sense. Apparently general itchiness of the skin is pretty normal. Fingers crossed it stops once my baby has arrived. Scratching in public is not a good look!"
Jen, 24, pregnant for the first time

"I was diagnosed with obstetric cholestasis (see pp.230–31) at 27 weeks and I'm 32 weeks now. The itching is really bad on the soles of my feet, but it's actually everywhere and I've made myself bleed with scratching. It drives me crazy. Long, cool baths and calamine lotion help to ease the itching. There's no cure for it, but I'm having extra antenatal checks to monitor my baby."
Shola, 27, pregnant for the first time

Getting ready for pregnancy

Staying safe and healthy

Your pregnancy diary

Birth and beyond

| FIRST TRIMESTER | SECOND TRIMESTER | THIRD TRIMESTER |

Your body at **25** Weeks

25 Weeks

❉ Hormone surges and the extra weight you're carrying can make you ache all over.

❉ Your growing bump may make it hard to get into a comfortable position to sleep.

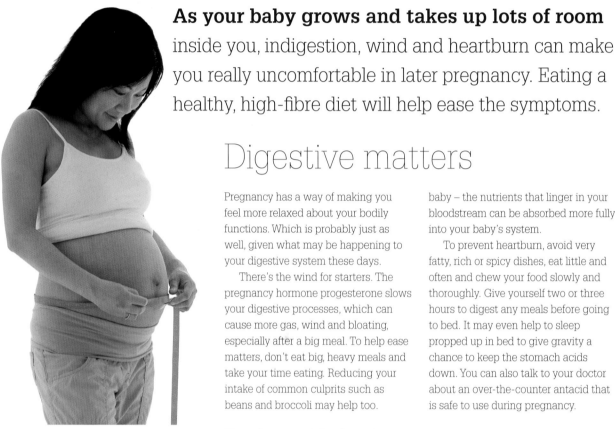

As your baby grows and takes up lots of room inside you, indigestion, wind and heartburn can make you really uncomfortable in later pregnancy. Eating a healthy, high-fibre diet will help ease the symptoms.

Digestive matters

Pregnancy has a way of making you feel more relaxed about your bodily functions. Which is probably just as well, given what may be happening to your digestive system these days.

There's the wind for starters. The pregnancy hormone progesterone slows your digestive processes, which can cause more gas, wind and bloating, especially after a big meal. To help ease matters, don't eat big, heavy meals and take your time eating. Reducing your intake of common culprits such as beans and broccoli may help too.

Heartburn and indigestion
You may experience heartburn and indigestion during your pregnancy. Heartburn causes a burning sensation in your upper chest. It happens because progesterone relaxes the valve that separates your food pipe from your stomach, allowing stomach acid to seep back up the pipe. Also, as your growing baby crowds the abdominal cavity, it can push acid up into your food pipe. Take comfort in the fact that the same process that causes you such discomfort may actually be of some benefit to your

baby – the nutrients that linger in your bloodstream can be absorbed more fully into your baby's system.

To prevent heartburn, avoid very fatty, rich or spicy dishes, eat little and often and chew your food slowly and thoroughly. Give yourself two or three hours to digest any meals before going to bed. It may even help to sleep propped up in bed to give gravity a chance to keep the stomach acids down. You can also talk to your doctor about an over-the-counter antacid that is safe to use during pregnancy.

Constipation
Constipation is another common problem in pregnancy: about 30 to 40 per cent of pregnant women get constipated at some point. The culprits

Fact: In later pregnancy, your growing baby crowds your abdominal cavity. This can slow down your digestion and pushes on your stomach, making you feel even more bloated when you've eaten.

▼ Your baby at **25** Weeks

Your baby now weighs nearly 660g/23¼oz and is about 34.6cm/13½in long.

❉ There's no air in her lungs yet – just amniotic fluid – but she's making movements that look like breathing. She's getting some baby fat, too. As this happens, her wrinkled skin will begin to smooth out. She's also growing more hair – if you could see it, you would be able to discern its colour and texture.

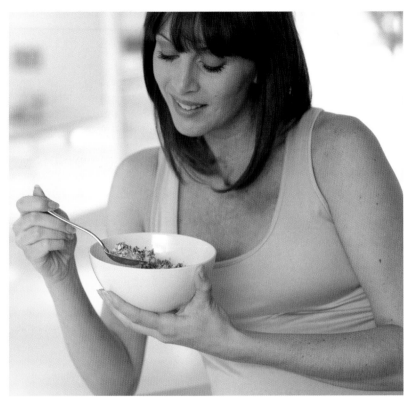

Constipation is a common pregnancy problem. Eating high-fibre foods such as wholegrain breakfast cereals, wholegrain bread and plenty of fresh fruit and vegetables can help prevent it.

Working mum

Office work brings special challenges for you and your ever-increasing bump.

"My bump and my desk appear to be having a fight at work – and I think the bump may be winning! I've really noticed it moving higher this week and now it's got to the point that the baby is really pushing against me and the desk. It's a bit uncomfortable to say the least. I wish there was a desk pillow that I could use as a buffer. Or even a special ergonomic desk for pregnant women with a bump-shaped cut-out!

I've already asked HR for a footrest. I'm starting to get swollen ankles too, so I'm hoping having something to raise my feet up will help. I try to get away from my desk every hour or so to stretch my legs, and I go out for a walk and some fresh air every lunch time. But the bigger I get, the more I look forward to maternity leave."

Sitting for long periods can cause backache, but more so if you're pregnant. You need plenty of breaks.

are the pressure of your growing uterus on your rectum, along with pregnancy hormones, which slow the transit of food through your digestive tract. Some iron pills can make constipation worse, so be aware of this side effect.

If constipation persists, do mention it to your doctor. If changes to your diet and lifestyle don't make a difference then your doctor or midwife can prescribe a laxative that is safe to use in pregnancy. Sometimes, constipation can lead to

"**High-fibre** foods and gentle **exercise** can ease **constipation**."

Eating high-fibre foods, such as wholegrain cereals, wholegrain bread, fresh fruit and vegetables every day, and drinking plenty of fluids, should help. Gentle exercise such as walking, swimming and cycling can ease constipation, too.

piles or haemorrhoids (see pp.237–8). These can be painful, itchy and uncomfortable but they can be treated with a range of creams and ointments to ease the symptoms. Haemorrhoids usually resolve themselves fairly soon after your baby is born.

Getting ready for pregnancy

Staying safe and healthy

Your pregnancy diary

Birth and beyond

FIRST TRIMESTER	SECOND TRIMESTER	THIRD TRIMESTER

▼ Your body at **26** Weeks

26 Weeks

✳ You may see a slight increase in your blood pressure. Don't worry: it's normal.

✳ Fend off constipation with fibre-rich foods like wholegrain breads and cereals, lentils and brown rice.

A birth plan is a useful part of your baby preparations. It gives you a chance to decide how you want your baby's birth to be managed. Having a written record will also give you confidence during labour.

Preparing your birth plan

Your baby at **26** Weeks

His eyes begin to open around now and his response to sound is more consistent.

✳ Towards the end of the seventh month, the network of nerves to your baby's ear is complete, which makes his response to sound better. He now measures about 35.6cm/14in from crown to heel and weighs a little more than 760g/1½lb. He is still continuing to take small breaths and, although he's only breathing in water and not air, it's still good practice for when he's born. If you are having a boy, his testicles are beginning to descend into his scrotum – a trip that will take about two to three days.

A birth plan is a method of communicating with the midwives and doctors who care for you in labour. It tells them about the kind of labour you would like to have, what you want to happen and what you definitely would like to avoid.

The best birth plans acknowledge that things may not go as expected. You need to write it in such a way that your midwife's hands aren't tied. She may need to recommend a course of action that isn't what you had hoped for, but which is in your baby's best interests.

Doing your research
Before you start writing get as much information as you can.
● **Go to antenatal classes** A good antenatal teacher will help you make the best choices for you.
● **Talk to other women** Women who have given birth at the hospital or birth centre you're going to or who've had a home birth, if that's what you'd like, can tell you how easy or difficult it was to get the kind of care they wanted.
● **Talk to your partner or birth companion** What kind of labour and birth would they like for you? Ask how they see their role. Then jot your "birth

wishes" down just as they come to mind. You can sort them out later.

Here is a list of headings that you might want to use in your birth plan. Have a look in your maternity notes and see whether there are any suggestions for birth plans in there as well.
● **Birth partner** Write down who you want to be with you in labour and whether this person should stay the whole time. There may be certain procedures or stages when you'd prefer him or her to leave.
● **Positions for labour and birth** Mention which positions you would like to use during labour and for the birth. For some useful positions, see pp.266–7. Also say how active you would like to be: would you like to remain upright and mobile for as long as possible, maybe using a birth ball, or would you prefer to be in bed?
● **Pain relief** Say what kinds of pain relief you want to use, if any, and in what order (for example, you might prefer to try Pethidine before an epidural). If you'd like to try for a natural birth (no pain-relieving drugs at all), make this clear.
● **Monitoring baby's heart rate** Say how you want your baby to be monitored during labour – whether you

Discuss your birth plan with your partner but remember, when the time comes, you will both need to be flexible in case anything unexpected happens.

would like your midwife to listen to your baby's heart intermittently using a hand-held device (Sonicaid) or whether you prefer to have electronic monitoring using a belt strapped around your waist.

- **Speeding up labour** If your labour slows down, you might want your midwife to use interventions to speed it up again, such as breaking your waters, or you may prefer to wait and see what happens naturally.
- **Birth pool** If your maternity unit has a birth pool, or if you are hiring one to use at home, make a note of whether you want to use it for pain relief as well as or instead of to give birth in.
- **Assisted birth** You might want to express a preference for forceps or ventouse if you need some help to deliver your baby.
- **Third stage (delivery of placenta)** You can choose to have an injection to speed up the delivery of the placenta, or you might prefer to have a natural third stage without drugs.
- **Feeding your baby** Be clear about whether you want to breastfeed or bottlefeed. Also be clear about whether

your breastfed baby may have any formula. If you definitely don't want her to have bottles, say so.

- **Unexpected situations** Some women say what they want to happen if their baby has to go to the special care baby unit (SCBU). They might want to care for him as much as possible themselves and be transferred with him to another hospital if that's needed. They might ask for their partner to stay with them at the hospital.

Special needs

You may have special requirements to mention in your birth plan. If you have a disability, write about the help you will need in labour. Say whether there is any special equipment you need.

If you have religious needs, be sure to include these. It might be important for certain rituals to be carried out when your baby is born. Or you might require a special diet during your hospital stay. Write all of these things down. Hospitals and health professionals are committed nowadays to being culturally sensitive and treating people as individuals.

Systemised mum

Make your birth plan as demanding as you like but prepare to be flexible, too.

"I have included as much detail as I possibly can in my birth plan. I would like my midwife to be clear on what I want to happen and what I want to avoid if possible. I'd like to have my husband and best friend in the delivery room with me, but I want Sophie to leave when it's time for me to actually push. I've also made it clear that I want to try for as little pain relief as possible and would like to use the birth pool for pain relief and relaxation. I want to breastfeed my baby as soon as I can and prefer him not to have any bottles of formula. I know I sound demanding, but I just want to have the best experience for me."

Laid-back mum

Your birth plan doesn't have be long. You may prefer to go with the flow and see how things develop.

"I've just written my birth plan and to be honest it's really short! I've pretty much only said who I want my birth partner to be and stated that if it's possible, I'd like to try for a water birth. When it comes to pain relief, I really don't know how high my pain threshold will be. If I can do it with as few drugs as possible then great, but if I'm suffering, I want them to hit me with everything they've got. I'm happy to be flexible about positions for labour. I'll just see what's comfortable at the time."

FIRST TRIMESTER | SECOND TRIMESTER | THIRD TRIMESTER

Your body at **27** Weeks

27 Weeks

✳ If you're unlucky you may discover the delights of leg cramps, haemorrhoids or varicose veins.

✳ If you're experiencing an odd rhythmic sensation, it may be that your baby is hiccupping.

Labouring and giving birth in water can be a very good experience. Being in water is relaxing and reduces the need for pain relief. It's also completely safe for mum and baby.

Planning a water birth

If you would like a water birth, the first thing to do is to talk to your midwife at one of your antenatal appointments. She can tell you if the hospital you are booked into has a pool available. About half of maternity units have facilities for water births, but some may be less encouraging about them than others. These days all maternity units should have midwives who are trained to care for women who want to labour or give birth in water. You can get an idea of how much experience your hospital has of water birth by asking the following questions:

● How many women each year use the birth pool for pain relief during labour?

● How many women give birth in the pool each year?

● How many midwives are trained in the use of the birth pool?

● Are there any times when the pool is not available?

If you are very keen on the idea of a birth pool and your local hospital hasn't got one, or hasn't got the staff to cover it on a 24-hour basis, you might consider transferring to another hospital. Another possibility is a home water birth. Your midwife should be able to tell you about local companies that hire out birth pools. Otherwise, try speaking to the supervisor of midwives at your maternity unit, or contact the local branch of the NCT. Alternatively, contact the Active Birth Centre, which hires out pools all over the country.

Researching water birth

There are several ways to find out more:

● Learn about other people's experiences: talking to women who have laboured and given birth in water is best. Talk to some who have used a birth pool just for pain relief and to some who have given birth in water. Ask them when they got into the pool, when they got out, what they found

---

Your baby at **27** Weeks

This week sees activity in your baby's brain as more of her brain tissue develops.

✳ At the same time, the characteristic grooves start to appear on the brain's surface. She now weighs nearly 875g/2lb and measures 36.6cm/14½in from head to toe. Her eyes open and close, and she sleeps and wakes at regular intervals. Some experts believe that babies begin to dream by the 28th week.

Fact: 1803 is the date of the first recorded water birth in Europe.

It happened in France when a mother whose labour had been extremely long and difficult was finally helped to give birth in a tub of warm water.

Many maternity units have a birth pool, but not all encourage their use. You should ask probing questions to gauge how much they're used.

helpful about being in water, and what they didn't like.

- Antenatal classes: these are a good source of information about water birth. When you book classes, ask whether they will include information about labouring in water. At the beginning of the course, your teacher will probably ask what topics to cover, so ask for water birth. Others in the group will almost certainly be interested as well!

- Books: most up-to-date books about pregnancy and childbirth will include a section on water birth.

Dads and paternity leave

If you're a dad-to-be, you'll probably be able to take up to two weeks' leave from work – paternity leave – immediately after your baby is born. You are entitled to paternity leave and pay if:

- You are the baby's biological father or the mum's husband or partner.
- You have (or expect to have) responsibility for the baby's care.
- You are an employee with a contract of employment.
- You've worked for your employer for at least 26 weeks by the end of the 15th week before the week the baby's due.

If you qualify, you can take either one or two weeks' leave. If you take two weeks, they must be consecutive.

Most dads will qualify for Statutory Paternity Pay (SPP). Dads who don't qualify for it may get Income Support while on paternity leave or other financial support – contact your local Jobcentre Plus office for advice.

If you're planning to take paternity leave, you must inform your employer in writing at least 15 weeks before the week when your baby is due. You can choose to start your leave immediately after your baby is born or in the following eight weeks.

Check your employment contract. Some employers have their own paternity benefits, which may suit you better than the statutory ones.

Dad's **Diary**

Timing paternity leave

"I've decided to take the full two weeks' paternity leave after our baby is born. It'll mean a bit of a financial sacrifice but I think we'll be able to manage. The only thing I haven't yet decided is when to take the time off.

Jenny's mum is coming to stay for a week or so after the baby's born, so, although I'd really like to be at home straight after the birth, it might be better for me to take the time off when she's gone back home. Otherwise, Jenny will be bombarded with support for the first fortnight and then left all alone soon afterwards. And I'm also thinking that it will give us the chance to spend time together as a new family, just the three of us. I can't wait."

Getting ready for pregnancy

Staying safe and healthy

Your pregnancy diary

Birth and beyond

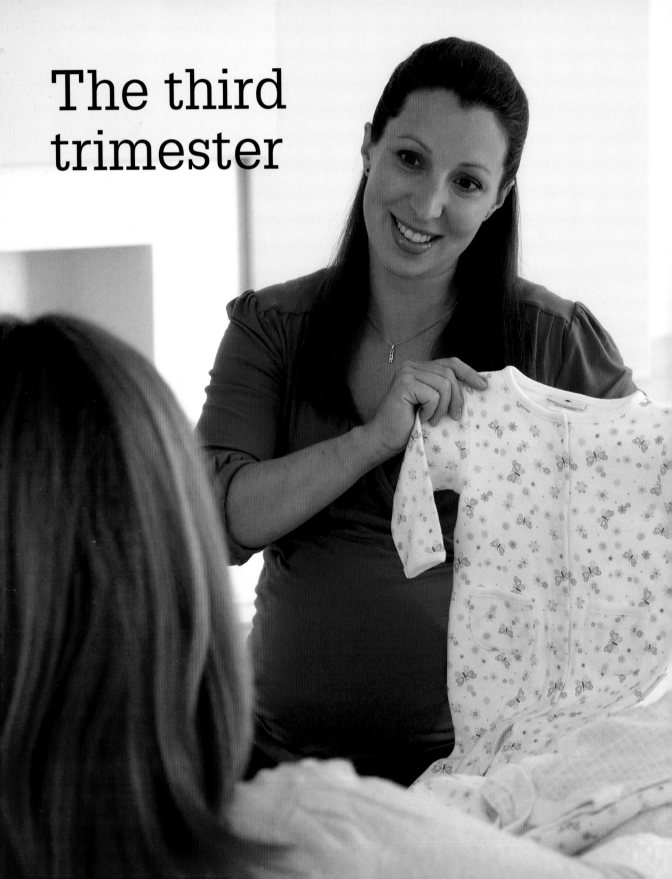

The third
trimester

The home stretch

You are probably becoming impatient to meet the baby whose squirms and kicks have become so familiar over the weeks. Indulge yourself by buying some little vests and nappies and daydreaming about the sleepless but happy time after your baby is born.

What to expect

At this stage you're probably veering from feeling "I've been pregnant for ever" one minute and "Help, I'm not ready for this!" the next. You're not alone. Swapping experiences with other women in your antenatal class can be reassuring.

Oh, the joys of pregnancy!

Sleep gets more difficult as your bump grows. Backache is a common problem, while some women also develop pelvic pain. Braxton Hicks contractions may become more intense or frequent. As early as 33 weeks your baby's head may engage (dip into the pelvic cavity in

The facial features of this baby are all well developed and his tiny fingers can be seen near his mouth.

preparation for birth), making you feel like you need to wee all the time. By 35 weeks your uterus is 1,000 times its original volume and has expanded up under your ribs. Together with hormonal changes, this causes heartburn in around 70 per cent of women in late pregnancy. Your feet, hands, face and ankles can become swollen too.

Your growing baby

At the start of the third trimester your baby can open his eyes and turn his head towards the source of any continuous bright light. His brain is growing rapidly and his lungs and digestive tract are maturing. From 32 weeks your baby gains around a third to a half of his birth weight, getting fattened up so he's ready for survival outside the womb. With six weeks to go, he could measure as much as 43.7cm (17¼in) long from top to toe. He's getting so big and snug in your uterus that you may notice he isn't moving around so much. By the end of week 36 your pregnancy will have come full term and your baby could be born at any time.

 Systemised mum

Now that you're on the final stretch, it's time to make sure you're on top of all the details.

"I've now gone completely list crazy. I'm so worried that I've forgotten to buy something vital that I've been carrying a notepad and pen around with me so I can jot things down as I remember them.

I've also got the contact details of all our close friends and family pinned to the notice board above the phone, and I'm planning to pack my hospital bag a couple of weeks before my due date, just so everything is ready.".

Make life easier

Now is the time to make sure you're organised for the home run. Stock up on shopping to save time and effort later. Make a list of important numbers – your midwife, doctor and the labour ward – and keep it by the phone or stored on your mobile. It's a good idea to have your hospital bag packed from 36 weeks onwards, so that you're not rushing around in early labour trying to get everything done.

Getting ready for pregnancy

Staying safe and healthy

Your pregnancy diary

Birth and beyond

FIRST TRIMESTER	SECOND TRIMESTER	THIRD TRIMESTER

Your body at **28** Weeks ▼

28 Weeks

❋ Your breasts may start producing colostrum – the concentrated early milk. They may leak a little.

❋ Most women will gain an average of 5kg (11lb) during the last trimester, which starts this week.

Congratulations – this week you enter your final trimester and you'll soon meet your baby. There will be more antenatal appointments now and, if it's your first pregnancy, one or two extra appointments.

Antenatal appointments from now onwards

You'll probably see your midwife or doctor more often from now on, but you don't have to wait for an appointment if you want to discuss anything – just ring. You may be offered more appointments if you have special problems such as a pre-existing medical condition, or if you develop problems during your pregnancy. Here's an idea of what antenatal appointments you can expect:

● **28 weeks** Your midwife will take a blood sample to make sure your iron levels are satisfactory and to check for antibodies in your blood. If you are low in iron, she may suggest you take iron supplements (see p.149). She'll also check your blood pressure and test your urine for protein, (its presence can be a sign of pre-eclampsia), and also for bacteria, which may increase your risk of giving birth too early. As with every appointment from now on, she'll measure your bump (see p.147) to check that your baby is growing well.

If you're rhesus negative (see p.233), you should be offered an anti-D injection to kill off any antibodies in your blood.

● **31 weeks (first pregnancy only)** At this appointment you will have the usual checks and a chance to chat through the test results from your 28-week appointment.

● **34 weeks** At this appointment you will again have the usual checks and, if this isn't your first pregnancy, you'll have a chance to chat through the test results from your 28-week appointment. If you're rhesus negative, you should be given a second dose of anti-D to kill off antibodies in your blood.

● **36 weeks** At this stage, your midwife will again do your routine checks and, if you've recently had a scan to check the position of your placenta, she will discuss the results with you. She'll also feel your bump with her hands to check the position your baby's lying in. If your baby is in a breech position (see pp.286–7), she'll offer to make you an appointment to have your baby turned – an effective technique known as external cephalic version (see p.287). If your anomaly scan at 18 to 20 weeks (see pp.156–7) showed that your

▼ Your baby at **28** Weeks

This week your baby can blink his eyes, which now sport lashes.

❋ He'll also turn in the direction of light if he notices bright light shining through the wall of your uterus. He now weighs a little over 1kg/2½lb and measures about 38cm/15in. His fat layers are starting to form as he gets ready for life outside the uterus. His bones are nearly developed, too, but they're still soft and pliable.

placenta was lying over the entrance to your cervix, you will have another scan now to make sure that it has moved out of the way.

● **38 weeks** At this stage, your midwife will check your blood pressure and urine, and measure your bump.

● **40 weeks (first pregnancy only)** At this stage, your midwife will again check your blood pressure and urine, and measure your bump.

● **41 weeks** If you haven't had your baby by 41 weeks, then at this appointment your midwife will offer you

a membrane sweep (see p.207), which might help to get your labour going. If you decide not to have a membrane sweep or if it doesn't make you go into labour, and if you are more than 10 days overdue, then you'll be offered an induction (see p.251).

How big will your baby be?

How big your baby will be depends on a number of factors. Probably the most influential factors are genetic. Big parents often have bigger babies.

Even your baby's sex can play a part, as boys are often bigger than girls. If your baby is overdue, he'll probably be bigger as he's had more time to grow.

Thankfully, you usually grow a baby to fit you. So even if your partner is much taller or heavier than you, your baby is likely to fit through your pelvis. It's not just size that matters – the position your baby is in influences

labour, so you can have a big baby in a good position and an easy birth, or a small baby who has managed to get into a difficult position that can make things complicated.

Some medical conditions are linked to an increased risk of a big baby. These include obesity and gaining a lot of weight during pregnancy. Unmanaged high blood sugar levels from gestational diabetes (see p.229) or diabetes mellitus (the chronic form of the condition) can lead to a bigger baby, as the baby uses the extra sugar to grow.

Factors that affect baby's birth weight

Many mums-to-be wonder how big their baby will be at birth. These factors affect the baby's birth weight:

● your height
● the baby's father's height
● your weight before pregnancy
● how much weight you gained during pregnancy
● the sex of the baby
● uncontrolled gestational diabetes
● whether you smoke while pregnant
● whether the baby is overdue (comes late) or premature (early)

Parents**Talk...**

"I loved my antenatal classes. It was so nice to be able to talk to women who were going through exactly the same as me. I could share my worries and concerns because they were all so supportive. One of the women I met there is my best friend now. We have such a strong bond because we're raising our children together."
Louise, 29, mum to two-year-old Tom

"What I learnt in my antenatal classes was invaluable. The relaxation techniques helped to keep me calm and feel more in control during labour. Rather than panicking

I could focus on getting my breathing right and telling my partner what kind of massage I needed and when."
Anna, 35, mum to six-month-old Joel

"Being informed about my pain relief choices helped me feel like I had some say in how my labour was going to go. I have a really low pain threshold, so just assumed that an epidural was the only way for me to get through it. But my antenatal teacher took the time to explain to me that this wasn't the case and that gas and air could be enough. It turns out she was right!"
Paula, 27, pregnant for a second time

You can easily strike up new friendships at your antenatal classes. It's good to share your worries with other pregnant women.

Getting ready for pregnancy

Staying safe and healthy

Your pregnancy diary

Birth and beyond

Diet in late pregnancy

As your pregnancy progresses you might be finding that, no matter how much or how often you eat, you still feel ravenous at all hours of the day and night. That's not surprising, because the rapidly growing baby inside you needs extra calories of his own.

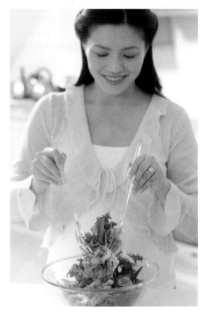

Keep a supply of salads, fresh fruit and vegetables at home, and you'll be less likely to snack on unhealthy foods.

Keep the calories in check

You may feel permanently starving these days but that doesn't mean it's a good idea to eat anything and everything. Remember, you're eating for yourself and a baby, not another adult!

Quality not quantity

As well as avoiding overeating, you should watch the quality of what you eat. When you have a craving for junk food, try to opt for a healthier choice. Help yourself to do this by keeping your fridge and cupboards well stocked with quick, healthy snacks, such as cottage cheese, boiled eggs, wholemeal bread, and fresh fruit and vegetables.

When you're going out and about, don't leave home without putting a bag of nuts and raisins or a piece of fresh fruit into your bag. You never know when you'll need a quick energy boost, and by tucking into something wholesome you'll hopefully be able to avoid the temptations of the nearest fast-food emporium.

You will of course already be following our useful advice on eating in pregnancy (see pp.48–51 and 120–21) but it bears repeating during this last trimester that you should also try to eat natural foods that have been processed as little as possible. For example, choose wholemeal bread or brown rice rather than white bread or white rice, and stick to fresh fruit as opposed to tinned fruit in syrup. We should all keep fatty foods and sweets to a minimum but the odd treat won't hurt.

Special needs of the last trimester

As your pregnancy progresses, heartburn becomes all too common. This is due to the hormonal and physical changes in your body. Although you may not be able get rid of it completely, you can minimise it. Try cutting out rich or spicy dishes, chocolate, citrus fruits, alcohol and coffee. Eat small, frequent meals, take small mouthfuls and chew your food well.

Top eating tips for the last trimester

During these last weeks, focus on not over-eating and on eating healthily.
- Stock up on healthy snacks – for example, boiled eggs and fresh fruit.
- Be prepared – carry healthy snacks when you are out and about.
- Avoid heartburn – eat small, frequent meals and chew your food well.
- Drink plenty of water.
- Get your vitamin K – from green beans, leafy green vegetables and cauliflower.
- Don't overeat – you only need about 200 extra calories a day at this stage. That's about the equivalent of a glass of milk and a banana.
- Don't forget your antioxidants – a diet rich in vitamins C and E may help prevent pre-eclampsia.

You need vitamin K in your last trimester because it helps blood to clot. If you have low levels of vitamin K you may bleed more at birth, and babies with low levels can also bleed internally. This is why babies are given vitamin K when they are born. Good sources include green leafy vegetables, cantaloupe melon, cauliflower, green beans, and wholemeal bread and pasta.

You may also be suffering now from swollen ankles and feet (oedema; see p.238). You can help to relieve it by drinking more water during the day and by cutting down on salty foods, such as olives and salted nuts.

Some experts believe that a diet that is high in antioxidants can help to prevent pre-eclampsia (see p.233).

Vitamins C and E are two important antioxidant vitamins. For vitamin C, eat citrus fruits, green and red peppers, melon, potatoes, tomatoes, strawberries, cabbage and broccoli. Foods rich in vitamin E include vegetable oils (especially corn, soya and wheatgerm oil), sunflower seeds, wheatgerm, sweetcorn, cashews, almonds, corn oil margarine and peanuts. Taking a general pregnancy multivitamin tablet may also help you to lower your risk of getting pre-eclampsia.

Make sure you spend the last few weeks eating well and getting plenty of rest. You can make life easier for yourself if you spend some time now making simple recipes that you can freeze and enjoy after your baby is born.

Active mum

Drinking plenty of water is essential, especially when you're exercising and pregnant.

"I've always found it difficult to drink plenty of water. When I got pregnant I knew I had to, not only for my sake – it can help prevent water retention – but for my baby's too. Whenever I have a glass, I add a wedge of lemon or a little fruit juice or squash to make it more interesting. If I have a day at home, I fill a big jug with water and aim to finish it by the end of the day. When I'm out, I always take a bottle of water to sip throughout the day."

Healthy main meals

In your last trimester, you're allowed an extra 200 calories a day to match your baby's growth spurt. But try to resist eating too many cakes, sweets and fast food snacks. Two hundred calories is less than you think – it's the equivalent of only two slices of wholemeal toast and butter. Try these healthy main meals to fill you up when you're hungry.

Ragu sauce
Serves four to six ● 500g/1lb 2oz lean minced beef ● 1 medium onion, finely chopped ● 1 clove garlic, crushed ● 100g/3½oz smoked bacon, cut into small pieces ● 4 sundried tomatoes in oil, drained ● 400g/14oz can chopped tomatoes ● 125ml/4¼fl oz red wine (optional) ● 1 tsp oregano

Gently heat the beef in a non-stick pan, stirring and breaking it up. Add the onion, garlic and bacon and increase the heat to fry gently. Cook for 5–10 minutes, stirring frequently, until the onion is softened. Chop the sundried tomatoes and add to the pan with the canned tomatoes, herbs and wine (if using). Bring to the boil, stir and reduce the heat. Cover and leave to simmer gently for 35–40 minutes, stirring frequently. Serve with any pasta.

Salmon with pine nuts and lime
Serves two ● cooking oil spray ● 2 salmon fillets ● juice and grated zest of 1 lime ● a little finely chopped lemongrass (optional) ● 1 tsp chopped parsley ● black pepper ● 2 tbsp pine nuts

Preheat the oven to 180°C/gas mark 4. Lightly spray two pieces of foil with oil. Place a piece of salmon on each piece of foil. Squeeze over half the lime juice. Sprinkle over the grated zest and lemongrass (if using). Sprinkle with parsley and season with pepper. Close the foil, place in the oven and cook for 15 minutes. Remove, open the parcel, sprinkle with the pine nuts and return to the oven to brown the pine nuts and finish cooking the fish (5 minutes). Pour the cooking liquid from the parcel over the salmon. Serve with new potatoes and steamed broccoli or green beans.

Getting ready for pregnancy

Staying safe and healthy

Your pregnancy diary

Birth and beyond

Your body at **29** Weeks

29 Weeks

❊ Be sure to get enough iron to help your baby make red blood cells. Eat meat and leafy greens.

❊ Are you feeling less pressure in your lower abdomen? If so, your baby has probably shifted position.

You don't need to give up on your workouts just because you're getting bigger; exercise prepares you for the hard work of labour ahead. But do make sure that you're not exercising too hard.

Exercise for the last weeks

Exercise does wonders for you during the last few weeks of pregnancy. It makes perfect sense: the better shape you're in, the stronger you'll be to cope with labour and the birth. Keeping physically active during pregnancy is also good preparation for the hard work of labour that lies ahead.

It also makes getting your body back in shape once the baby's born much easier. If you've managed to maintain your strength and muscle tone all through your pregnancy by staying fit, your body will have an easier time bouncing back after you give birth.

What is more, any type of aerobic exercise helps increase the body's ability to process and use oxygen, which is important for you and your baby.

Importantly, exercise at this stage will help you sleep better, too. When you're carrying all that extra weight in front of you, you'll quickly see that finding a comfortable position to sleep in at night can be a real challenge (see p.198). Exercise will help you work off any excess energy, and will tire you enough to lull you into a deeper, more restful slumber.

Don't go for the burn

Staying active doesn't necessarily mean going for the burn. Your body releases a hormone called relaxin during pregnancy which loosens your joints in preparation for delivery, so you need to take care with the choice of exercise and pay attention to technique. It's important to find exercises that won't injure you or harm the baby.

As you grow bigger, you'll be better off avoiding activities that could put you at risk of slips and falls, such as cycling, rollerblading, horseriding, and skiing, although people who take part in these sports competitively often continue well into their pregnancies.

However, most pregnant women should stick to gentle, low-impact exercise such as walking, yoga (see p.59) and Pilates (see p.57). Swimming is great, too. It improves circulation and builds muscle tone, strength and endurance – while the water supports your weight (see p.57). Whichever form of exercise you choose, you should always start slowly, stretch well before and after, warm up and cool down gradually, and don't over-exert yourself.

▼ Your baby at **29** Weeks

This week your boy baby's undergoing some changes to his sex organs.

❊ His testicles now descend from near the kidneys through the groin en route to the scrotum. In girls, the clitoris is rather prominent because it's not yet covered by the still-small labia. These will grow to cover it in the last few weeks before birth. Your baby now weighs around 1.1kg/2½lb and measures about 38cm/15in.

Getting up from lying down is harder the bigger you get. Start by rolling onto one side, with one or both knees bent.

Push down on your arms to come up fully, then unbend your knees. You can reverse the process when you want to lie down.

Help me get up!

Getting out of bed won't be a problem until your belly starts to bulge in your second or third trimester. Then you need a safe, comfortable way to get up, especially if you have back pain.

● **Getting out of bed** Roll onto your side with your knees bent up, drop your feet over the edge of the bed and push yourself up sideways with your arms. Reverse the process when you lie down. If rolling onto your side is too painful, try the following technique: lying on your back, bend both knees up as far as they will go and separate them to clear your bump. You may need to use your hands to help pull your legs up. Put your chin on your chest, and use your arms to pull yourself directly up, keeping your knees bent up as high as you can. This may work for you but you may find that your bump is too big or your tummy muscles too weak to perform this manoeuvre.

● **Getting out of the bath** Roll onto your side in a sitting position and move onto your hands and knees. Lean on the sides of the bath to stand and perch on the edge. Holding firmly onto the sides of the bath behind you, arch your back and lift one leg at a time over the bath sides. Use a bath mat to prevent slipping.

Umbilical stem-cell collection

Your baby's umbilical cord contains special cells called stem cells. These will eventually develop into – among other types of cell – blood cells that fight infection, carry oxygen around the body and help with blood clotting. These are the same blood cells that are affected in diseases such as leukaemia and other cancers affecting the blood. Stored cord blood would provide a perfect match in the event that your child needed a transplant, and possibly for a sibling, too.

Cord blood may be stored by freezing. The blood has to be prepared soon after delivery of the baby. In the UK there are only a handful of hospitals that will carry out this procedure under the NHS. If you are interested in umbilical stem-cell collection, you may have to consider using a private service.

ParentsTalk...

"I had backache when I was pregnant; it was really painful in the third trimester. I found the gentle exercises and stretching I learned at prenatal yoga very helpful, though. Swimming worked wonders, too – just gentle walking in the pool helped to relax the muscles."
Fran, 26, first-time mum

"I joined a pregnancy yoga class when I was 20 weeks pregnant and I love the way it makes me feel afterwards. It also made realise how stiff I am in certain places. I'm sure the exercises will help me prepare for labour, too."
Mica, 24, seven months pregnant

"I love nothing better than a soak in a warm bath, but getting out has become a bit of a palaver now that I'm bigger. I have to get onto all fours and hold on to the sides. My partner is usually there to help me, too. I even bought a bath mat to make sure I don't slip."
Magdalena, 31, first-time mum

Getting ready for pregnancy

Staying safe and healthy

Your pregnancy diary

Birth and beyond

Your body at **30** Weeks ▼

30 Weeks

❄ Do you misplace your car keys and forget your appointments? Don't worry – pregnancy is to blame.

❄ Don't be alarmed if you feel breathless. It's just your uterus pressing against your diaphragm.

By this stage you may have come to love your increasing size, but not the clumsiness it causes. Do remember, though, that annoying symptoms like this will disappear after your baby is born.

Clumsy and forgetful?

▼ Your baby at **30** Weeks

At this stage it is believed that your baby can probably distinguish light from dark.

❄ This week he will continue to open and shut his eyes, and if you shine a light on your stomach, he may well reach out to try and touch it. While he may soon slow up growing in length (by now he measures about 40cm/15¾in from crown to toe), he will continue to gain weight steadily until the time he's born. Right now there's about 1 litre (1¾ pints) of amniotic fluid surrounding your baby, but that volume will decrease as he gets steadily bigger.

Feeling graceful and dextrous isn't part of the pregnancy package and you may be a little clumsy from now on. You may find that your memory isn't what it was, either. It's all perfectly normal.

Clumsiness should come as no surprise if you consider what your body's going through: you're carrying more weight, your centre of gravity has changed and many of your joints are loosening up. You may even experience numbness and weakness in your arms as your posture changes.

Be reassured that, if you were to take a tumble, your baby would be well protected by your pelvis and the waters he floats around in. Even so, try not to get into situations where you have a high risk of falling, like climbing steep steps or walking on wet, icy or uneven surfaces. And don't carry anything that you can't safely drop. If you do fall, you should contact your doctor or midwife just to make sure everything is all right.

If your clumsiness is accompanied by sudden swelling of the hands or feet, headaches, blurred vision, vomiting or upper abdominal pain, contact your doctor or midwife immediately. These can be signs of pre-eclampsia (see p.233).

Are you forgetting things?

Becoming forgetful in pregnancy is pretty common, too. If you get forgetful, it's not something you need to worry about and isn't a medical problem, although it may well have a physical cause. Several small-scale studies have suggested that the size of women's brains can alter during pregnancy.

Forgetfulness may also stem from feeling a little overwhelmed by the huge life changes you are about to experience. And expectant mothers often have a lot going on, what with planning for birth and life with a baby, and maybe moving house as well.

Forgetfulness may be your cue to simplify your life but meanwhile, devise strategies to help you remember what's important and so reduce frustration:

● Carry a small notebook in which you can jot down reminders.
● Keep a detailed daily calendar.
● Assign items you use often, such as keys, to one place.

You don't absolutely have to wallpaper that room right now or clean out your cupboards just because a new baby is arriving. This sort of self-imposed stress can lead you to forget things, so do cut yourself a little slack.

Specialist antenatal monitoring

If you've got special problems, such as a pre-existing medical condition like diabetes or epilepsy, or if you develop a problem during your pregnancy, you'll probably find yourself under the care of an obstetrician. You'll then see a doctor at most of your antenatal visits, and may need to go for more regular check-ups than other mothers-to-be.

If your blood pressure starts to rise towards the end of pregnancy, the results of your regular urine test will be crucial to what happens next. If your urine has protein in it, you may be in the early stages of pre-eclampsia, and you'll need more frequent antenatal checks.

If your midwife finds that your baby is small or large for dates she may wish to refer you for an extra ultrasound scan just to make sure. This is a much more accurate way of measuring your baby's growth than using a tape measure.

If you do have a problem in late pregnancy, such as a rise in blood pressure or your waters break but labour hasn't started, you may find yourself referred to a Day Assessment Unit. This means you can have regular antenatal checks and tests as an outpatient.

If you have a pre-existing condition or develop a problem in pregnancy, you'll be invited for extra antenatal checks.

Fact: Smoking in pregnancy greatly increases the risk of cot death.

Statistics suggest that this risk is four times higher if you smoke between one and nine cigarettes a day during pregnancy, rising to eight times higher if you smoke 20 cigarettes or more daily.

ParentsTalk...

"I was really struggling to give up the cigarettes until I had my scan picture. I uploaded it onto my computer and used Photoshop to put a cigarette in my baby's mouth. It was such a disturbing image that something in my brain finally clicked into place."
Tina, smoker from the age of 20

"It took a few months into my pregnancy but I did eventually stop. Patches work, good thoughts about your baby's health work, support from your husband or partner works, too."
Agnes, smoker from the age of 16

Determined to stop smoking now you're pregnant? Nicotine patches help.

ParentsAsk...

My last baby was premature. Will the same thing happen in this pregnancy?

If you have already had one premature birth, you do have a greater chance of having another, but you should try not to let this worry you. Most women whose first baby was premature go on to have their next baby after they are 37 weeks pregnant, or at full term.

There is about a one in five chance that your next baby will be premature, so you have a four in five chance that you will not have another premature baby.

The earliness of your last birth seems to influence your chances of having another premature birth. If you gave birth very early, when you were between 20 and 31 weeks pregnant, you'd have a much higher chance of having another premature birth than if you'd given birth when you were between 32 and 36 weeks pregnant.

Knowing that you are at increased risk of having another premature birth can be a frightening thought. However, the fact that you have already been through it means you'll be well-placed to monitor your pregnancy.

Getting ready for pregnancy

Staying safe and healthy

Your pregnancy diary

Birth and beyond

Your body at **31** Weeks

31 Weeks

❋ Is your bump giving you backache? Switch to low-heeled shoes and avoid heavy lifting.

❋ Gaining 450g (1lb) a week is normal during the last trimester as your baby has a final growth spurt.

It could be your partner, your mum or your friend. Whoever you choose to be with you, having a trusted companion by your side during labour will help you to feel calmer and more relaxed throughout.

Birth partners

As your pregnancy progresses, you may start to feel worried about how you'll cope during labour and childbirth. A birth partner, who stays with you throughout it all, will help to make the experience less scary and bolster your confidence. He or she can also provide practical help and can communicate on your behalf with hospital staff.

Since the 1970s, fathers have tended to attend births but they don't have to. If your partner doesn't want to be there, decide what's right for both of you. If he isn't going to be there, you may want to enlist the services of a close friend, your sister, your mother, or a paid birth companion called a doula (pronounced "doola"; see p.194).

Attending antenatal classes with you is a good way for your labour partner to prepare. So, too, is talking through together what you're hoping for at the birth. If you write a birth plan (see pp.174–5), your birth partner should be aware of its contents. It's also a good idea for your birth partner to meet the midwife or midwives who may attend you during the labour and birth.

Your labour partner's job is to encourage, reassure and assist you in

 Your baby at **31** Weeks

If your baby isn't moving so much now, don't worry. She's running out of space!

❋ Her arms, legs and body are still filling out – and at last they are proportional in size to her head. In fact, she is looking more like a newborn. She's now weighing in at about 1.5kg/3¼lb and measures about 41cm/16in from crown to toe. It's no wonder that she's running out of space in your uterus.

Dad's **Diary**

Military route planning
Our route to the hospital has been planned with almost military precision. I have two routes planned: one for a rush-hour hospital dash – that's my newly found rat runs and traffic light-free roads, and one for an off-peak, middle of the night run. I'm pushing (excuse the pun) for the latter – although when the time comes, I don't think I'll have a lot of say in the matter.

It's useful to practise positions you might use with your birth partner.

any way you find comforting and useful. You can practise some of the ways your partner can help – massaging your lower back, for example, and sorting out the TENS machine (see p.272) – but you both need to keep an open mind about what needs to be done, because you won't really know what you want until you go into labour.

Another useful role for a labour partner is that of prompter – for example, you may forget about how important it can be to keep moving around in labour and your partner can remind you if necessary. If a medical intervention is suggested, your partner can help to ensure that you are as aware as possible about what is going on.

Flexibility is key during labour and birth and it's essential that your partner is as aware of this as you are. It's important for him to remember that things can change quickly and that you may have to change your mind or make a new decision about some aspect of your care or treatment. So it's important that he doesn't cling to something you said before the event, not realising that your views have now changed. He must be aware that you have the final word; although he might want to help you in making a decision, or in communicating that decision to your care-givers, your views are what count.

Top tips for labour partners

Preparing yourself to be a birth partner? Follow these succinct tips to be sure of being the best.
- Ask questions.
- Bring a few things for yourself, such as a clean T-shirt and some food.
- Know what to expect – labour isn't the right time to be flipping through a birth manual.
- Be flexible.
- Find useful distractions for your partner, such as rhythmic breathing.
- Be a one-person support team – you are her main emotional and physical support.
- Be prepared to take charge of the situation.
- Be aware of what you're ready to do and what to leave to the professionals.
- Be there – just showing up is the most important thing of all.

Backache in late pregnancy

Back pain can be divided into two categories. True back pain happens when ligaments, muscles, discs and joints are placed under strain from poor posture, bad lifting technique, weak or tight muscles or injury. It often gets worse towards the end of the day or if you have spent a long time on your feet.

The second type of pain is pelvic pain (see p.231). Most women who seek help because of back pain in pregnancy have this type of pain.

Research shows that you can reduce your chances of developing back pain in pregnancy by taking weekly exercise, having a good upright posture and avoiding heavy lifting (see p.150).

Below are a range of other measures that may also help:
- Massage to the lower back can often help tired, aching muscles. Try leaning forwards over the back of a chair or lying on your side.
- A warm bath, a hot pack or a warm jet of water from a shower head can all help with back pain.
- A physiotherapist may recommend a special back support to take some of the weight of your baby off your tummy muscles and back.
- Sleeping on your side with a wedge-shaped pillow tucked underneath your tummy can help to reduce back pain.

If you have backache it might be helpful to use a special pregnancy support to take the weight of your baby off your back.

Getting ready for pregnancy

Staying safe and healthy

Your pregnancy diary

Birth and beyond

FIRST TRIMESTER	SECOND TRIMESTER	THIRD TRIMESTER

Your body at **32** Weeks

32 Weeks

❋ Pressure on your bladder may mean frequent loo trips – which can make a good night's sleep difficult.

❋ Constipation, increased blood circulation and the pressure of your uterus may give you piles.

Breastfeeding is the most natural way to feed your baby, but it doesn't always come naturally. If you're planning to breastfeed your baby, now is a good time to find out as much as you can about it.

Preparing for breastfeeding

Breastfeeding gives all the nutrients your baby needs to thrive for the first six months of life, and alongside other foods after this time, it's an important and healthy part of the diet.

The health benefits

Research shows that breastmilk contains antibodies that protect your baby against infection – including gastroenteritis, respiratory illness, urinary infections, and ear infections. In addition, it reduces the risk of childhood diabetes and leukemia.

As well as the anti-infective properties that are always in breastmilk, the breastfeeding mother makes specific antibodies when she comes into contact with an infection. These transfer to her milk, ready for the baby to receive as soon as he next comes to the breast.

Breastfeeding is the healthiest choice for mothers, too. It gives them a reduced risk of pre-menopausal breast cancer, ovarian cancer, and of fractures caused by osteoporosis.

As long as you're healthy, there's not much more you can do to prepare your body for breastfeeding. But you can

prepare your mind. Learn as much as you can about breastfeeding before your baby is born. Talk to other breastfeeding mothers, read books to familiarise yourself, and contact local breastfeeding support organisations.

Try to attend a breastfeeding class or preparation for breastfeeding session (offered by many hospitals and by the NCT as part of their antenatal courses) some time during your last few months of pregnancy. The more you know about the mechanics and the benefits of breastfeeding, the more likely you are to succeed at it.

Whether you think about it or not, your pregnant body is busy preparing itself for breastfeeding. That's one reason why your breasts get so much bigger during pregnancy – your milk ducts and milk-producing cells are developing, and more blood goes to your breasts than before.

But don't worry. Breast size has nothing to do with the ability to breastfeed successfully – even if you stay small-breasted, that will not reduce your chances of being able to feed your baby yourself.

 Your baby at **32** Weeks

By now your baby may have a full head of hair – or perhaps just a few wisps.

❋ He now weighs approximately 1.7kg/3¾lb and measures about 42cm/16½in long from head to toe. Although his lungs won't be fully developed until just before birth, your little one is busy inhaling amniotic fluid. This is to exercise his lungs and practise breathing for after he's born.

Escape routes

If you're starting to feel a little, well, bored of being pregnant, you're not alone. What was exciting and new during the first few weeks and months of pregnancy can become pretty tedious by the sixth or seventh month.

Sometimes you need a break from all things baby-related. So, take on tasks and dabble in activities that a new mum couldn't possibly squeeze into her busy schedule. Below are some ideas:

- **Make dates with friends** Take time to enjoy a good natter with your pals over a lunch or coffee.
- **Streamline your space** Clean out your files, sift through the kitchen drawers, or put those boxed-up photos in the loft into photo albums.
- **Connect with your partner** Enjoy some romantic dinners together and focus on each other while you can.
- **Set up time-savers** Make an appointment for a new, easy-to-manage haircut, collect takeaway menus from restaurants near your home, set up an online bank account so that you can manage your finances easily, hire a cleaner if you can afford to and don't have one already, and learn to master online grocery shopping.
- **Pamper yourself** If you can possibly afford it, a pregnancy massage at a spa is well worth the money.
- **Indulge in some retail therapy** Treat yourself to a pretty new maternity bra or some elegant ballet pumps to wear in late pregnancy.
- **Do some exercise** Go for a gentle swim at your local pool and enjoy the sensation of weightlessness! If swimming isn't your thing, go for a stroll in the fresh air instead.
- **Escape to another world** Tuck into a nice big novel or rent a few DVDs that sweep you off to another place for a little while.

Ask your partner for a massage. It will help him to feel involved, will help you to relax and will give you extra time together.

An online bank account is a real time-saver for new mums. Setting up one will give you a break from thinking about your pregnancy.

ParentsAsk...

My hips are sore at night. How can I relieve the pain?

Hip pain is common in pregnancy and is often a problem in bed at night. Try sleeping on your side with legs bent and a pillow between your knees supporting the whole length of your leg. A pillow under your bump is also helpful to stop you rolling forwards. An extra layer of padding, such as a sleeping bag or quilt, under your bottom sheet can improve matters. You may also find gentle heat on your hips – a hot water bottle or a wheat bag – helpful. Avoid activities that seem to aggravate the pain, too.

You will probably find that your pain is worse if you have had a busy day. Try to spend time resting on an exercise or birthing ball or on your hands and knees. This takes the weight off your hips and gives them a rest.

Do I need to toughen my nipples or do anything else before I can breastfeed?

The hormonal changes pregnancy brings to the breasts are sufficient preparation for most women. You don't need to use creams to soften your skin beforehand or express colostrum either. In particular, don't rub or scrub your nipples – this will only hurt you and make breastfeeding difficult. The best preparation for breastfeeding is getting your partner to support you in your decision to breastfeed, so that you and your baby can get off to a good start. Research shows that you are more likely to breastfeed for longer if your partner is well informed.

The other thing you can do to help breastfeeding is make sure that your midwife or doctor who attends you during your baby's birth knows that you would like plenty of skin-to-skin contact with your baby when he or she is born. Skin-to-skin contact has been shown to increase the length of time that women breastfeed for.

Getting ready for pregnancy

Staying safe and healthy

Your pregnancy diary

Birth and beyond

FIRST TRIMESTER   SECOND TRIMESTER   THIRD TRIMESTER

Your body at **33** Weeks ▼

33 Weeks

❋ Mild, irregular contractions, known as Braxton Hicks, may become more noticeable around now.

❋ You may notice that your feet, hands, face, and ankles have become a bit swollen.

It's hard to imagine how life will be once your baby's born. One thing is sure, though – it's going to be busy. Making preparations now will make life easier in those sleepless early days.

Stocking up

As you head into the final weeks of pregnancy, it's time to make life easier for yourself. In the first weeks after your baby's birth, it may not be so easy to pop out to the supermarket, so it's worthwhile stocking up on basics – everything from tins to toilet paper – before shopping becomes a real chore.

Buying in bulk is good advice – the prices really are better, so you'll save yourself some money, too. But if you're not careful, you can also spend a lot on items you don't need or that will go bad before you can eat them. Below are a few bulk-buying tips:

● Make a list of things you use a lot, such as washing powder or bottled water. These are perfect to buy in bulk.

● Concentrate on non-perishable and long-life items, such as tinned soups and vegetables, grains and dried pasta and tea and coffee.

● When you get home, repackage perishables into smaller quantities. Big packages of steaks or chicken breasts,

for example, can be divided into daily portions and frozen until needed.

● Don't forget to stock up on non-food products too – you won't want to run out of washing up liquid or tissues.

Feed the freezer

It's also a great idea to start cooking extra portions to freeze as ready meals for the early weeks. This will prove to be a godsend when you're getting to grips

Cooking extra meals and freezing them for later use will be a life-saver once you're in the throes of new motherhood.

 Your baby at **33** Weeks

She might be positioning herself for birth now – upside down and head down.

❋ Your doctor or midwife will be paying careful attention to your baby's position during the coming weeks. Although she may be perfectly positioned now, some babies do decide to turn around again. She now weighs in at about 2kg/4½lb and measures approximately 44cm/17½in from head to toe.

with caring for your new baby. So, for example, the next time you make a lasagne, a stew or casserole, make double the batch, then freeze half of it. It won't just save you time when the baby's born; homemade meals are also much healthier and more nutritious than fast food and ready meals that you buy from the supermarket.

Nutritious homemade soups are also freezable, and get into the habit of putting leftovers into the freezer rather than the fridge. Milk and bread can be frozen, too, so keep a couple of cartons of milk and a few loaves in the freezer. And remember, frozen vegetables are just as nutritious as fresh, and will be more convenient once the baby is born.

Still commuting?

The journey to and from work can be the most stressful and tiring part of your day, especially if you have to stand for long periods. While travelling as part of your job can be assessed for possible risks to you or your baby (see p.62), unfortunately the commuting part can't. But there are strategies that you could try to improve matters. For example, you could suggest to your employer that you change your working hours so that you are travelling outside the rush hour. It wouldn't affect the number of hours you work, but it might mean you get a seat on the bus or train. Or would your employer consider letting you work from home for one or two days a week to help reduce the strain on you?

Ask your employer if you can change your working hours to avoid commuting in the rush hour so you might get a seat.

"Try changing **your working hours** to avoid **rush hour**."

You could also talk to your doctor, who might suggest that you take a period of sick leave if the commuting is affecting the wellbeing of you or your baby. However, remember that your Statutory Maternity Pay is assessed on your income during pregnancy, so if your salary drops, you could be affected by this after your baby is born.

If you really find it too much, and you are not too far away from giving birth, could you perhaps consider starting your maternity leave earlier than you had originally planned? The earliest time that you can start your leave is 11 weeks before your baby is due, but ask your employer and you may be able to take some annual leave as well.

Active mum

Bored by the last few weeks of pregnancy? Most mums are, especially if they're usually active.

"I'm in my third trimester and can categorically say that the novelty of being pregnant has well and truly worn off! I'm used to being fit and active so I hate having to roll out of bed sideways just to get up.

I've worked hard in the gym to get a physique that I'm happy with, so to have people constantly commenting on my size, not to mention touching my stomach, is getting really tedious.

And I'm bored by the fact that everyone assumes that all I want to talk about is the baby and my pregnancy. I am open to other topics! I don't think there's been a single non-work related conversation with any of my colleagues that hasn't been centred round children for months!"

Green mum

Cloth nappies plus eco-friendly disposables are a greener choice and kind to your baby's skin.

"I'm happy to say I've bought some shaped one-size cloth nappies. As well as being economical and made from organic cotton, they'll be soft and gentle on my baby's skin. I'll wash them carefully, too, to protect the environment. For holidays and day trips I'm getting some eco-friendly disposables. They're a little bit more expensive than ordinary disposables, but they're made from renewable materials and are greener to produce, so I feel happier about using them."

Getting ready for pregnancy

Staying safe and healthy

Your pregnancy diary

Birth and beyond

Your body at **34** Weeks

34 Weeks

❉ If you notice a tingling sensation or numbness in your pelvis, it's the pressure of the baby on the nerves.

❉ Try the relaxation, positions and massage learned at antenatal classes to help relieve any discomfort.

The big day is only a few weeks away. If you're one of the many women whose mother has offered to come and help, you can start to make plans now. Otherwise, a doula may be for you.

Mums and doulas

Most women need someone they can count on for support, strength and guidance during childbirth, as well as their midwife or doctor. Usually this special person is their partner, but for others it will be a close friend or their own mother. Although lots of mums want to support their daughters during labour, only you can decide if having your mother in the delivery room with you will be a help or a hindrance. You may feel you can't give birth without her, or you may prefer to keep it as a special time for just you and your partner. Don't rush or be pushed into a decision and, if you don't want mum there, let her down gently.

Another alternative is to employ a doula. She is an experienced woman who offers emotional and practical support before, during and after childbirth. The idea is to "mother the mother", nurturing her during pregnancy, birth and the early days as a new mum.

A doula is trained in childbirth and has a good knowledge of female physiology, but she isn't a replacement for the midwife or medical staff. You can

find out if there is a doula in your area and details of costs from the website for Doula UK (www.doula.org.uk).

In many cultures, women rest for up to 40 days after giving birth. In the West, however, social pressures mean that mums are rushed back into normal day-to-day activities much sooner. If your partner has taken paternity leave, he is likely to return to work when your baby is still only one or two weeks old. It can feel overwhelming to look after a newborn on your own, particularly if you've had stitches or a caesarean. With the help of your mum, close friend or postnatal doula, you can enjoy some of the benefits of a prolonged "lying in" period, giving you the chance to bond with your new baby and spend extra time with your other children.

66% of new mums think that their parenting style is more like their own mother's than they thought it would be – even though they were sure they'd do things differently!

▼ Your baby at **34** Weeks

Now your baby's building his fat layers to help keep him at the correct temperature.

❉ These fat layers show in the way he's gradually filling out and getting rounder. The fat helps him to regulate his body temperature after birth. He now weighs more than 2.2kg/5lb and is around 45cm/17¾in long. If you don't already talk to your baby, this is a good time to start – by 35 weeks his hearing's fully developed.

As well as getting on with the everyday chores that you haven't got the time or energy for – the shopping, cooking and cleaning – mums can help by preparing some home-made meals and putting them in the freezer for you to enjoy when you need them. As all mums know, good nutrition is vital to a speedy recovery after the physical demands of pregnancy and labour. A little forward planning goes a long way!

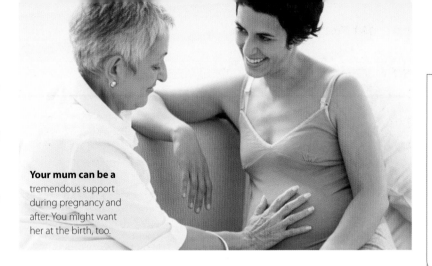

Your mum can be a tremendous support during pregnancy and after. You might want her at the birth, too.

Go shopping: nursing bras

When you are breastfeeding your boobs expand enormously, but that doesn't mean you have to settle for a bra that would look better on your granny. You can look good as well as be comfortable.

A good nursing bra needs to be flexible, allowing extra room for when the milk comes in and when your breasts reduce in size (usually after 12 weeks or so). It almost goes without saying that the cups should open and close easily, preferably using only one hand. The opening should allow plenty of room for your baby to feed and never constrict or squeeze your breast as this can lead to blocked ducts or mastitis.

When it comes to comfort, the same tips apply as to maternity bras (see p.92). Make sure you go for a professional fitting service. When trying on, make sure that the cups fit snugly and cover most of the breast. The centre seam should lie comfortably against your breastbone. Also make sure your maternity bra has:

- four hook and eye fastenings
- wide non-slip shoulder straps for extra support
- broad side and back for extra support
- deep centre at the front for extra support
- drop-cup feature

Systemised mum

There's no doubt that your life and your partner's is about to change. It pays to prepare well.

"My partner Dan and I have been chatting about how our lives will change after our baby is born. It's hard for us to imagine now how different things will be after the birth, but I've been speaking to friends and trying to plan as much as I can.

Dan thinks that our lives will carry on as before, but I know that it will be hard for us to travel and go out as much as we do now, especially in the early days when I'm sore and we're feeling exhausted.

I've been reading lots of books about babycare and I'm going to try and get my baby in a gentle routine as soon as possible, so that hopefully she'll sleep better and we'll be able to get our lives back on track. I really want to breastfeed too, so I've been reading up on how to do it and going to some breastfeeding preparation classes. I think I'm quite prepared now (Dan jokes that I have a degree in parenting!) but I fear my darling partner is going to have more of a shock in store."

ParentsAsk...

I'm 34 weeks pregnant and my breasts are leaking. Is it normal?
Leaking breasts late in pregnancy are perfectly normal, so don't worry. What they are leaking is called colostrum (see p.93). Some women leak quite a lot before their babies are born and others don't leak at all. There doesn't seem to be any link between how much you leak before the baby's birth and how much milk you manage to produce afterwards.

This leaking can be embarrassing for you or your partner if you leak when you are making love. But you should both be assured that this is quite normal.

When you are out and about, wearing breast pads inside your bra will help prevent wet patches on your tops. You should change the pads at regular intervals during the day to keep you feeling fresh and comfortable. This will also help to prevent any smell of stale colostrum.

FIRST TRIMESTER	SECOND TRIMESTER	THIRD TRIMESTER

Your body at **35** Weeks ▼

35 Weeks

❋ You may feel that you've run out of room – your uterus has expanded to 1,000 times its original volume.

❋ Don't be surprised, but you'll gain little or no more weight from now until your due date.

As you head towards your baby's birthday, now is a good time to try to encourage your baby into a good position for birth. Here are a few techniques you can try.

Positioning baby for birth

▼ Your baby at **35** Weeks

Do you see the occasional protrusion from your tummy? That might be baby's foot.

❋ When she stretches and squirms about, your baby's elbow, foot or head may now protrude from your stomach. She weighs about 2.4kg/5¼lb and measures around 45cm/17¾in. Soon, as the wall of your uterus and your abdomen stretch thinner and let in more light, she will develop daily cycles of sleeping and waking. Your little one is now sporting full-length fingernails and toenails and has a fully developed pair of kidneys.

The best position for your baby to be in when you start to go into labour is head down, with the back of her head slightly towards the front of your tummy. In this position, it's simple for her to move gently downwards during labour, so labour is nearly always shorter and easier. Your midwife describes a baby in this position as being in an anterior position.

But Nature isn't always so helpful. Some babies go down into the pelvis with the back of their heads towards their mothers' spines. This is called a posterior position and it can lead to several things happening:

● Your waters are more likely to break at the beginning of labour.

● You have a lot of backache during and in between contractions.

● Labour is slower.

● You may need forceps or ventouse to help you give birth to your baby.

There are some accepted techniques to get a baby to enter the pelvis in an anterior, rather than a posterior, position. This is called "optimal fetal positioning" and should be done from about 35 weeks of pregnancy. It's all about making sure that your knees are always lower than your hips:

● Sit on a cushion in your car to lift your bottom up.

● Check that your favourite chair doesn't make your bottom go down and your knees come up.

● Take regular breaks and move around, especially if your job or leisure activities involve a lot of sitting.

● Watch television kneeling on all fours for 10 minutes every day.

● Scrub all your floors and skirting boards – our grannies used to say that washing the kitchen floor was a good way of preparing for labour. And they were certainly right! When you are kneeling on all fours, the back of your baby's head can't help but swing to the front of your abdomen.

Sometimes women have a lot of niggly pains for several days before labour really starts. These pains might well be due to the fact that your baby is trying to turn from a posterior position into an anterior one. If this happens to you, get as much rest as possible during the night, and during the day try to remain upright and active, leaning forwards while you are having the pains. Don't despair. This is Nature's way of getting your baby into the best position, ready for birth.

Presentation positions

By around eight months, there's not much room in the uterus. Most babies settle in head down, in what's known as a cephalic presentation. When labour begins at full-term, nearly 97 per cent come out head first. Most of the rest are breech, but there are several other presentation positions.

Anterior position The best position for labour, with the back of baby's head slightly towards the front of your tummy.

Posterior position Your baby has the back of her head towards your spine. You are likely to have a slow backache labour.

Breech position Your baby is bottom-down. Vaginal delivery is usually attempted, but you may need a caesarean.

Brow presentation Your baby's head is extended slightly. Unless it flexes, it is very unlikely you'll have a vaginal delivery.

Transverse Your baby is lying horizontally across your uterus. In this position your bump will feel tight and firm.

Oblique Your baby is lying diagonally across your uterus. In this position you're likely to have a caesarean.

Anterior position   Posterior position   Breech position

Brow presentation   Transverse   Oblique

Baby car seats

A car seat is one piece of equipment you really need before your baby is born. If you are having your baby in hospital and are going home by car, you are legally obliged to put her in a car seat.

Choosing the right car seat for your baby's age and weight is very important. You must also make sure that the seat is properly installed. Some seats work better in some models of cars than others, so do try before you buy. If a car seat doesn't seem to fit your car perfectly, or if it seems difficult to fasten in place, do not buy it. The seat should

be held tightly by the seatbelt with very little sideways movement. Practise putting the empty seat in and tightening up the seatbelt. If the seat moves around, it's not safe.

Rear-facing car seats should never be used on a front seat if there are airbags in the car. To make sure that your car seat is safe, have it checked by a professional. Call your local council's road-safety team and ask to have your car seat checked or ask at car dealerships, as some are happy to do a free check.

When choosing a car seat for your baby, make sure it's right for your baby's age and weight, and that it's correctly installed.

Getting ready for pregnancy

Staying safe and healthy

Your pregnancy diary

Birth and beyond

Sleep in late pregnancy

Is a good night's sleep nothing but a distant memory now?
Lots of women have trouble sleeping as the birth gets closer, and maybe some rather strange dreams, too. Find out here what to expect sleep-wise during your third trimester, and why it's happening.

Meeting the challenge

Most women have trouble sleeping at some stage of their pregnancy and often remember a good night's sleep as a distant memory as the birth gets closer.

During your third trimester, just lying down comfortably might be a challenge.

Your bump is now simply too big. If sleeping on your left side with pillows wedged between your legs and behind your back doesn't help, try settling in a comfy chair instead. In the final four to six weeks, you may find that you get

your best rests by sleeping sitting up.

And if that weren't enough, remember during your early pregnancy days when it seemed as though you spent more time in the bathroom than out of it? Well here we are again. This

---

Comfortable sleep positions

Finding it impossible to get comfy in bed? Try curling up or stretching out on your left side with a pillow between your legs. (And keep returning to that position if you wake up at night on your stomach or back.) You can buy a number of different maternity pillows, although you may find that your usual pillows work just as well. Arrange them between your legs, under your bump, and behind your back for extra comfort and support.

You might find that wearing a sleeping bra and a maternity belt gives you extra support and aids sleep.

Finally, if lying on your side puts too much pressure on your hips, sleep on a piece of soft foam. The foam layer goes on top of your mattress and under the sheet for added comfort and air circulation. You should be able to buy soft foam in a range of sizes at most large department stores.

Lying stretched out on your left side with a soft pillow between your legs can be comfortable at this late stage.

Bending your knees with a pillow between them is another sleeping position that many women like.

Imagining yourself lying in the grass or enjoying a beautiful view is using guided imagery. This technique can help you get off to sleep.

time it's thanks to your growing baby, who's putting pressure on your bladder. You can try to reduce the number of trips to the loo by cutting back on fluids in the late afternoon and completely emptying your bladder on every trip to the toilet by leaning forward when you pee. Another technique is to rock back and forth while you are peeing, or to stop, wait for 30 seconds, then squeeze again to get out any last drops.

Heartburn and other sleep stealers

Don't be surprised if heartburn, leg cramps, restless leg syndrome, and snoring, not to mention your baby's kicking and squirming, keep you awake at night during your third trimester. Studies show that pregnant women during their third trimester have fewer periods of deep sleep and wake up more often during the night. In short, the quality of your sleep is heading towards an all-time low.

Try to catch up during the day if the opportunity arises. Otherwise you can become really run down and exhausted. This can become a bit of a vicious circle

though, since cat naps during the day will reduce your requirement for sleep during the night. Nevertheless, this pattern of needing less sleep at night will continue when you are dealing with night feeds so it may be some time before you will need to get back to a normal diurnal (asleep at night and awake during the day) rhythm.

Bizarre dreams

Are you having strange dreams now you're in the third trimester? Many mums-to-be find that during pregnancy, their dreams become more bizarre than ever before. It's all down to the changes taking place with your hormones, perhaps combined with mixed feelings about your changing shape – and maybe the added ingredients of anxiety and excitement about the prospect of becoming a mother.

A taste of things to come

Although you can ease or avoid some of these sleep disturbances, it's likely that you will have to endure some sleepless nights. Think of this time as a dress rehearsal for life after your baby is born!

Dad's **Diary**

Neither of us can sleep now!
Sleep is a real problem for Karen as she nears her due date. She struggles to get into a comfortable position and then, when she does, she finds that she's too hot and the stretch marks on her tummy start itching like crazy. I wake up in the middle of the night shivering to find that she's opened the window to let in the freezing autumn air. Of course, I can't complain, so I just find the nearest blanket and try to go back to sleep.

Getting ready for pregnancy

Staying safe and healthy

Your pregnancy diary

Birth and beyond

36 Weeks

❋ More pressure in your lower abdomen? Your baby is dropping as his head engages ready for birth.

❋ By now, you may feel as if you need to go for a wee all the time as your baby presses on your bladder.

Your baby could arrive any day, so fill the car with petrol and make sure you know where to park when you get to hospital. If you're planning a home birth, other children will need to be looked after.

Be prepared

As your due date approaches, make sure you've got the practical preparations in place for the day (or night) you go into labour. Make sure your partner (or whoever will be driving you) memorises the route to the hospital. If you're in the throes of labour in the passenger seat, your partner may not be in a fit state to navigate. So do a dry run and make sure you know the route as well. It's also a

else lined up to take you to the hospital; maybe one of your parents, or a friend or relative. You probably won't need their help but it'll give you peace of mind that you're prepared for any last-minute changes to your plans.

If you have a child already, arrange alternative care for her for when you go into labour. A trusted friend or relative will need to be able look after her at the

"Your partner **has to be ready** for that **'drop-everything' call**."

▼ Your baby at **36** Weeks

Congratulations! By the end of this week, your pregnancy will be full term.

❋ Your baby can safely be born any day now and is not classed as premature. Your baby is still gaining weight – about 28g/1oz a day. She now weighs nearly 2.7kg/6lb and is about 47.4cm/18½in long. At this stage you may feel increased pressure in your lower abdomen as your baby engages in your pelvis, ready for birth.

good idea to plan a few alternative routes in case there are obstacles when the big day arrives. Keep the car filled with enough petrol to get you there. A last-minute stop at the petrol station is the last thing you need when you're battling through the contractions.

Make sure that you can contact your partner no matter where he is when you need him. He has to be ready for that "drop-everything" call. In the unlikely event that your partner isn't around when you go into labour, have someone

drop of a hat. Even if you have a home birth, you'll need someone to come and look after her, or to take her to their home. If the care giver is someone who has never spent the night with your child, it might be helpful to have a practice run first – especially if you'll be sending her to stay in the care giver's house. Arrange a sleepover party sometime before the birth with games or other simple, fun activities so that she'll have happy memories of spending the night with this person.

ParentsTalk...

"When my due date was a week away, the reality of what was about to happen set in. I felt like I was going to run a marathon and hadn't done enough training."
Bella, 34, mum of six-month old Anna

"I'm most scared about the pain. I'm not planning on having pain relief, but I'm worried that it'll be so agonising I'll ask for it anyway."
Rani, 33, first-time mum

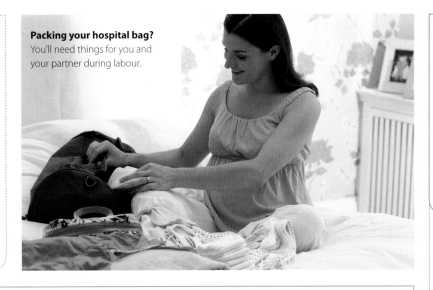

Packing your hospital bag?
You'll need things for you and your partner during labour.

Getting ready for pregnancy

Staying safe and healthy

Your pregnancy diary

Birth and beyond

Packing for hospital in preparation for labour

This is the final stretch, with only a few weeks to go before your due date. Now's the time to pack a bag for all the essentials you'll need during labour and after your baby is born.

Check what the hospital provides and what you can bring yourself, but be aware that hospitals can be short on space – there may be only a small cabinet by your bed for your things.

What to pack for labour

- Your birth plan and medical notes.
- Dressing gown, slippers and socks.
- An old nightdress or a T-shirt to wear in labour.
- Massage oil or lotion.
- Lip balm.
- Snacks and drinks for while you are in labour, or some glucose tablets.
- Watch with a second hand – to time contractions.
- Digital camera or camcorder (not all hospitals allow camcorders in delivery rooms, so do check with them before).
- Relaxation materials – books, magazines, portable DVD player, hand-held games console and games.
- TENS pain relief machine – if you are planning to use one.
- Toiletries.
- Water spray – or a hand-held fan.
- Music to listen to – on a CD or MP3 player, but check with the hospital in case they won't let you plug anything in to re-charge it, in which case you'll need to take a battery-operated machine.

For your birth partner

- A change of clothes.
- Snacks and drinks.
- Book or games console.

For after the birth

- Going-home outfit and loose, comfortable clothes to wear while you're in hospital.
- Nursing bras and breast pads.
- Maternity pads – a couple of packs.
- Nightshirt or T-shirt – front-opening shirts are useful for breastfeeding.
- Toiletries.
- Towels, hairbrush, toothbrush and toothpaste.
- Old knickers/cheap knickers/disposable knickers – don't bring your best ones as they will get messy.

- Arnica tablets which may help with bruising after the birth.
- Ear plugs, in case you end up on a noisy ward!
- Address book – unless all your numbers are stored on your mobile phone.
- Fully charged mobile phone and charger (if allowed in hospital).
- Coins/card for using hospital phone.

For your baby

- Towel.
- Infant car seat.
- One outfit for the trip home.
- Two to three babygros and vests for baby to wear while you are in hospital.
- Baby blanket (a warm one if the weather is cold).
- Nappies.
- One pair of socks or booties and a hat.
- Jacket or snowsuit if you are having a winter baby.
- Muslin squares.

FIRST TRIMESTER	SECOND TRIMESTER	THIRD TRIMESTER

Your body at **37** Weeks

37 Weeks

❋ If you need help to conquer the late pregnancy blues, read up on what your newborn will be like (see pp.302–309).

❋ It may be harder than ever to get to sleep at night. Take it easy during the day if you can.

The next couple of weeks are a waiting game.
Try to enjoy this time before your baby arrives – eat well and get plenty of rest. And if you already have a little one, make the most of this special time together.

Coping with a toddler

Your toddler may become anxious in the month or so before you give birth. As you get bigger, less energetic, and more focused on the labour, he may become clingy, develop new fears and even regress slightly. This is normal. Acting like a baby may be just his way of exploring how babies behave and what it felt like to be your baby. Lots of love and affection during this time will help him regain his confidence.

Try to avoid any other major changes that might unsettle your toddler, such as moving or starting a new nursery. Now isn't the best time to pressure him to complete potty training or ask him to give up security items such as his dummy, either. Keeping to his regular routine as much as possible is key in helping him to feel secure.

Spend as much time with your child as possible in the last few weeks of your pregnancy. It's likely that you're going to be pretty busy with the baby when she arrives, so make the most of your time together. He will really appreciate it and remember this special time when he had you all to himself.

How will we manage in the early days and weeks?

It will be hard at times, but it won't be impossible. Below are our top tips on how you can cope.

● Make your toddler aware from the very start that the baby is interested in him, is watching him and loves him. Say things like, "She's following your game with her eyes" and "She's very interested in what you're doing".

● Involve him in games with the baby from the earliest days, and always tell your toddler how much you value his help and assistance at bathtime, or fetching a clean nappy, and so on.

● Buy a few small presents for him, wrap them up and leave them by the door so that visitors with gifts for your newborn can also give him something.

60% of mums think that 18 months to three years is the best age gap to have between siblings. Just 10 per cent think that 18 months or less is ideal, while eight per cent think the age gap doesn't matter.

Your baby at **37** Weeks

With baby's head now in your pelvis, she has more room for her growing legs.

❋ If your baby's head has engaged (see pp.204–5) and is cradled in your pelvis, she will now have a bit more room for her 2.8kg/6¼lb body and her 50cm/19½in length. Many babies now have a full head of hair, which may be around 2.5cm/1in long. But don't be surprised if her hair isn't the same colour as yours.

Your last antenatal appointment

If you've had a baby before, your last antenatal appointment will take place at 38 weeks. If this is your first pregnancy, you'll also have a check-up at 40 weeks. During this appointment, your midwife will check your blood pressure and urine, and measure your bump. She'll examine your abdomen to determine your baby's position and growth, and listen to your baby's heartbeat.

If you haven't had your baby by 41 weeks, your midwife will offer you a membrane sweep to try to kickstart labour. If you choose not to have a membrane sweep, or if it doesn't make you go into labour, you'll be offered an induction. Your midwife will also carry out the usual blood pressure and urine checks, and measure your bump.

Before your last appointment, make a note of any questions you'd like to ask your midwife. It's an ideal time to raise any last-minute worries or fears you have about the labour, or about your preparations for caring for your baby after she's born. Your midwife will be able to reassure you and offer you help and advice during these last few days.

Finally, remember that due dates aren't always accurate. Though you think you're overdue and may start worrying, you may not be overdue at all.

"Your midwife will **reassure you** during these **last few days**."

ParentsTalk...

"When my breech baby simply refused to turn, I was booked in for a caesarean. I was OK about it until I got into the operating theatre. All of a sudden, after a day of just relaxing, watching TV and chatting to my husband, the reality of what was about to happen just hit me. I was trying hard not to cry, but as they gave me the epidural I burst into tears! It wasn't until the midwife reassured me that everything would be fine that I started to calm down and enjoy the whole experience."
Mags, 30, first-time mum

"During my caesarean I asked for the curtain to be lowered so I could see my twins being born. It was a weird experience but totally incredible. It's something I'll always remember and will tell the twins about when they're older."
Jenna, 37, mum to Rosie and Harriet

"Having a caesarean doesn't make you any less of a mum or woman. Remember that how you give birth isn't the measure of being a good mother – it's what you do afterwards that really counts."
Sheena, 24, mum to two-year-old Josh

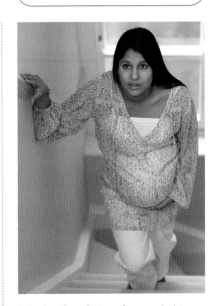

During these last weeks even climbing the stairs can be an effort. Tell your doctor if you develop any worrying symptoms.

Getting ready for pregnancy

Staying safe and healthy

Your pregnancy diary

Birth and beyond

FIRST TRIMESTER	SECOND TRIMESTER	THIRD TRIMESTER

Your body at **38** Weeks

38 Weeks

※ Your due date is right around the corner and your baby's just waiting for the right time to be born.

※ Take it easy during the final week or so – this may be your last opportunity to relax for a while.

You may now feel more pressure in your lower abdomen and notice that your baby is gradually dropping. This is called lightening, or engagement. Your lungs and stomach now get a chance to expand.

Rules of engagement

Your baby at **38** Weeks

Baby is still growing and laying down the fat stores that regulate body temperature.

※ Although your baby is still growing, boys tend to have a slightly heavier birth weight than girls. The average baby at 38 weeks weighs about 3 to 3.2kg/6½ to 7lb. Your little one's organ systems are now fully developed, but his lungs will be last to mature, which is why premature babies need help breathing.

Towards the end of pregnancy, the shape of your uterus, your liver and intestines encourage your baby's presenting part (usually his head, but sometimes his bottom) to dip down into your pelvis. This can occur as early as 33 or 34 weeks of pregnancy, but may not happen until labour starts.

If your baby engages in the pelvis early this does not mean that you will give birth early. Usually he will engage in the pelvis by 37 to 38 weeks, but this process can also be affected by lots of other things:

● If you are very sporty and have well-toned abdominal muscles, this may mean that your tummy is held in tighter, which changes the angle of the baby's body and presenting part to the pelvic brim. In this position it is harder for him to engage in the pelvis. To encourage his head to engage you need to relax your tummy muscles and "dangle your belly" out at the front.

● If you spend a lot of time sitting down at work, in a car, or in soft easy chairs or on squidgy sofas to watch TV, your baby is more likely to be lying in a posterior position – that is with his back to your back. In this position it is harder for him

to enter your pelvis. This is not the best position for an efficient labour, partly because the presenting part of the baby remains high for so long. Make sure to sit leaning forwards whenever you sit down, with your knees below your hips. This will help your baby to turn his back towards your front and move down. A kneeling chair is ideal for you to adopt this position.

● If you have had several babies before, your tummy muscles may be loose, which makes it easy for your baby to move and change position frequently. Sometimes he may lie across your tummy (transverse) or at an angle (oblique). If he gets into one of these positions (see p.197), it is less likely that he will manage to engage in your pelvis before the start of labour.

● Your baby may be a large one. If this is the case, he may not be able to descend into your pelvis until your contractions start.

● Sometimes the entrance to your pelvis is narrow. If that is the case, it may take a long time for your baby's presenting part to enter your pelvis but, once he is in position, birth is generally rapid because the pelvic outlet usually tends to be roomy.

Enjoying the last weeks together

If you're expecting your first baby, your relationship is facing one of its toughest tests. Going from being partners to parents is a steep (some would say perpendicular!) learning curve. No one can predict how you will cope, but one thing is for sure: nothing will be the same again. That's why you and your partner should make the most of your last few weeks alone together.

First there were two

With the excitement of your imminent new arrival, it's easy to lose track of where it all began: your relationship with your husband or partner. Take time out to remind yourself of your shared history and how you've dealt with life's ups and downs so far. Taking stock like this gives you confidence that you will manage whatever life throws at you. It's also an opportunity to discuss your plans for the future.

A kiss and cuddle

Research shows that sharing affection every day boosts the chances of a partnership lasting. Like children, adults who do not get hugged, praised or supported start to feel cut off and out of touch with others. Regular shows of affection deepen the bonds between you and set you up for the challenges of parenthood that lie ahead.

You can show that you love and care for each other in little ways every day. Cuddle up on the sofa together, or hold hands as you walk along. Try a peck on the cheek when you make them a cup of tea, put a loving note on the fridge or in their pocket, or buy a small surprise gift to show that you've been thinking about them during the day. Remember, too, that sex is not a replacement for affection, and that when it comes to lovemaking, it's quality, not quantity, that's important.

Invest in your relationship

Investing in your relationship as a couple will be just as important once your baby is born. The demands of parenthood, work and social life can often mean that partners start to take their relationship for granted. If that happens, you may begin to lose sight of what you both want and need from each other. So you should always make sure to find regular time for just the two of you throughout the coming weeks, months and years.

60% of new mums say that having a baby has strengthened their relationship with their partner. It takes time for a couple to adjust to their roles as parents but for many it strengthens the bond they share.

Engagement

During these last few weeks of pregnancy, your baby's head will drop down into your pelvis, ready for the birth.

A sense of relief

As your baby's head engages, you'll find that eating and breathing become easier as your baby frees up space for your lungs and stomach. However, walking may become increasingly uncomfortable – some women even say it feels as if the baby is going to fall out. (But don't worry, it can't happen.)

You may also feel as if you need to go to the loo more as your baby squashes on your bladder. Practising your pelvic floor exercises (see p.135) can help.

Your bump is at its maximum height

Your bump has now visibly lowered

The baby's head is at the brim of your pelvis

The baby has dropped into your pelvis

Not engaged

Engaged

FIRST TRIMESTER	SECOND TRIMESTER	THIRD TRIMESTER

Your body at **39** Weeks

39 Weeks

❋ These last few days will probably drag as you wait impatiently for the arrival of your baby.

❋ You and your partner might try relieving the tension with a little love-making. It might get labour started.

With your baby about to arrive any day, it's an exciting time, but you're probably a bit apprehensive too. How will you know when you've started labour? What will happen if the baby comes suddenly?

Last-minute fears

It's perfectly normal to feel anxious as the big day draws near. You may have heard some childbirth horror stories, or believe that all labours start a certain way and progress at a certain rate. The truth is, every single birth is different.

Feeling in control

Some of the most common fears women have about childbirth are worrying about being able to cope with the pain, losing control during labour and problems arising that might require medical intervention. That's why it's a good opportunity to use these last few days to review your birth plan in case you've missed anything out. Make sure it's clear in your head and talk to your birth partner about it, too, so he's sure about his role during the birth.

If you still have any last-minute worries about the forthcoming birth, speak to your midwife – she is the most qualified to put your mind at rest.

The countdown continues…

You're probably as big as you're going to get now, and likely to be feeling tired and uncomfortable with it. Your uterus fills your entire pelvis and abdomen and, with all the excitement of baby's imminent arrival, you may be finding it increasingly difficult to sleep at night. Try to make up for it during the day, and put your feet up whenever you can.

Remember, too, that the days leading up to the birth can be a confusing time for any other children you may have. Involve them as much as possible in the preparations and excitement to help manage their natural feelings of jealousy (see p.219).

Finally, don't worry if by the end of this week you're still waiting – only a tiny proportion of babies are born on their due date, many are born later. You and your partner might try relieving the tension with a little lovemaking – sex has been known to get labour started. It is thought to stimulate the uterus during orgasm into triggering the release of oxytocin, the "contraction" hormone. Semen also contains a high concentration of prostaglandins which help to prepare the neck of the womb for labour. But if passion is the last thing on your mind, don't worry – your baby will be born in her own sweet time.

▼ Your baby at **39** Weeks

Your baby's about to greet the world! But don't worry if you're still waiting.

❋ Only 5 per cent of babies are born on their due date and a whopping 75 per cent are born later. She's still building a layer of fat and is shedding the greasy, white substance which has been protecting her skin. It's likely she already measures about 20in/51cm and weighs a bit over 7lb/3.2kg – a mini watermelon.

Suddenly feeling the urge to clean every surface in sight could mean that your baby's birth is just around the corner.

Signs of labour

Pregnant first-time mums often worry they won't know when they're in labour. Here are the signs you should watch out for:

- Persistent lower back or abdominal pain, often accompanied by a crampy premenstrual feeling.
- A bloody show (a brownish or blood-tinged mucus discharge).
- Painful contractions that occur at regular and increasingly shorter intervals and become longer and stronger in intensity.
- Broken waters, but you're actually in labour only if it's accompanied by contractions that are making your cervix dilate.

The nesting instinct

As well as the physical signs of labour (see Signs of labour, above right) a common clue that labour is just around the corner is the sudden emergence of the "nesting instinct". If you're close to your due date and find yourself frantically cleaning out drawers, organising cupboards and dusting like crazy, it may be that you'll soon be welcoming your baby into the world.

Nesting is probably prompted by your pregnancy hormones and the instinctive desire to prepare the "nest" for the new arrival. In the animal kingdom female animals and birds have similar patterns of cleaning and preparation before they give birth. By having the house spotlessly clean, your baby's room ready and all her clothes organised, you are ensuring that she will have the best chance for growth and survival once she is born.

Don't worry if you haven't had a nesting instinct – many women are simply too tired and worn out by now! But if you do find yourself packing and repacking your hospital bag, cleaning every room or sorting out your kitchen cupboards, don't push yourself too hard. Rest frequently and eat regular, healthy meals. Remember, you'll need your energy for labour and the wakeful nights that lie ahead…

Meanwhile, plan something good to do each day so you have something (else!) to look forward to.

ParentsAsk...

I've heard about a membrane sweep. What is it?

Membrane sweeping can be a useful way of bringing on labour. It's done by your midwife or doctor while she examines you internally. She simply "sweeps" a finger around your cervix. The aim is to separate the membranes around your baby from your cervix. This releases hormones called prostaglandins, which may help to kick-start your labour.

If it's your first baby, you're normally offered a membrane sweep at your 40-week antenatal appointment and again at your 41-week appointment. If this isn't your first baby, then you should be offered a membrane sweep at your 41-week antenatal appointment.

A membrane sweep can be uncomfortable as the cervix is often hard to reach. It doesn't increase the risk of infection to you or your baby.

FIRST TRIMESTER	SECOND TRIMESTER	THIRD TRIMESTER

Your body at **40** Weeks ▼

40 Weeks

❋ After months of anticipation, your due date rolls around, and... you're still pregnant.

❋ You still have a couple of weeks before you're considered to be having a "prolonged pregnancy".

Congratulations! You've made it to the end of your pregnancy. If the last nine months have flown by, be prepared for time to slow down drastically as you count down the days to your baby's birth.

Your due date's arrived

So you've made it to your due date but there's no sign that your baby is on his way. You may not only be just plain fed up with the whole, long, drawn-out process, but also worried in case there is anything wrong. Well, first of all, calculating the due date isn't an exact science, so although you may think you're now overdue, you may not be yet.

But if you want to get labour going, there are a few old-fashioned remedies that you could try to kickstart your contractions. Unfortunately there is no research to show that any of these is effective, but there's probably no harm in trying a hot curry, a long walk or making love (see p.206). If nothing else, they might well help you to relax.

 Your baby at **40** Weeks

His skull bones won't fuse until after he's born to help him through the birth canal.

❋ Mother Nature thinks of everything. Those unfused skull bones will be able to overlap a bit when he's going through the birth canal. This is the reason your baby's head may look a little cone-shaped after birth. Rest assured, it's normal and only temporary. The average newborn weighs 3.4kg/7½lb and is 51cm/20in long.

Parents**Talk...**

"As my due date came and went without so much as a hint my baby was on its way, I used the time to prepare for the chaotic weeks after the birth. I stocked up the freezer with dinners, spent lots of time with my feet up, went to the hairdressers (as there was no way I'd have time for the next couple of months!) and enjoyed one or two last romantic evenings out with my partner before we were transformed into fatigued and dishevelled versions of ourselves."
Chris, 34, mum to six-month old Ben

"When I got to 39 weeks I got obsessive about trying to bring on labour. I had as much sex as I could manage, ate fresh pineapple and hot curry, drank raspberry leaf tea and walked and swam. And by 41 weeks it happened – a few days before I was due to be induced!"
Pritty, 32, first-time mum

"I ended up being induced at 42 weeks. If you're overdue, don't worry – just take it easy and make the most of some time to yourself."
Frances, 28, mum to one-year old Alex

Still going strong

If you're still pregnant by 41 weeks, you'll have an antenatal appointment with your midwife or doctor. She will examine your bump to check the position and size of your baby and will do an internal examination to see if your cervix feels ready for labour. If you haven't had one already, she may offer you a membrane sweep (see p.207) to see if this triggers labour. She'll discuss with you whether or not you want to be induced if the membrane sweep doesn't work. As an alternative to induction she may offer that you have your pregnancy monitored on a regular basis (see p.250).

By 42 weeks obstetricians usually recommend that you have an induction.

5%

of babies are actually born on their expected due date, while a whopping 75 per cent are born later. So if you've gone beyond 40 weeks, don't worry. You're in the majority.

The reason for this is that the very small number of babies who die unexpectedly while they are still in the womb increases after 42 weeks of pregnancy, and again after 43 weeks. However, do not be alarmed as the numbers are still extremely small.

Take your mind off things

For the time being, it's a good idea to try to have something planned for every day. Don't stay at home wondering whether you can feel anything happening. Get out of the house – but don't go too far! Make an appointment with the hairdresser and ask for a nice long head massage, or book yourself in for a pedicure. If you haven't already stocked up the freezer, do so now. Tell friends and relatives not to ring every day to find out what's happening – say you'll call them when the big event has taken place.

A visit to the hairdresser will help to take your mind off the fact that you've been pregnant for weeks and weeks and weeks!

If you can manage it, go for a few walks; it might get things started. Enlist the help of friends and family to keep you entertained – meet up for lunch, or invite them over for coffee.

But above all, rest, rest, rest. Labour requires a great deal of energy and stamina, so make the most of your last few days by putting your feet up whenever you can.

Getting ready for pregnancy / Staying safe and healthy / Your pregnancy diary / Birth and beyond

Your full-term baby

The average baby measures about 51cm (20in) long from head to toe and weighs approximately 3.4kg (7½ lb) at birth, but anywhere between 2.5 and 3.8kg (5½ and 8½lb) is a healthy range for newborns. Your amniotic fluid, once clear, is now becoming pale and milky as your baby sheds the vernix caseosa (the waxy coating that was protecting his skin). The outer layers of his skin are still continuing to slough off as new skin forms underneath.

In TV soaps, labour always begins with the waters breaking – in the middle of a crowded room, of course – just before contractions start. If you've been worrying that this scenario will happen to you, you can stop.

Membranes rupture in less than 15 per cent of pregnancies and, when they do, the baby's head tends to act as a cork at the opening of the uterus. You should stay calm – it may be hours before you feel your first contraction – and call your doctor or midwife right away. Your body will produce more amniotic fluid until the baby is born, so your carers may suggest you wait at home until contractions are under way or may suggest an induction.

ParentsAsk...

What's a post-maturity assessment?

If you go past your due date you will have an antenatal appointment at 41 weeks. Your midwife or doctor will check that your due date is correct. She will then check the position and size of your baby and will carry out an internal examination to see whether your cervix feels "ripe" for labour (that is, soft and stretchy). She may also offer to sweep your membranes to see if this will trigger labour (see p.207). Finally, she will discuss whether it would be better for your baby to continue inside the uterus if the membrane sweep doesn't work, or if you want to be induced.

Common concerns in pregnancy

It's natural to worry

Worrying is a way of coping with major life changes. Share your concerns with your partner, midwife or doctor. Talk with other mothers at the same stage of pregnancy as you. They will understand how you feel.

Reassurance needed

Many pregnant women fret about how they'll cope with labour and whether their baby will be born healthy. It's normal to spend a few nights tossing and turning as you ponder best and worst-case scenarios. Your worries may continue during the day too.

But if your anxiety starts to become all-consuming and regularly disrupts your sleep, then it's time for you to find a better way to deal with it. Share your fears with your partner – he's probably harbouring similar concerns. Turn to friends or family for support. And of course, talk to your midwife or doctor, who should be able to reassure you.

If you're feeling extremely anxious or have a particular reason to be concerned about your baby's health, you may be able to arrange to have an ultrasound scan. Although this can't detect every potential problem, you may find it comforting to see even a fuzzy outline of your growing baby.

"Remember that **most babies** are born **completely healthy**."

Of course, if your scan suggests there is a problem, you will naturally be very worried. A whole range of specialists, from paediatricians to physiotherapists, will be on hand to support and guide you through the options available. The hospital will also put you in touch with community organisations and specialist charities that can help.

But do remember that most babies are born completely healthy, so relax and enjoy your pregnancy!

Having an ultrasound scan can help to allay any particular fears you may have. It's reassuring to see how your baby's growing.

Parents**Ask...**

If I have a high-risk pregnancy do I have to stay in hospital or stop work early?

Not necessarily. A high-risk pregnancy is one in which you or your baby are at higher-than-average risk of experiencing complications. For example, this might be if you have a pre-existing medical condition such as a heart problem, previous pregnancy-related complications (such as cervical weakness), or a history of pregnancy loss.

Your pregnancy will be more closely monitored than usual and extra tests may be recommended. If complications do arise – or seem likely to arise – you may be advised to avoid strenuous activity and to rest as often as possible.

Dad's **Diary**

Is it "sympathetic pregnancy"?

"I've been feeling easily exhausted and sick to my stomach on and off for weeks. Friends say I should stop eating in dodgy restaurants, but could this be a sign of couvade syndrome or 'sympathetic pregnancy'? I've heard it's a controversial topic, as there hasn't been much scientific research on it. Of course, I don't want the doctor to scrutinise my body as well as Karen's, but maybe, on some level, I would like to be involved as much as possible in her pregnancy."

Getting ready for pregnancy

Staying safe and healthy

Your pregnancy diary

Birth and beyond

Baby-safety worries

Some drugs can be harmful to you and your unborn baby, but try not to fret if you took a headache pill or a cold remedy before you knew you were pregnant. Chances are your baby will be absolutely fine – just exercise a little caution from now on.

Could I have harmed my baby?

It always pays to think twice before you take any medication while you're pregnant, but you may worry about medicines you took before you actually knew you were pregnant. These might include the pill.

Active mum

It's great to stay fit but you should always listen to your body and don't overdo it.

"I've always been a bit of a fitness fanatic. Looking good and feeling healthy are both so important to me. Before I fell pregnant, I went to the gym at least five times a week for an hour and a half. I'd feel guilty if I missed a session. When I found out I was expecting, I dropped down to four workouts a week but still really went for it. That's until my ninth week of pregnancy, when I woke up one morning to find I'd bled a little in the night. My doctor asked me if I'd been over-doing it and I realised that I had. I spent the next three days in bed and, thankfully, the bleeding stopped and baby is well. I've since substituted the gym for the much more relaxing yoga."

In the past, when doses of hormones in the pill were higher, there used to be worries that getting pregnant while taking the pill, or just after stopping, would be harmful to the developing embryo. But more recent research has found no evidence of an increased risk of abnormalities.

Aspirin and ibuprofen aren't usually recommended in pregnancy, but if you have taken them – or cold remedies containing them – without knowing that you were pregnant, they are unlikely to

If you took the pill before you knew you were pregnant, don't worry. There's no evidence that it will cause any problems.

have harmed your baby. Paracetamol is considered safe to take throughout pregnancy, as long as you stick to the recommended dosage and only use it occasionally.

Likewise, doctors advise against taking some of the ingredients in cough remedies, such as codeine, ephedrine and dextromethorphan, while you are pregnant. But they are unlikely to have harmed your baby if you have taken them unknowingly. From now on, though, just stick to a simple honey-and-lemon linctus.

Treatments to avoid
However, there are some treatments that are known to be potentially harmful to unborn babies. These include:
- Isotretinoin, which is used to treat acne.
- Psoriasis drugs, such as acitretin and methotrexate.
- Mebendazole and other drugs used to eliminate threadworms.

If you have taken any of these drugs while unaware that you were pregnant, or if you are taking drugs for an ongoing condition, such as epilepsy or diabetes, do talk to your doctor. The chances are that your baby is fine, but she can reassure you and arrange for extra checks if necessary.

Has my baby stopped growing?

Sadly, just over one in 200 pregnancies ends in stillbirth in the UK. One of the first signs that something might be wrong is if you notice that your baby is moving significantly less than he was previously or has stopped moving completely. You may also have vaginal bleeding. In some cases, the first sign that there is a problem is going into premature labour. If any of these things happens, you should contact your midwife or doctor straight away.

More than half of stillbirths are classified as "unexplained", which means that doctors are unable to identify the exact cause of death. However, some of the things that are known to cause stillbirths include a genetic or physical defect in the baby, placental abruption (when the placenta begins to separate from the uterus; see p.232), pre-eclampsia (see p.233) and infections, such as listeriosis, salmonella or toxoplasmosis. When a baby dies before birth and premature labour doesn't occur, labour may have to be induced. Some parents decide that they want to have the induction as soon as possible; others prefer to wait for a few days so that they have time to take in what has happened and to see if the labour starts naturally. Depending on the circumstances of your loss, you may be asked if you would like to see, touch or hold your baby. Many parents find this extremely helpful.

Measuring the height of the fundus (the top of the uterus) is one of the methods used for checking that your baby's growing.

Note: If you've had an unexplained stillbirth, it may be comforting to know that there is no increased risk of it happening again. However, if your baby was affected by a genetic abnormality, you may be referred for genetic counselling to assess the risks and discuss future options.

After a stillbirth

It may seem cruel that, at this time of shock and grief, there is paperwork to be done. However, some parents appreciate the formal recognition of their baby's existence and treasure the certificates that they receive.

● **Registration** You are legally obliged to register a baby stillborn at or after 24 weeks of pregnancy. Hospital staff will issue a Medical Certificate of Stillbirth, which should be taken to the nearest office of the Registrar for Births, Marriages and Deaths within six weeks (21 days in Scotland and five days in Northern Ireland).

● **Certificate for burial or cremation** Once you've registered the stillbirth, the registrar will give you a certificate for burial or cremation. By law, a baby must be buried or cremated if he was stillborn at or after 24 weeks. Either you or the hospital can make the arrangements. Don't feel pressured to make decisions too quickly. Your baby's body will be kept safely by the hospital until you have decided what arrangements you wish to make.

● **Saying goodbye** There is no obligation on you to hold a service before burial or cremation. You can say goodbye to your baby in almost any way you choose. This could mean letting the hospital make all the arrangements for you, or holding a religious or non-religious, traditional, or personally designed ceremony.

Dad's **Diary**

Anxious times

"There's nothing worse than suddenly thinking there might be something wrong with your baby. We had a worrying time at around 22 weeks when Laura hadn't felt the baby move for a couple of days.

She tried lying down on her side in a quiet room – nothing. She tried drinking a very cold drink – still nothing. We called the midwife and she reassured us that the baby might have shifted to a position where his movements wouldn't be felt. But to be on the safe side, she also booked us in to see her the next day so that she could listen to the baby's heartbeat. Everything was absolutely fine – but it was an anxious wait before the appointment."

Getting ready for pregnancy

Staying safe and healthy

Your pregnancy diary

Birth and beyond

Worries about birth defects

Discovering that your unborn baby has a birth defect is devastating, but it does give you and your doctors the chance to plan her care before she's born. Some defects may be corrected soon after birth, but others have lifelong implications for your baby and your family.

It's a shock to have a baby with Down's syndrome but support groups offer help and put you in touch with other parents.

Fact: Spina bifida is becoming an increasingly rare condition – mainly because pregnant women are now advised to take folic acid supplements (see p.49) to prevent neural tube defects.

Will my baby be normal?

Every parent-to-be worries at some point about whether or not their baby is going to be born normal. Luckily, serious birth defects are rare and antenatal care is so good now that problems often get picked up well in advance of your baby's birth. But, although serious defects are rare, it's wise to be aware of the kind of problems that can affect babies. Below are some of the more common ones.

Heart defects

Some heart problems are detected during an antenatal ultrasound scan. Others are picked up during your baby's newborn examination when the doctor hears a heart murmur – unusual sounds that blood makes as it passes through the valves and blood vessels of the heart.

Most heart murmurs are completely normal or "innocent" and cause no symptoms. However, some are a sign of a heart defect. Serious heart defects may need surgery. Many children make a complete recovery and can lead a normal life afterwards. Others may need further surgery when they are older.

Cleft lip and palate

A cleft lip is a split in the upper lip between the mouth and nose caused because separate areas of the face did not join properly during pregnancy. A cleft palate happens when the roof of the mouth has not joined completely. Clefts sometimes run in families.

A cleft lip is usually repaired by surgery by the time a baby is two to three months old. A cleft palate is usually repaired by the time a baby is one year old. Like the lip repair, the operation is carried out under general anaesthetic.

Babies born with clefts can have problems with latching on to the breast or sucking on a teat, which can make feeding difficult. However, a feeding specialist should be able to help you feed your baby successfully.

Down's syndrome

Down's syndrome is a genetic condition that affects just over one in every 800 babies born in the UK. We do not know what causes Down's, but there is a definite link with older mothers.

Children born with Down's syndrome all have a degree of learning disability, but this will vary from child to child. They also have certain physical characteristics. For example, your baby may have looser muscles and joints than other babies and she may possibly have a lower than average birth weight.

Strawberry marks are thought to be caused by abnormalities in the way blood vessels have developed. They are harmless.

Many babies are born with "stork marks" or "angel kisses". They're nothing to worry about and will eventually disappear.

Babies with Down's often have eyes that slant upwards and outwards. Their eyelids may have an extra fold of skin that appears to exaggerate the slant. Many babies with Down's have a single crease on their hands which runs right across the palm.

Spina bifida

Spina bifida happens when the spinal cord does not fully close, leaving a gap. There are three types of spina bifida: spina bifida occulta (hidden) is the commonest and mildest form, myelomeningocele is the most serious form, while spina bifida meningocele is less serious than meningomyelocele and is the rarest form.

It is estimated that approximately 5 to 10 per cent of people may have spina bifida occulta without realising it. Around one in 1,000 babies is born with myelomeningocele, the most serious form of spina bifida.

Spina bifida can be picked up either during a routine ultrasound scan or following a blood test. Babies with severe spina bifida will need surgery during the first two days after birth to repair the gap in the spinal cord. Some doctors do not use surgery but let the area heal on its own.

Birthmarks

Birthmarks are markings on your baby's skin that may be permanent or fade away over time. The most common are caused by tiny blood vessels just beneath the skin. These small red, mottled spots are sometimes called "stork marks" or, when they're on the forehead or eyelids, "angel kisses". They are harmless and usually disappear in a few months but, sometimes, over years. Other birthmarks can be caused by abnormalities in the blood vessels.

The most common types of birthmark are strawberry marks – a raised, crimson mark which develops on about five per cent of babies – and port-wine stains – flat red or purple marks ranging in size from a few millimetres to several centimetres in diameter. About three in 1,000 babies are born with this type of birthmark, often on one side of the face. Port-wine stains can be made lighter with laser therapy.

Congenital moles are another type. They can be brown in fair-skinned babies, ranging to almost black in dark-skinned babies. Some are raised or hairy.

Most birthmarks don't cause any physical problems, but it's worth showing the birthmark to your doctor or midwife to monitor it.

 ## Systemised mum

Finding out your baby has a heart defect is a shock, but there is lots of help at hand.

"We discovered that our baby had a heart defect at our 20-week anomaly scan. The sonographer told us that he suspected she had a ventrical septal defect – a hole in the heart. We were referred to a cardiac specialist, who confirmed the diagnosis. Fortunately, we were told that the hole was quite a small one, which might heal by itself once our baby was born. But she'll need regular check-ups to make sure the hole is getting smaller and there's also a chance that she might need heart surgery to correct the problem when she's a little older.

It's really frightening to be told that your baby has something wrong with her heart. I found it much easier to cope once I knew all the facts. Our doctor gave us some information to take home with us and there are lots of websites and support groups for parents of children with heart defects. It also helped to talk online to other parents in a similar situation."

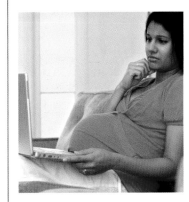

Most parent support groups will have a website and a helpline to give you information and advice.

Getting ready for pregnancy

Staying safe and healthy

Your pregnancy diary

Birth and beyond

Worries about labour day and after

Whatever stage of your pregnancy you're at – but especially in those last weeks – your head is bound to be full of worries about what exactly will happen on labour day and how you'll cope. This is all perfectly normal. The key is always to be well prepared.

Parents**Talk...**

"I got very excited a week before my due date when I started to have some contractions. These felt different to, and stronger than, the Braxton Hicks contractions. After roughly five hours, they were about five minutes apart and becoming more painful. I phoned my partner at work and told him to come home straightaway. An hour later I was at the hospital. And that's when the contractions stopped! My cervix hadn't dilated at all. The midwife said it was just my body getting ready to have my baby. I gave birth two weeks later."

Kim, 28, mum to two-month-old Ryan

"I'd been having strong contractions for about two hours when Ken and I got in the taxi. Then I suddenly had an overwhelming urge to push. Even the panic in the driver's eyes wasn't going to stop me! He pulled over and he and Ken made me as comfortable on the back seat as they could while they called an ambulance. I gave birth before the paramedics arrived, though."

Helena, 32, second-time mum

Worries about the day

If you're having a hospital birth, you may well be wondering whether or not you'll reach the hospital or birth centre on time. Providing that you've prepared well, you'll have nothing to fear. Those preparations include making sure that your hospital bag is packed (see p.201) and that your car has a full tank of petrol. Also check that your partner or friend has worked out the best route to the hospital, and if you're planning on taking a cab, make sure you've set your phone to speed-dial the taxi company number. The last thing you want to do is rummage around trying to find the number between contractions.

And if you're planning a home birth, rest assured that your baby is unlikely to arrive before the midwife does! That only happens in very few cases. To be

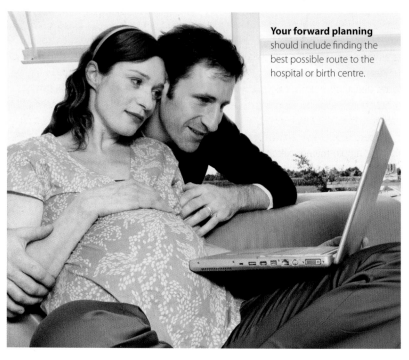

Your forward planning should include finding the best possible route to the hospital or birth centre.

on the safe side though, all mums-to-be should read pp.292–3 for tips on how to cope if your baby decides he's in a hurry to make an appearance.

Labour and after

You may also have worries about the labour itself. Will you be able to cope with the pain? Will you make a fool of yourself in labour? How will your partner manage? Will they follow your birth plan? What happens if you have complications and need a caesarean? How long will you stay in hospital?

When worries strike, take a few deep breaths and just visualise yourself holding your new baby. If you find that hard, take a look at those tiny baby clothes you have ready. That will remind you why you are on this journey.

Will my breasts do the job?

If you're not generously endowed in the boob department, don't worry about your ability to breastfeed. Most differences in breast size are down to the different amounts of fat in the breasts. You need milk-producing and storing tissue to make milk, and this is laid down in pregnancy. Most women find this means their breasts do get bigger, especially towards the end of their pregnancy. Even with this extra growth, some women still have smallish breasts at the end. They are just as likely as anyone else to breastfeed effectively.

Flat or inverted nipples shouldn't cause difficulties with breastfeeding, either, though you may find you are a little sore in the early stages. Preparing your breasts before birth with breast shells or nipple-rolling exercises seems to make little difference. In any case, you often find that flat nipples stand out when your baby feeds because of the drawing-out action of his jaws.

Like all new mums, you'll need help latching your baby onto the breast for the first few feeds. He has to learn how to open his mouth wide so that he draws in a deep mouthful of breast. Discuss this with your midwife before you have your baby, to be sure you get the right help once he is born.

Flat or inverted nipples can sometimes be drawn out if you use a breast pump before feeds.

If you do experience problems, using a breast pump before feeds may help to draw out inverted nipples. And avoid engorgement as far as possible so that your baby can "practise" while your breasts are soft. Speak to your midwife or breastfeeding counsellor if you need help with this.

10% of women have flat or inverted nipples but this won't prevent you from breastfeeding. If one nipple is flatter than the other, your baby may prefer the more accessible side, but persevere.

ParentsAsk...

What's my risk of getting MRSA in hospital?

Despite many mums' worries, the risk of being infected by a superbug such as MRSA in a maternity unit is very low. MRSA infections are more likely to occur in hospital patients who are elderly or seriously ill, or who have an open wound from an operation. Maternity ward patients tend to be young and healthy.

If you're planning to have a caesarean, or if you end up having an emergency caesarean, you may be offered a swab test to see whether you're carrying MRSA. If you're found to be a carrier, you'll be treated with an antibacterial wash and special nose cream to get rid of the bacteria and reduce your risk of a wound infection.

You may also be screened for MRSA if your baby is likely to need care in the neonatal unit. This is to reduce the risk of MRSA spreading among babies who are already vulnerable.

If you are a carrier, there is no chance that your baby can catch MRSA from you in the womb, and it's very unlikely that he'll pick up the infection from you when he's born. Only sick or premature babies, or babies who have had surgery, are more susceptible to infection.

In hospital, you can take precautions to reduce the risk of infection.

Getting ready for pregnancy

Staying safe and healthy

Your pregnancy diary

Birth and beyond

Different mums, different worries

Becoming a parent isn't always easy. And if you are a young parent, you may find that the changes ahead are even more challenging. Make sure you build a strong support network around you and take up any offers of help (including financial) that you are given.

Concerns of very young mums

If you're still only in your teens, one of the most difficult aspects of pregnancy is the sense of isolation. Your parents' first reaction to the news may have been shock or rejection, rather than delight. You may also be the first in your group of friends to be pregnant and feel as if you have little in common with them any more, which can make you feel very lonely. Pregnancy can be scary and confusing at the best of times. But having no one to confide in and share the experience with can make coping with the big physical and hormonal changes doubly difficult.

Not only that, but expecting a baby in your teens can disrupt your school or college studies. It could even force you to postpone or abandon your career dreams. If you have a partner, you might also worry that having a baby on the way will put too much pressure on your relationship, and that your partner may leave you to bring up the baby alone.

But with the right support you can overcome many of these challenges. Often, after the initial shock, parents come around to the idea of their own "baby" being pregnant. A supportive mum or dad helps to ensure you get the right antenatal care. Teachers, too, can push for special provision to help you continue your studies if possible. And

Financial help for young mums

One of your concerns if you're very young and pregnant may well be money. Don't despair. Financial help is available if you know where to look for it.

● **Income Support** If you're aged over 16 and under 19, you can apply for Income Support. This kicks in 11 weeks before your baby is due and you may be able to apply earlier if you've been ill. You'll also qualify for the Sure Start Maternity Grant.

● **Benefits while continuing in education** If you're continuing your education you may be entitled to some benefits. These include Education Maintenance Allowances. The government's Care to Learn programme

also provides childcare and additional travel-cost benefits for 16 to 19-year-old parents who are still in education.

● **Child maintenance** If you're a single parent, you can apply for child maintenance. Visit the Child Support Agency's website to find out more. The One Parent Families website has a useful online helpdesk and also prints a Lone Parent Handbook. If you're single parent living in Scotland, One Parent Families Scotland has its own website.

● **Where to go for help** If you can't understand the system, you can ask for help from independent and council-run welfare rights advice agencies, disability organisations, and law centres.

Single mum

If you're single and pregnant, you may feel lonely and worried. Try turning to a best friend.

"Being single and pregnant is really scary. I always imagined I'd be sharing this experience with someone I loved, and who loved me. I've been feeling very lonely and have been panicking about money as well. I've got some savings and a job that'll provide good maternity pay, but I'm still concerned I'll struggle while I'm on leave. Above all, I'm terrified of being alone when I go into labour. Luckily, my best friend has offered to move in with me for the last couple of weeks of my pregnancy."

Parents may be shocked at first, but most will eventually offer the support you need.

your friends and partner can help by just listening and being there for you through your emotional ups and downs.

Remember – all new mums struggle. But with youth on your side, you probably have more energy than most to cope with the physical demands of pregnancy and having a child!

Parents**Talk**...

"I dreaded telling my mum and dad I was pregnant. Having a baby at 15 certainly hadn't been part of my life plan. I couldn't believe my parents' reaction, though, when they found out. They just hugged me and told me not to feel anxious because they were going to support me every step of the way."
Mae, 17, mum to two-year-old Ben

"My mum and dad weren't best pleased when I told them I was pregnant at just 16. When they'd had time to take it all in and realise how scared I was, though, they became much more supportive. They were with me at every scan and my mum was my birth partner. I just know that I couldn't have got through it without them."
Bella, 17, mum to three-month-old Dee

"I fell pregnant at 18 and was so worried I was going to lose my friends because all our nights out revolved around drinking and clubbing. They were amazing, though, and organised more DVD nights and lunches, specially for me. Now my son is here, one of my friends will often offer to babysit so I can have a night off and go out with the others."
Sophie, 19, mum to four-month-old Josh

"I was absolutely terrified as I was expected to take my GCSEs the week my baby was due. My form tutor was amazing, though, and arranged it with the exam board so I could take them a year later. I'm pleased to say I now have nine GCSEs and, thanks to mum's help with my lovely baby, I'm doing A levels!"
Amy, 17, continuing in education

Concerns of second-time mums

If you're already mum to a toddler, you may wonder how he's going to take to being an older sibling. It can be hard for him but you can ward off upsets by telling him about the coming birth.

Four or five weeks before is a good time to talk to your toddler. Explain what will happen once the baby arrives, and get him involved in the preparations. For example, invite him to help you make simple decisions, such as whether he thinks the baby would prefer bunnies or ducks on the nursery curtains.

Once your baby comes home, try to involve your toddler in looking after her. He can help you hold towels or fetch

nappies. When she cries, he can sing or talk gently to her. Ask him for advice and help, too: "Do you think the baby would like to wear her red hat or her white one?" And set aside some time each day to do something just with him, even if it's only a few minutes of drawing or building with blocks.

Your toddler will sometimes feel jealous. Don't be surprised if he hits or throws something at his new sibling. Make sure you prevent him from hurting the baby, and encourage him to talk about how he feels. Tell him that it's natural to feel this way, but make it clear that trying to hurt the baby is not OK.

Inviting your toddler to get involved in preparing for your new baby's arrival can help him get used to the idea.

Getting ready for pregnancy

Staying safe and healthy

Your pregnancy diary

Birth and beyond

Recurring pregnancy problems

It's very normal to feel anxious at certain points in your pregnancy, particularly if you experienced problems last time round. Do bear in mind that every pregnancy is different and you and your baby will almost certainly be fine. If you do feel concerned, talk to your midwife.

I've had a problem pregnancy before

If you had difficulties with your last pregnancy or birth, it's natural to feel a little anxious this time around. Try to remember that this experience is different. Stay positive and look forward to your future with this baby.

Miscarriage

Most women who have had a miscarriage (see pp.42–3) go on to have healthy pregnancies. Even women with unexplained recurrent miscarriages (three or more in a row) have about a 75 per cent chance of having a healthy pregnancy next time.

When you have had a miscarriage, it's normal to worry that you might lose this baby, too. It may be particularly stressful up to the stage where you lost your baby last time. You will probably feel more sad and anxious as the date approaches, and that's perfectly normal and understandable. Don't be too hard on yourself for not feeling happy all the time, especially during the first weeks. Allow yourself to vent your feelings; a good cry now and then will help to relieve a lot of tension.

Stillbirth

If you've had an unexplained stillbirth, it may be comforting to know that there is no increased risk of it happening again. But of course you will want to take every precaution possible to make sure this baby is healthy. Eating well (see pp.48–51, 120–21, 148–9 and 182–3), giving up smoking, drugs and alcohol (see pp.118–19) and looking after yourself are the best ways there are of protecting your baby. You may have extra antenatal appointments and tests as well, partly to reassure you and partly to pick up any problems early. And your midwife and doctor will understand if you need to check out any twinges or spotting straight away.

Caesarean

If you had a caesarean section (see pp.288–91) last time, you may wonder about a vaginal birth this time. Occasionally there is a recurring problem (such as having a very small pelvis), which means you have to have another caesarean.

Parents**Talk...**

"I had a miscarriage six months ago when I was nine weeks pregnant with my first child. I was so scared when the bleeding started and, as the hours ticked by, it gradually became heavier and heavier. I called my doctor and a scan revealed that I had lost my baby. I never even knew if I was having a boy or a girl, although for some reason I feel strongly that it was a boy. I'm now in the early stages of my second pregnancy and I feel so nervous that I'm going to lose this one, too."
Renée, 28, pregnant for a second time

"I had high blood pressure when I was pregnant and, at 30 weeks, they found protein in my urine. I had to have an emergency caesarean and Kieran was whisked off to the Special Care Baby Unit. I found it hard to bond because it was ages before I could hold him. I'm scared it'll end up the same this time round. I took plenty of exercise and got my diet on track before I fell pregnant this time, though, and, so far, thank heavens, my blood pressure has been fine. Fingers crossed!"
Joanna, 31, mum to Kieran

About 75 per cent of women who choose to have a vaginal birth after a first baby by caesarean (VBAC) go on to have a successful vaginal birth. If you've had a previous vaginal birth, you will have an even higher success rate of up to 90 per cent.

You also have a better chance of a vaginal birth if you previously had a caesarean for one of these reasons as they are unlikely to reoccur:

- Your baby was in the breech position (see pp.286–7).
- Your baby was becoming tired and distressed during labour.
- Your labour happened very slowly.
- Your induction failed.
- You requested a caesarean.

Midwives and doctors do tend to be a bit more cautious during labour if you have had a caesarean section. This is because of a very small risk (one in 200) of the scar from your last caesarean tearing during contractions. This is called uterine rupture. It will probably mean that you and your next baby will be monitored closely during labour.

Premature baby

If you have had a premature baby (see pp.280–81) before, you are slightly more at risk of having another premature baby. That can be a worrying thought,

but the risk only increases a little. The general rate of premature births for all women is about 10 per cent, but if you have had a premature baby before, it rises to about 20 per cent. But, of course, you may be one of the lucky 80 per cent of women who do not go on to have another premature birth.

Having had a premature birth already means that your increased awareness of what might happen will play an important role in monitoring your new pregnancy, particularly when you get to the same stage in pregnancy when your last premature labour started. And that increased awareness also means that you can take extra care with your diet, avoid smoking and other risky activities, and make sure you get to all your antenatal appointments.

If you've had a premature birth, there is a slight risk that you will have another one. You'll be better prepared the second time.

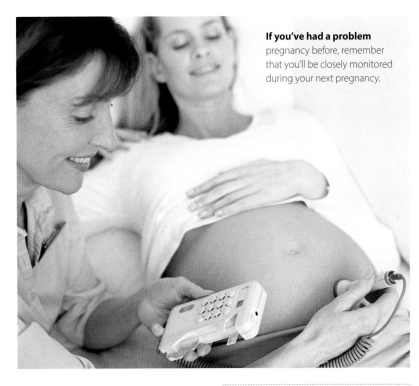

If you've had a problem pregnancy before, remember that you'll be closely monitored during your next pregnancy.

Dad's **Diary**

Fourth time lucky?

"After having three miscarriages (two in the second trimester) in the past two years, my partner and I can't help but worry that this pregnancy might end the same way. Leandra had a vaginal scan early in this pregnancy and it revealed that she may have a weakened cervix. The doctor advised us to have a cervical stitch inserted as a precautionary measure after 14 weeks. We know it doesn't work for everyone, and that there are risks involved, but it has made us feel more positive that we'll carry this baby to full term.

We're still extremely cautious, though. It's hard for Leandra – and me! – not to worry about every twinge or if she gets any vaginal discharge. We're regularly in touch with our midwife. She's given us lots of support, and we're not afraid to call her if we're at all worried."

Getting ready for pregnancy

Staying safe and healthy

Your pregnancy diary

Birth and beyond

Genetic disorders

Having a genetic disorder may mean that you need extra care during pregnancy. It could also mean that your baby is affected by the same disorder as you, so you and your partner will have some serious thinking to do. Your doctors and midwives will support you with this.

I've got a genetic disorder

If you have a genetic disorder, you may feel anxious about whether or not your baby will be affected. You are probably already an expert on your condition. Talk with your specialist, midwife or doctor to see if it may affect your baby.

Thalassaemia

Thalassaemia is a genetic blood disorder that causes the body to make fewer healthy red blood cells and less haemoglobin (the iron-rich protein in red blood cells). If you have thalassaemia during pregnancy, you might be more prone to iron-deficiency anaemia (see p.229). Certain kinds of thalassaemia can affect blood test results, causing them to indicate that your iron stores are low when they are not. As a result, you should have additional blood tests to confirm that you are iron-deficient before you take iron tablets. If you have thalassaemia, you will also benefit from taking 5 milligrams (mg) of folic acid a day.

Your baby can be tested for thalassaemia during pregnancy using a diagnostic test, such as chorionic villus sampling (CVS; see p.136) or amniocentesis (see p.147). If you or your

---

ParentsAsk...

Should I seek genetic counselling?
You may want to talk to a genetic counsellor before you try for a baby if you, your partner, your children, or any other family member has an inherited condition, such as cystic fibrosis or sickle cell anaemia.

A genetic counsellor is a medical professional who can help you sort through complex information about your chances of having a child with a genetic disorder or birth defect and about the testing, treatment and other options available. The counsellor's role is to explain the technical and scientific information you need to understand to make informed choices.

If you are already pregnant and your baby has been diagnosed with a genetic disorder through antenatal testing such as CVS (see p.136) or amniocentesis (see p.147), there will be a counsellor available to offer you support and guidance. Genetic counsellors are trained to work with you and your family to help you absorb, digest and understand information. They can put the risks in perspective by giving you information and helping you articulate your feelings.

Genetic counsellors won't make any decisions for you, nor will they suggest that you follow any particular course of action. A good counsellor will explain to you the outlook for a child with an abnormality and will describe the treatments that might be necessary, both immediately after birth and throughout the child's life. Once you have understood all the facts, it will be up to you to decide what to do.

Carrier screening

Carrier screening is a special type of testing that's done to ascertain if you or your partner carry a genetic mutation that could cause a serious inherited disorder in your baby. Some of the more common disorders that are screened for include cystic fibrosis, sickle cell disease and thalassaemia.

These disorders are recessive, which means that a person must inherit a defective gene from each parent to have the disease. If you're a carrier of a defective gene for a recessive disorder, that means you have one normal copy of the gene from one of your parents and one defective copy from the other. (Carriers don't usually have any symptoms of the disease.)

If both you and your partner are carriers of a disorder such as cystic fibrosis or sickle cell disease, your child will have a one in four chance of inheriting one defective gene from each of you and of having the disease. This is why some people choose to find out if they are carriers for certain diseases.

Risk factors include having a family member with the inherited disorder (or a family member who's a known carrier) or being part of an ethnic group at increased risk for the disease.

If you opt for this kind of screening, you'll probably be asked to give a blood or saliva sample first. Then, if you're found to be a carrier, your partner will be screened as well. (Both partners may be screened at the same time to get the results faster.)

You can have a screening test to see if you are a carrier of a genetic mutation that might be passed on to your baby.

---

baby is tested for thalassaemia, you will be offered counselling to help you to make the necessary informed medical and personal decisions.

Cystic fibrosis

Cystic fibrosis (CF) is an inherited condition that affects the internal organs, especially the lungs and digestive system, by clogging them with thick, sticky mucus. This makes it hard to breathe and digest food.

If you have CF, pregnancy shouldn't adversely affect your health provided your CF is mild to moderate. If it is severe, you are more likely to develop pregnancy complications. It is important to continue your treatment for CF throughout your pregnancy to get the best outcome for both you and your baby. Sign up for antenatal care as soon as possible so an appointment with an obstetric team that has experience in CF can be made for you early on. They will monitor the growth and

development of your baby, and will review and adjust your medication if necessary. If both you and your partner are known to be carriers or affected by CF, you will usually be offered a diagnostic test, such as CVS (see p.136), during pregnancy, to see if your baby is also affected.

Sickle cell anaemia

Sickle cell anaemia is an inherited condition. People affected by it have abnormal haemoglobin, which causes their red blood cells to become misshapen or "sickled". These sickled cells then get stuck in the tiny blood vessels, blocking the flow of blood and producing pain.

For sickle cell anaemia to affect your child, both parents must carry the gene responsible for sickle cell, and are usually Asian, African, Caribbean, Mediterranean or from the Middle East.

It is possible to test an unborn child for sickle cell from as early as 11 weeks

50%

is the chance that a baby who has one parent with thalassaemia minor has of inheriting the gene defect from the parent and of also being a carrier. Babies who inherit the gene disorder from both parents have a double dose of the gene and can sometimes have thalassaemia major.

of pregnancy by using tests such as amniocentesis (see p.147) and CVS (see p.136). Fetal blood sampling is usually carried out between 15 and 23 weeks of pregnancy, but it may be carried out at any time up to delivery. Your doctor will be able to give you more information.

If your baby has sickle cell, he may need to take penicillin every day to prevent infections. Children with sickle cell disorder also need folic acid to help them make blood and prevent them from becoming run down.

Getting ready for pregnancy

Staying safe and healthy

Your pregnancy diary

Birth and beyond

Medical problems in pregnancy

Some women bloom during pregnancy, feeling better than ever, but for others it can be a time of discomfort and worry. You and your baby are vulnerable to common infections, and your body may no longer feel your own, as you adapt to the physical changes of pregnancy.

There are many physical conditions that are linked with pregnancy that are neither serious nor lasting, but which can make life when you're pregnant a bit of a drag. During pregnancy your body has to adapt to the changes in your hormone levels, your circulation, and the increasing weight that you're carrying. These changes are great for looking after your baby, and preparing for labour, but some of them may not feel quite so great for you.

Physical changes

Inside your abdomen, everything shifts to make room for your growing baby. Your organs and bowels are squashed up or pushed to one side, and you'll feel extra pressure on your bladder or stomach depending on your baby's position. It's amazing how your body adapts but it can be an uncomfortable experience, causing pain, indigestion and incontinence.

The blood volume in your circulation increases during pregnancy and the tissues in your muscles and joints also take on more fluid. You may notice some swelling in your ankles and other parts of your body.

The hormone relaxin (see p.74) makes your ligaments and joints more mobile and flexible, so there is room for your baby to move through your pelvis during labour. The down side to this is that it can make some parts of your body too loose, resulting in pain, and problems with your pelvis and other joints. Pregnancy hormones also have an effect on the walls of your veins and arteries, which is why varicose veins and piles are another common complaint of pregnancy. All these physical changes can be uncomfortable, painful and embarrassing, but most of them will clear up in the hours, days or weeks following your baby's birth.

Infections in pregnancy

Infections can be much more significant during pregnancy. First, your immune system doesn't work so well so you're more vulnerable to them. Second, you may find it harder to get rid of an illness. Third, you're more likely to develop complications with some infections, which you'd have sailed through if you weren't pregnant. Finally, an infection that is fairly harmless to you may be dangerous for your growing baby.

Some infections only cause a problem if you catch them at a certain stage of pregnancy. For some infections, there are treatments that can reduce the risk of harm to your baby while, for others, you just have to wait and see if your baby is going to be OK. In many cases, there are things that you can do to prevent you getting an infection in the first place, such as avoiding certain foods (see pp.52–3) and following good personal hygiene. You may also already be immune to some infections, so your baby will be protected by the antibodies in your blood.

The changes in your body during pregnancy help your developing baby, but may make you feel unwell.

Infections

Chickenpox

Chickenpox is a mild but highly infectious disease that usually affects children. If you had it as a child, you probably have no reason to worry. Your body will have developed antibodies to the virus, making you immune to further infection. However, if you think that you've never had the virus before, you should avoid contact with people with chickenpox. This is because the virus can lead to serious complications for you and your baby. You also need to be aware that you can catch chickenpox from someone who has shingles, which is a related condition caused by the same virus as chickenpox.

Causes Chickenpox is an illness caused by the varicella-zoster virus (VZV). It usually spreads via sneezes and coughs from an infected person.

Symptoms The commonest symptom of chickenpox is a red rash. Other symptoms may include nausea, fever and aching, painful muscles. Chickenpox can be more severe if you catch it while pregnant, and you are more likely to develop dangerous complications, such as pneumonia.

There are other potential problems if the virus affects your baby during pregnancy or as a newborn. These may include eye problems and shortened limbs. Possible neurological problems may also mean your baby is slow to reach his developmental milestones.

Treatment Your doctor may offer you acyclovir, an anti-viral treatment that reduces the severity and duration of chickenpox, but only if it is given within 24 hours of you developing a rash. If you are less than 20 weeks pregnant, doctors probably won't recommend it because there's a risk it will affect your baby.

Amniocentesis can show whether there are signs of the virus in your amniotic fluid, but this does not necessarily mean that your baby was infected. Your doctor may arrange for you to have a detailed ultrasound scan to check that your baby's vital organs look healthy.

Cytomegalovirus (CMV)

At least 50 per cent of women already have antibodies to CMV before they become pregnant, meaning they were previously infected. Most people with CMV don't develop any symptoms, so you probably wouldn't know if you'd ever been infected.

Causes CMV is a common virus that is part of the herpes family of viruses. It's spread through bodily fluids such as saliva and urine, and can be transmitted from person to person through close bodily contact.

Symptoms Most people don't know when they have a CMV infection. Those who do know tend to have symptoms such as fever, swollen glands and a sore throat. You may also feel tired and achy.

CMV is the virus most frequently passed to babies during pregnancy. About 1 to 4 per cent of previously uninfected women have a first (or primary) CMV infection during pregnancy. Among these women there's about a 30 to 50 per cent chance that the baby will become infected in the uterus.

Most babies won't have any symptoms at birth or develop any CMV-related problems later on. However, some babies born with CMV are very ill at birth and may end up with a number of long-term problems. Others may seem fine initially but develop hearing loss or other complications months or even years later.

Treatment There are blood tests to check for CMV, but you would only have one in certain circumstances, for example, if you suspect you've recently been exposed to CMV. If the blood tests show that you've had a recent infection, you'll get a thorough ultrasound to look for CMV-related abnormalities in your developing baby or the placenta. You may also have amniocentesis to see if your baby has CMV, but this test won't tell you whether your baby will develop health problems from the infection.

Flu

Flu (or influenza) is a viral disease of the lungs and upper airways. The symptoms of flu – fever, headaches, chills, achiness, fatigue and loss of appetite – can really lay you low when pregnant. This is your body's way of telling you that you need to take it easy.

Causes The flu virus is usually spread in the small droplets of saliva coughed or sneezed into the air by an infected person. Direct contact can also spread infection. It takes an average of two days to go from being infected to having the full symptoms.

Symptoms The main symptoms are a high temperature that comes on quickly, and general aches and pains. You may also experience a loss of appetite, nausea and a harsh dry cough. Your symptoms will usually peak after two to three days and you should begin to feel much better within five to eight days.

Treatment If you develop flu-like symptoms, speak to your midwife or doctor. It's important to keep your temperature as normal as possible while you are pregnant, so avoid the temptation to sweat it out snuggled under a duvet.

Paracetamol helps to lower fever and is safe to take at the recommended dose. Make sure you drink plenty of water and juice, get plenty of rest and give yourself time to recover completely. Always ask your pharmacist's advice before buying over-the-counter cold and flu remedies since some are not suitable for pregnant women.

The flu jab used in the UK is prepared from an inactivated virus and there is no evidence that it's harmful to unborn babies. However, as with all drugs in pregnancy, it's recommended that you don't have it unless there is a clear medical indication, for example, if you have asthma.

Genital herpes in pregnancy

If you suffer from genital herpes there is a very small risk that your baby will catch the infection and, if she does, the results can be serious. That's why it is important to tell your midwife if you or your partner have ever had genital herpes. Extra care can then be taken of you and your baby.

Causes Genital herpes is usually caused by herpes simplex virus type 2 (HSV-2). It's usually spread during sexual activity.

Symptoms Most people with the herpes simplex virus (HSV) do not experience any symptoms when they are first infected. If you do get symptoms, they may include:

● Painful sores over your genitals and buttocks.

● Itching.

● Stinging when passing urine.

● Vaginal discharge.

● Swollen glands in the groin area.

● Flu-like symptoms including fever, headache and aching muscles.

With a second or later infection you may get no symptoms at all, or just a small area of irritation.

Treatment If you catch genital herpes for the first time in the first or second trimester of your pregnancy, there is a slight risk of complications such as miscarriage, intrauterine growth retardation (IUGR) and premature labour. Your doctor will probably give you a five-day course of an anti-viral medicine, usually acyclovir. This is safe to use in pregnancy.

Your baby is at greater risk if you catch genital herpes for the first time in late pregnancy. She can catch the virus through direct contact with an active sore during birth. If you suspect you have an active genital herpes infection in the last trimester of pregnancy it is vital that you tell your midwife or doctor. You may be advised to have a planned caesarean section to minimise the risk of transmitting the virus to your baby. If you caught herpes early in your pregnancy, and it has been successfully treated, you will still be able to have a vaginal birth.

Group B Streptococcus

Group B streptococcus, also known as group B strep or GBS, is one of the many bacteria that normally live in our bodies. In certain rare cases GBS can cause serious illness and even death in newborn babies.

Causes Approximately one third of the population "carry" the GBS bacterium in their intestines without even knowing. About a quarter of all women also have it in their vagina. Most don't know it is there, but it can spread to your baby during birth and can cause a serious infection.

Symptoms Because GBS usually causes no symptoms, pregnant women often find out that they have it by chance, perhaps when they have a vaginal swab taken to check for something else.

Most babies exposed to GBS before or during birth also suffer no ill effects. However, around one in 2,000 babies in the UK develops a GBS infection. Sadly, about one in 10 of these babies die. GBS infections in babies usually happen within seven days of birth, with 90 per cent occurring within 12 hours of birth. Typical signs of GBS in newborns include: grunting when breathing, poor feeding, lethargy, irritability, low blood pressure and an abnormally high or low temperature, heart rate or breathing rate.

Treatment If you are found to be carrying GBS, talk to your midwife or obstetrician and agree a pregnancy and birth plan that will protect your baby from the infection. Women in higher-risk situations – for example, those who go into labour prematurely – can be given intravenous antibiotics either from the start of labour or from when their waters break (whichever comes first) until their baby is born.

If your baby is at higher risk of developing a GBS infection, a paediatrician should examine him immediately he is born. He may be put on intravenous antibiotics until he's given the all clear.

Hepatitis B

Hepatitis B is a virus that can cause chronic inflammation of the liver. It can also be transmitted to your baby at birth. If you have an acute attack of hepatitis B during pregnancy, or if you are a carrier, you will be at risk of premature labour.

Causes Hepatitis B is spread via the blood or body fluids from someone who has the virus. Many people with hepatitis B do not even realise that they are infected. Because hepatitis B is transmitted through blood and body fluids and especially during sexual intercourse, those most at risk are people who have had unprotected sex with several different sexual partners, drug users who use intravenous drugs, people who have been tattooed with dirty needles and health professionals who may come into contact with the blood of an infected person.

Symptoms An infected person may be jaundiced so that their skin and the whites of their eyes have a yellowish tinge. Sometimes the symptoms are simply loss of appetite and tummy pain, which are difficult to distinguish from flu or a mild bout of food poisoning.

Treatment When you go for your booking visit, your midwife will probably take a blood test for hepatitis B. If it shows that you are a carrier, you may be referred to a specialist for advice. Since carriers are at risk of liver disease, you should continue to receive follow-up appointments after you have given birth.

Your baby will be washed thoroughly after he is born to remove all traces of your blood and he will then be treated immediately with hepatitis B vaccine. These precautions almost always prevent the infection from being passed to your baby. If he is not treated, your baby risks going on to develop serious liver disease.

HIV and AIDS in pregnancy

HIV stands for human immunodeficiency virus. Most people who have HIV do not have any symptoms and the only way of telling they are infected is by testing their blood for antibodies. AIDS stands for acquired immune-deficiency syndrome. People develop AIDS when their immune system has been so damaged by the HIV virus that they start to catch lots of other infections.

Causes The HIV virus is passed from person to person during sex and through body fluids, such as blood and breastmilk. It can also be passed from a woman to her unborn baby during pregnancy and birth.

An unborn baby has about a one in four chance of catching HIV if his mother is HIV positive and does not receive any treatment or interventions to stop the virus.

Symptoms When you first catch the HIV virus you may experience symptoms such as a fever, sore throat, tiredness and swollen glands. These symptoms are often very mild, so it is easy to mistake them for another condition, such as a cold. After these initial symptoms, you will probably have no other symptoms for years.

Eventually, though, the virus will damage your immune system, leading to symptoms such as chronic tiredness, night sweats, weight loss, diarrhoea and shortness of breath.

Treatment In the UK, most women who are HIV positive are identified before or during pregnancy. If you are HIV positive, you will be offered specialist care and regular check ups while pregnant. You will also be offered treatment in the form of anti-retroviral drugs. These interventions can greatly reduce the chance of your baby catching the infection from you during pregnancy and birth.

Having a caesarean reduces the risk of your baby catching HIV during the birth, but if your HIV is well managed then a vaginal birth may not increase the risk to your baby.

Rubella (German measles)

Although rubella is a relatively mild illness, it's very dangerous for a pregnant woman as it can lead to all sorts of problems in your baby. Fortunately in the UK, the majority of women in their child-bearing years are immune to the disease, either because they were vaccinated against it as a child or because they have already had the illness. Since immunisation was introduced, the number of pregnancies complicated by rubella has shown a significant decrease.

Causes Rubella is a very infectious disease. The virus is passed on via droplets in the air from the coughs and sneezes of infected people. It used to be common in young children.

Symptoms Rubella causes a pinkish-red rash that first appears on the face and then spreads elsewhere on the body. Other symptoms – which usually appear before the rash – include a temperature, conjunctivitis and swollen glands. Up to half of people don't get any symptoms.

When an unborn baby is affected, it has what is called congenital rubella syndrome (CRS). This can lead to:

- Cataracts and other eye defects.
- Deafness.
- Heart abnormalities.
- A smaller head than normal (microcephaly).
- Restricted growth.
- Damage to the brain, liver, lungs and bone marrow.

Luckily, due to the high uptake of the rubella vaccine, CRS is now very rare.

Treatment If you know that you are not immune to rubella, you should, if at all possible, be vaccinated before you become pregnant. If your lack of immunity has been picked up from a blood test in early pregnancy, you'll have to wait until you've had your baby before you can be vaccinated.

Unfortunately, if you do catch the disease during pregnancy, there's nothing that can be done to protect your baby. Your midwife will talk to you about what tests can be done to find out whether your baby has been damaged. Sadly, you may want to consider terminating the pregnancy.

Getting ready for pregnancy

Staying safe and healthy

Your pregnancy diary

Birth and beyond

Slapped cheek syndrome

The chances are that you've already had slapped cheek syndrome, since most people are exposed to the virus in childhood some time between the ages of three and five. Slapped cheek syndrome is also called erythema infectiosum or fifth disease.

Causes Slapped cheek is passed from person to person in saliva, through close contact or via the air, such as through coughing and sneezing. It is highly contagious and can spread quickly through schools or nurseries.

Symptoms In children, slapped cheek disease may cause mild respiratory symptoms, which are sometimes accompanied by a temperature. A distinctive blotchy red rash may begin to appear on the face, which gives the appearance of "slapped cheeks". Once the facial rash has appeared, the disease is no longer contagious.

Adults may have no symptoms at all, or they might experience a sore throat, headache, itching or fever. Very occasionally, slapped cheek disease causes painful joints.

It's rare but, if caught between nine and 20 weeks of pregnancy, the virus can cause a condition called hydrops fetalis in unborn babies. This is when an unusual amount of fluid builds up in a developing baby's tissues and organs, and it can be picked up by an ultrasound scan. Sometimes a baby can recover from this condition on her own and is born healthy but, occasionally, she may need a blood transfusion to improve her chances of survival.

Treatment A blood test will be able to determine if you're immune, but can't tell whether you have been exposed to the disease during your pregnancy or many years ago.

If your blood test proves positive and you're in the first 20 weeks of your pregnancy, you will be offered extra ultrasounds because your risk of miscarriage is higher. If your baby develops hydrops fetalis, a blood transfusion in the uterus may help.

Urinary tract infections (UTIs)

About 50 per cent of women will have at least one UTI during their lifetime. If left untreated, UTIs can be quite painful – and even dangerous because the infection can travel upwards and reach the kidneys. If a kidney infection is left untreated during pregnancy it could make you very ill and could lead to your baby being born with a low birth weight or being born prematurely.

Causes A UTI is caused when bacteria infect the urinary system. The changes your body goes through during pregnancy make you more susceptible to UTIs. Progesterone relaxes the muscles of your ureters, the tubes that connect your kidneys to your bladder. This slows down the flow of urine from your kidneys to your bladder. Your enlarging uterus has the same effect. This is an ideal opportunity for bacteria because they have more time to grow before they're flushed out.

Symptoms Indications of a UTI include pain when passing urine, a feeling that you are unable to urinate fully, a raised temperature and a frequent need to go to the toilet. Signs that the infection has spread to your kidneys might include a high temperature and constant pain in the area of one or both of your kidneys.

Treatment UTIs can be safely treated with antibiotics during pregnancy. You will probably be prescribed a three to seven-day course. Talk to your doctor or midwife as soon as you notice any symptoms because an untreated UTI can lead to a kidney infection, which may in turn cause premature labour. To reduce the risk of getting a UTI, wipe yourself from front to back after going to the loo to prevent bacteria from the back passage being spread to the front passage. Drink plenty of fluids, and empty your bladder completely when you go to the toilet. Wear cotton pants and avoid tights.

Certain infections don't put your baby at risk. You may just need to rest, drink plenty and keep your temperature down. Check any medication is safe with your doctor.

Conditions in pregnancy

Anaemia (iron deficiency)

During pregnancy, you need extra iron to keep you and your baby healthy (see p.121). If you don't have enough iron for both of you, you may develop iron-deficiency anaemia. One in five women develop this when they are pregnant.

Causes Women who have a diet that is low in iron (see p.149) are likely to become anaemic. You are also more likely to have iron-deficiency anaemia in pregnancy if your body's iron supplies have already been depleted, perhaps because you've had two or more pregnancies close together, or you had heavy periods before you became pregnant. If you're carrying more than one baby then the demands of each baby can also increase your risk of getting anaemia.

Symptoms You may not be aware that you have become anaemic, although fatigue and breathlessness are common signs. However, these are symptoms also experienced by many pregnant women who are not anaemic.

Headaches, tinnitus and palpitations are other symptoms of anaemia, along with unusual food cravings. Your eyelids, nail beds and tongue may also look pale.

Unless you are severely anaemic, you don't need to worry about your baby's health. Your body will make sure that your baby gets her quota of iron before you get yours.

Treatment You shouldn't need to take iron supplements if you take care to have a diet rich in iron. This means eating lots of dark green leafy vegetables, wholemeal bread, iron-fortified cereals, lean red meat, raisins, prunes and pulses.

Vitamin C helps your body absorb the iron in your diet. Try drinking plenty of orange juice or eating fruit or vegetables that are rich in vitamin C when you have an iron-rich meal. This is particularly important if you don't eat meat as the iron in meat is easily absorbed, but iron in vegetables is not. Tea and coffee make it difficult for your body to absorb iron, so it's best not to drink them at mealtimes.

If your iron levels drop very low your doctor will prescribe iron supplements.

Gestational diabetes

Gestational diabetes is diabetes that develops for the first time during pregnancy. It affects somewhere between 2 and 14 per cent of pregnancies. Unlike other types of diabetes, gestational diabetes usually resolves itself after your baby is born.

Causes Diabetes develops when the body can't produce enough insulin, a hormone made by the pancreas. Insulin regulates the sugar in the blood. During pregnancy your body has to produce extra insulin to meet your baby's needs. If your body can't manage this, you will have too much sugar in your blood and may develop gestational diabetes.

You are in a high-risk group for developing diabetes in pregnancy if your body mass index (BMI; see pp.72–3) is above 30.

Symptoms Gestational diabetes often doesn't produce any symptoms, but you may experience the following:

- Tiredness.
- Excessive thirst.
- Passing a lot of urine.
- Blurred vision.

The main problem with having too much sugar in your blood is that it crosses the placenta to your baby, which means that there is a small risk that he could grow very large. A big baby may make labour and birth more difficult and you may end up needing to have a caesarean section.

Babies affected by too much blood sugar during pregnancy may have low blood sugar (hypoglycaemia) or jaundice after birth. Babies born to mothers with diabetes are also more prone to obesity and type 2 diabetes later in life.

Treatment In most cases, you can manage the condition by changing your diet and taking regular exercise. In about 10 to 20 per cent of cases of gestational diabetes, the condition can't be controlled by diet and exercise and you'll either need to take medication to control your blood sugar levels or to inject insulin.

Gestational hypertension

If you develop high blood pressure after 20 weeks of pregnancy and you don't have protein in your urine, you will be diagnosed with gestational hypertension (high blood pressure in pregnancy, as distinct from chronic hypertension). Gestational hypertension is usually diagnosed if you have two consecutive blood pressure readings of above 140/90.

Causes Caused by the extra stress that pregnancy places on your body, gestational hypertension is usually mild and probably won't cause any obvious problems for you or your baby.

Gestational hypertension is more common in women who are overweight. Around 10 per cent of obese women (BMI of 30 or above; see pp.72–3) will have gestational hypertension, compared with around 4 per cent of women with a BMI of 19 to 25.

Symptoms You probably won't notice

Getting ready for pregnancy · Staying safe and healthy · Your pregnancy diary · Birth and beyond any symptoms. However, the earlier in pregnancy it sets in, the greater your risk of having a small-for-dates baby, or of it developing into pre-eclampsia (see p.233) The risk of pre-eclampsia is increased if you are obese or overweight, and have put on a lot of weight during pregnancy.

Treatment It's very important to attend all your antenatal appointments, as your doctor or midwife will take your blood pressure at each visit. If you have either gestational or chronic hypertension, they will monitor your health closely, and your doctor may prescribe drugs (which won't harm your baby) to lower your blood pressure.

If your blood pressure was normal before you became pregnant, it will most likely return to normal within 12 weeks of your baby being born. If it doesn't return to normal, then the original diagnosis of gestational hypertension will have been wrong. After performing investigations, your doctor may then start treating you for chronic hypertension.

Hyperemesis gravidarum

Hyperemesis gravidarum literally means "excessive vomiting in pregnancy". Hyperemesis starts early, usually before week five of pregnancy. It may lessen around week 16 and end around week 20. Hyperemesis occurs in between approximately 0.5 and 2 per cent of pregnancies.

Causes As with nausea and vomiting (see p.237), a variety of factors are likely to be involved, including hormone changes. You are at greater risk of hyperemesis if you:
● Are expecting twins or more.
● Are the daughter or sister of a hyperemesis sufferer.
● Had hyperemesis in a previous pregnancy.

● Have a history of travel sickness or migraines.
● Have liver disease.
● Have thyroid abnormalities.

Symptoms You are said to have hyperemesis if you are vomiting many times a day, are unable to eat and drink without vomiting, and if you are losing weight. The usual treatments won't have helped, and you'll be struggling with normal life.

Treatment Your doctor may prescribe anti-sickness medicine that is safe to use in pregnancy.

If you cannot keep food or fluid down, swallowing pills is also likely to be difficult. Some anti-sickness medication is available as a suppository, in buccal form (dissolved between upper lip and gum), or it can be injected.

It can be a matter of trial and error to find the drug that works for you. Antihistamines are usually given first, as they have the strongest safety record in pregnancy. If these don't help, you may be offered phenothiazines, such as Stemetil, or a drug called metoclopramide. Steroids (such as dexamethasone) are sometimes given for hyperemesis.

You may be admitted to hospital to for re-hydration and/or tube feeding if you cannot drink or eat, and continue to lose weight.

Low amniotic fluid (oligohydramnios)

Oligohydramnios means having too little amniotic fluid in your uterus. About 8 per cent of all pregnant women are found to have low amniotic fluid at some point, usually in their third trimester.

Causes Experts don't always know what causes low amniotic fluid. The most common cause is your waters breaking early. Oligohydramnios is more common in summer months so may be

due to maternal dehydration. It has been found that drinking plenty of water may boost levels of amniotic fluid. You'll also want to take care to eat well and rest.

There are other causes of oligohydramnios, which may include placenta problems and fetal abnormalities. Each individual case requires its own treatment.

Symptoms Your doctor or midwife may suspect this problem if:
● You are leaking fluid.
● Your baby is "small for dates".
● On examination, the outline of your baby is easily felt.
● You have had a previous baby whose growth was restricted.
● You have chronic high blood pressure.
● You have diabetes (see p.23).
● You have lupus (see p.23).
To find out what's going on, she'll send you for an ultrasound.

Treatment Oligohydramnios is most commonly diagnosed later in the third trimester, when it usually requires nothing more than keeping a close watch on things. You may need to have your baby's heart rate monitored regularly and ultrasound scans to closely watch your baby's development until you give birth. If your waters have broken early you may need antibiotics to reduce the risk of infection.

If your doctor is concerned about your baby's growth, it may be safer for your baby to be born early than to remain in the womb. If you are near your due date and your doctor thinks your baby's growth is poor, she may decide to induce labour.

Obstetric cholestasis

Obstetric cholestasis, sometimes called OC, affects the liver and causes intense itching. This itching usually begins during the last 10 weeks of pregnancy, although it can start much earlier.

Women describe it as constant and sometimes intolerable.

Causes It seems that, in some women, the liver is oversensitive to pregnancy hormones. Bile is produced in the liver and normally it flows down into the intestines. If you have OC, the flow of bile is reduced and so bile salts build up in your blood.

If you have a family history of OC and your mother or sisters were affected, you are more likely to suffer from it yourself.

Symptoms The main symptom is itching, which is usually worse at night so can result in fatigue and insomnia. It often begins on the palms of the hands and the soles of feet and can become generalised. Less commonly, women can develop jaundice. The itching completely disappears within a couple of weeks of giving birth.

Careful management of OC is important to prevent stillbirth. In the past, the stillbirth rate for women with OC was about 15 per cent higher than in normal pregnancies but, if well managed, the risk can be reduced to about the normal rate of 1 per cent.

Treatment Two drugs are currently used to manage OC. Ursodeoxycholic acid is favoured in the specialist centres for OC. It appears to eliminate or reduce the itching and can result in the liver function and bile acid results returning to normal. Steroids (in particular, dexamethasone) can also be considered, but need careful management.

Mothers with OC may be at risk of bleeding after the baby is born. This is because bile is needed to absorb vitamin K from food, and vitamin K helps the blood to clot. For this reason, in some hospitals, the mother is given vitamin K daily by mouth until delivery to protect her from this small risk of bleeding. The baby is also protected by the vitamin K.

Pelvic pain

The joint at the front of your pelvis may be more mobile during pregnancy, causing inflammation and pain. This is known as symphysis pubis dysfunction or SPD. This loosening may also lead to related conditions, including diastasis symphysis pubis (DSP), in which the gap in the pubic joint widens too far, and pelvic girdle pain (PGP), which is thought to be caused by instability of the sacroiliac joint at the back of the pelvic girdle.

Causes It's thought that pelvic pain in pregnancy is due to the effects of the pregnancy hormone relaxin. This softens the ligaments of your pelvis to help your baby pass through the birth canal as easily as possible. Unfortunately, this loosening effect can also cause instability, inflammation and pain.

Symptoms Pain in the pubic area and groin are common symptoms. But you may also have:
- Back pain, pelvic girdle pain, or shooting pains in your buttocks or down the backs of your legs.
- Weakness in your legs.
- A grinding or clicking sensation in your pubic area.
- Pain down the insides of your thighs.
- Worse pain at night.

Treatment Treatment of pelvic pain in pregnancy may include exercises, especially for the tummy and pelvic floor muscles. These are designed to improve the stability of your pelvis and back. You may need some gentle, hands-on treatment, such as osteopathy or physiotherapy to correct any stiffness or imbalance. Exercise in water can sometimes be useful and a pelvic support belt can also give quick relief. You should also be given advice on how to make your everyday activities less painful and on how to make the birth of your baby easier.

You should not take any medication during pregnancy unless you have checked it is safe for you and your baby.

Acupuncture, chiropractic and osteopathy may also help, but you must make sure that your practitioner is trained and experienced in working with pregnant women.

Placenta praevia

Placenta praevia (sometimes called low-lying placenta) is when the placenta covers part or all of the cervix after 20 weeks. About one in 200 pregnant women have this problem. If you have an ultrasound scan in early pregnancy and the placenta seems to be near, or even covering, the cervix, don't be too alarmed. As your baby grows, your expanding uterus usually pulls the placenta away from your cervix.

Causes Women who are having their second or subsequent baby are more at risk of placenta praevia than women having their first. Also slightly more at risk are women who have had a caesarean, or who have previously had

Getting ready for pregnancy · Staying safe and healthy · Your pregnancy diary · Birth and beyond a pregnancy with placenta praevia, or who smoke. However, most women with placenta praevia do not have any obvious risk factors.

Symptoms Painless vaginal bleeding during the last three months of pregnancy is often a warning sign and you should call your doctor or midwife immediately if this happens. However, there may be no warning signs at all and the fact that you have placenta praevia may only be discovered during a routine ultrasound scan.

Treatment The treatment you will be given depends on whether you're bleeding and how far on in your pregnancy you are. If the condition is diagnosed after 20 weeks, but you're not bleeding, you'll probably just be advised to take life easy. If you're bleeding heavily, you will be admitted to hospital so that the bleeding can be monitored.

Uncontrolled bleeding (haemorrhage) is life-threatening for both mother and baby, although this is rare. If the bleeding doesn't stop, or if you go into premature labour, your baby will need to be delivered by caesarean section even if your due date isn't for quite a few weeks.

Placental abruption

A placental abruption is a serious condition in which the placenta partially or completely separates from the lining of your uterus before your baby is born. Placental abruption happens in about one in 200 pregnancies. It is most common during the third trimester of pregnancy.

Causes No one knows exactly what causes placental abruption, but there are certain conditions that make it more likely, including having had an abruption in a previous pregnancy, high blood pressure (hypertension), pre-eclampsia and too much amniotic fluid (polyhydramnios).

Symptoms Usually, you will have some vaginal bleeding, ranging from a small amount to an obvious and sudden gush. The bleeding is usually dark, without blood clots. Sometimes, though, the blood stays in the uterus behind the placenta, so you might not see any bleeding at all. You're likely to have some abdominal or back pain and your uterus will feel tender.

Call 999 immediately if you're losing a lot of blood or have any signs of shock – if you feel weak, faint, pale, sweaty, or disoriented, or your heart is pounding.

When you get to hospital, your baby's heart rate will be monitored and you'll probably have an ultrasound scan.

Treatment If you're near your due date, your baby will need to be born straight away, even if the abruption is minor, because the placenta could separate further at any time. In most cases you'll have a caesarean. If the abruption is severe you may have lost a lot of blood. You'll be given oxygen, extra fluids and a blood transfusion through a drip in your vein.

If your doctor suspects that you have a minor abruption and your baby is very premature, you may be able to delay the birth a bit, as long as you and your baby are doing well and there is no further active bleeding.

Polyhydramnios

Polyhydramnios means having too much amniotic fluid in the uterus. It occurs in less than one per cent of pregnancies in the UK.

Some medical conditions don't have any symptoms, but are picked up during your regular antenatal examinations.

Babies regularly swallow the amniotic fluid and it is passed out of their bodies as urine. In this way, your baby controls the volume of amniotic fluid around her. When this delicate balance is disturbed, the amniotic fluid can increase rapidly.

Causes It can be difficult to identify the cause of polyhydramnios and, sometimes, no cause can be found. It may be that the extra fluid is due to a problem with the baby, or with the placenta or with you, the mother. Possible causes include having diabetes, being pregnant with twins or infections, such as rubella.

Symptoms Polyhydramnios usually starts from about the 30th week of pregnancy. You may feel that your tummy is getting too large too quickly and that your skin is stretched and shiny. You might feel so breathless that it is hard to climb a flight of stairs. Other symptoms include abdominal pain, severe heartburn and constipation, swollen legs and varicose veins.

Treatment If you are not known to have diabetes, you'll be given a glucose tolerance test to check your blood sugar levels. If these are high, you may be referred to a diabetes specialist who can help to get your blood sugar levels down. This will reduce the amount of fluid.

Ultrasound scanning can help spot any problems with your baby. If a detailed scan shows nothing untoward, your baby is almost certainly fine and the polyhydramnios is caused by something else. There are other laboratory tests for investigating polyhydramnios if it is thought that it might be due to infection. In severe cases, it may be possible to drain away some of the amniotic fluid.

Pre-eclampsia

Pre-eclampsia is a pregnancy-induced condition, which usually occurs in the third trimester. It is characterised by high blood pressure, swelling that happens suddenly along with rapid weight gain due to fluid retention, and protein in the urine. Since it reduces the flow of blood to the placenta, pre-eclampsia can be quite dangerous for your unborn baby.

Causes The cause of pre-eclampsia is not known but there are recognised risk factors. You're more likely to get pre-eclampsia in a first pregnancy or if there is a big gap, usually of at least ten years, between this and your last pregnancy. You are also more at risk if you are 40 or older, were very obese at the start of your pregnancy, or have a chronic problem that affects your blood system, such as kidney disease.

Symptoms Occasionally pre-eclampsia develops very quickly. Don't hesitate to call your doctor or midwife if you have any of the following symptoms in the second half of pregnancy or in the first few weeks after birth:

● Sudden swelling of your face, hands or feet.
● Intense headaches.
● Blurred vision or flashing spots before your eyes.
● Severe pain in the upper part of your abdomen.
● Vomiting.

Treatment If your blood pressure is moderately raised, you will simply be advised to have as much bed rest as possible, lying either on your left-hand side because this improves the flow of blood to the placenta, or sitting well-propped up. Your midwife will probably visit you on a daily basis to check your blood pressure.

If your blood pressure becomes very high, you might be admitted to hospital so that your condition can be monitored. You may also be given magnesium sulphate injections.

Rhesus incompatibility

People who are rhesus positive, or RhD positive, have a protein known as D antigen on their red blood cells. Those who don't have the D antigen are known as RhD negative. Rhesus status only matters if an RhD-negative mother is carrying an RhD-positive baby. If your baby's blood gets into your bloodstream, your immune system may react to the the D antigen in his blood.

If you become pregnant again and your new baby is also RhD positive, the antibodies you now have in your system can attack your new baby's blood cells, causing anaemia, jaundice or, in severe cases, heart or liver failure in your baby.

Causes You may have antibodies in your blood if you have had a termination or an ectopic pregnancy (see pp.44–5) or if you have had vaginal bleeding or a miscarriage after 12 weeks of pregnancy. There is a chance that your and your baby's blood may come into contact during chorionic villus sampling (CVS; see p.136), amniocentesis (see p.147), external cephalic version (ECV; see pp.286–7) or after suffering a hard blow to your tummy.

Your blood will almost certainly come into contact with your baby's at the birth, particularly if you have a traumatic birth, a caesarean or a manual removal of the placenta.

Symptoms You will not usually notice any symptoms.

Treatment Rhesus antibodies can be prevented by anti-D immunoglobulin, which is usually injected into your shoulder. It destroys the fetal blood cells in your circulation before you can make any antibodies. All pregnant RhD-negative women should be offered anti-D routinely at 28 and 34 weeks of pregnancy. Anti-D only stays in your system for about six weeks, which is why you need to have it more than once.

Getting ready for pregnancy

Staying safe and healthy

Your pregnancy diary

Birth and beyond

Minor/temporary complaints

Backache and back pain

Backache is a problem for many people, but during pregnancy it can be caused by pregnancy hormones that have a relaxing effect on your joints and ligaments. Supporting the weight of your bump also means there's more strain on your back.

What can I do?

- Avoid heavy lifting.
- Improve your posture.
- Don't sit or stand in one position for long periods.
- Wear a well-fitting, supportive maternity bra.
- Wear comfortable shoes.
- Avoid crossing your legs.
- Leave your desk regularly at work and get some fresh air.
- Make yourself comfortable when you are driving.
- Take gentle exercise, such as walking, swimming and yoga.
- Do pelvic floor exercises.
- Use a hot pack.
- Try a support pillow in bed.
- Sleep on your side.
- Use a support belt.

What can my doctor do?

- Refer you to a physiotherapist, if necessary.

Bleeding gums

Bleeding, sensitive gums are also known as gingivitis. During pregnancy, the pregnancy hormones play a part. They can make your gums swell and become inflamed. Then, when you floss or brush, your gums may bleed.

What can I do?

- Continue to floss and brush regularly, but gently.
- Use a soft brush.
- Brush your teeth twice a day for two minutes using fluoride toothpaste.
- Use an electric toothbrush – the action of an electric brush is more effective at removing plaque.
- Floss or use inter-dental brushes at least three times a week.
- See your dentist regularly.
- Give up smoking.
- Use a mouthwash (check with your doctor or pharmacist for one that's safe to use in pregnancy).

What can my dentist do?

- Refer you to a dental hygienist so you can have your teeth properly scaled and polished to remove plaque.

Breathlessness

During pregnancy you may find you are short of breath, particularly when you exert yourself physically. It is a problem that can start in the first trimester, but sometimes not until the second trimester. Later, as your baby grows, he pushes up against your diaphragm, which can contribute to your breathlessness as well. Don't be alarmed. Breathlessness in pregnancy is completely normal and harmless. In the early stages, it is thought to be caused by changes in the levels of carbon dioxide that occur in your system during pregnancy.

What can I do?

- Try getting some light exercise – if you are unfit, you are more likely to feel breathless.
- If you notice any other alarming symptoms, such as chest pain, palpitations, a racing pulse, or clamminess in your fingers and toes, call your doctor or midwife.

What can my doctor do?

- Test you for anaemia.
- Adjust your asthma medication if you have asthma (see p.22).

Constipation

Difficulty in passing a bowel movement is a condition that can strike at any time, whether you are pregnant or not. If you suffer from it during pregnancy, it is likely to be caused by the pregnancy hormone progesterone. This hormone has a tendency to relax and slow down the movement of your intestines.

What can I do?

- Always go to the toilet when you first feel the urge.
- When going to the toilet, give yourself plenty of time and privacy.
- In the morning, or half an hour after a meal, are good times to try to pass a bowel movement.
- Don't take iron tablets.
- Avoid drinks that make you want to pass more urine, such as tea or coffee.
- Drink at least two litres of water a day.
- Start the day with a cup of warm water with a slice of lemon in it.
- Begin each meal with a salad or fruit.
- Eat high-fibre foods, fresh fruits and vegetables daily.
- Take gentle exercise, such as walking, cycling and yoga.

What can my doctor do?

- Advise you on your antenatal vitamins, especially if they contain iron.
- Prescribe a laxative that is safe for you to use, if necessary.

Which complementary therapies can I try?

- Acupressure
- Acupuncture
- Aromatherapy
- Chiropractic
- Homeopathic remedies, such as nux vomica, sepia, lycopodium or graphites
- Osteopathy
- Reflexology
- Tai chi

Dizziness

You may feel dizzy and possibly nauseous in the first and second trimesters of your pregnancy. This is caused by normal changes that occur in your circulation during pregnancy. In the second trimester, your growing uterus can put pressure on blood vessels and this can contribute to your dizziness. You might also feel dizzy if you haven't eaten for a while, if you've become overheated or if you stand up too quickly.

What can I do?

- Sit down!
- If you're in a stuffy office or a crowded train, try to get some fresh air.
- If you haven't eaten for an hour or two, a quick, healthy snack will help boost your blood sugar levels.
- Try drinking some water or juice.
- Get up slowly and smoothly, instead of springing up from a chair or bed.

What can my doctor do?

- Check you in case you have an underlying problem, such as anaemia or low blood pressure.

Fatigue

Tiredness and exhaustion are common during pregnancy as your body works hard to develop your baby. They are also caused by your changing hormone levels and metabolism. Low blood pressure and blood sugar levels can be factors, too.

What can I do?

- Basically, get as much rest as you can, when you can.
- Take catnaps and go to bed early.
- Eat a well-balanced diet with plenty of fruit, vegetables and protein.
- Try not to skip meals, especially breakfast.
- Have regular healthy snacks.
- Eat foods that are high in iron, such as red meat and dark green vegetables.

- Avoid energy-sapping junk food.
- Drink at least eight glasses of water a day.
- Ask your family to help with the housework.
- Shop online.
- Get plenty of gentle exercise and fresh air.
- Socialise with your friends at lunchtime, instead of in the evenings.

What can my doctor do?

- Unfortunately, nothing, although he may check for anaemia. The tiredness should pass after the first trimester, but may return in the third.

Which complementary therapies can I try?

- Aromatherapy
- Massage
- Reflexology
- Shiatsu

Finger pain and numbness (carpal tunnel syndrome)

You may feel some pain and numbness in your hands, fingers and wrists. This is caused by swelling and weight gain.

What can I do?

- Don't sleep on your hands.
- Hang your hands over the edge of your bed during the night.
- Shake your hands until the pain or numbness reduces.
- Flex your wrists and fingers regularly throughout the day.
- Dip your hands in ice-cold water or apply an ice pack.
- Massage from your hands and wrists upwards.
- Avoid jobs that require repetitive hand movements.
- Eat a well-balanced diet to avoid excessive weight gain.
- Drink at least eight glasses of water a day.
- Eat five portions of fruit, salad and vegetables daily.

- Have a small amount of protein with every meal.

What can my doctor do?

- Provide wrist splints.
- Advise you on an antenatal vitamin rich in B6 that could help.
- Organise surgery after your baby's born, if necessary.

Which complementary therapies can I try?

- Acupressure
- Aromatherapy
- Chamomile tea
- Chiropractic
- Homeopathic remedies, such as apis, causticum, lycopodium or calcerea carb
- Osteopathy
- Reflexology

Frequent urination

Often needing to run to the toilet is common in early pregnancy. It's mostly because your volume of blood increases, leading to extra fluid being processed and ending up in your bladder. In late pregnancy (especially when your baby's head has engaged), there's less room for your bladder, so its capacity is reduced. Pregnant women also often find that they can't empty their bladder completely.

What can I do?

- Try drinking less for the hour or two before bedtime to cut down on night-time trips.
- Keep drinking at least eight glasses of water during the day.
- Talk to your doctor or midwife straightaway if you feel pain or burning when you urinate, or a sense of urgency while being able to produce only a few drops at a time.

What can my doctor do?

- Test you for a urinary tract infection (UTIs; see p.228) – if this is left untreated, it can lead to a kidney infection and this, in turn, can increase your risk of premature labour.

Getting ready for pregnancy / Staying safe and healthy / Your pregnancy diary / Birth and beyond

Headaches

We all suffer from headaches sometimes. If you find you get more headaches than usual during pregnancy, don't worry. They are caused by changes in your hormones and blood pressure and there is a lot you can do to help yourself. Remember too that a headache is very different to a migraine. Migraines affect fewer people.

What can I do?

- Apply a compress.
- Take a cold shower.
- Get lots of fresh air.
- Ask your partner or a friend to give you a head massage.
- Take regular, gentle exercise, such as swimming, walking or yoga.
- Improve your posture at work and when you're driving the car.
- Avoid bright lights and noise.
- Eat little and often.
- Eat a wide variety of foods of all types and all colours.
- Drink eight glasses of water a day.
- Cut down or avoid caffeinated drinks and alcohol.
- Get plenty of rest.
- Have an early night or a lie-in every now and then.
- Paracetamol is considered safe if taken in moderation.

What can my doctor do?

- Make sure that your headaches aren't a sign of something more serious, especially if you are still getting them in your third trimester.

Which complementary therapies can I try?

- Acupuncture
- Aromatherapy
- Chiropractic
- Homeopathic remedies, such as aconite or chamomilla
- Osteopathy
- Reflexology
- Shiatsu

Heartburn

This common problem during pregnancy gives you a burning sensation that often extends from your lower throat to the bottom of your breastbone. It is caused by the pregnancy hormone progesterone, which relaxes the valve at the top of your stomach, allowing a small amount of stomach acid to surge upwards.

What can I do?

- Eat small, frequent meals.
- Avoid spicy dishes, chocolate, citrus fruits, alcohol and coffee.
- Take your time over food.
- Eat your main meal of the day at lunchtime.
- Don't drink with your meals.
- Wear loose and comfortable clothing.
- If you smoke, stop.
- Keep an upright posture, particularly during and after meals.
- Don't eat or drink anything in the three hours before going to bed.
- Sleep in a propped-up position.

What can my doctor do?

- Suggest an over-the-counter antacid.
- Recommend a different treatment if none of the above strategies works.
- Make sure that nothing else is wrong.

Which complementary therapies can I try?

- Acupuncture
- Chamomile, ginger or peppermint tea
- Garlic capsules
- Homeopathic remedies, such as nux vomica or pulsatilla
- Osteopathy
- Reflexology

Indigestion and wind

During early pregnancy, high levels of the hormones oestrogen and progesterone circulating in your body relax your gastrointestinal tract. The result of this is the slowing down of your entire digestive system. This is thought to benefit your baby as it gives your body more time to absorb essential nutrients from your food as it makes its (slow) way through your system. However, it may also give you bloating, indigestion and heartburn, especially in the third trimester when your baby starts to push your stomach up towards your oesophagus.

What can I do?

- Avoid putting extra pressure on your stomach while it's digesting: sit up straight and make sure you wear loose, comfortable clothing.
- Wait at least an hour after meals before lying down.
- Bend at your knees instead of from your waist.
- Don't eat big meals. Instead, eat several small meals throughout the day, take your time eating, and chew thoroughly.
- Avoid rich, spicy and fatty foods.
- Avoid drinks containing caffeine or alcohol, which can aggravate your indigestion.
- Don't smoke, as this can relax the valve between your stomach and your oesophagus.
- Avoid meals within three hours of your bedtime.
- Sleep with your upper body propped up with several pillows.

What can my doctor do?

- Prescribe a safe remedy to help ease your symptoms.

Itchy skin

Many pregnant women suffer from some kind of itchiness of the skin. The experts believe that changes in your hormones, together with your stretching skin, are probably to blame. In addition, about two-thirds of all pregnant women will get red and itchy palms and soles, a condition that is believed to be caused by an increase in oestrogen.

What can I do?

- Apply moisturiser or try a warm oatmeal bath (some chemists sell ready-made oatmeal bath products).
- Wear loose cotton clothing and avoid going out in the heat of the day.

What can my doctor do?

- Prescribe a cream that will ease intense itching.
- In the third trimester, your doctor can test you for the rare liver problem, obstetric cholestasis (see pp.230–31), which causes itching.

Leg cramps

These are a type of muscle contraction that give you a sharp pain in your legs. They are probably caused by the extra weight you are carrying during pregnancy and the pressure that puts on your legs. It is also thought that too much phosphorus and too little calcium and potassium in the diet can be factors.

What can I do?

- Stay as active as possible by taking gentle exercise such as walking, swimming and yoga.
- Incorporate foods into your diet that are high in magnesium, calcium and vitamin C (see p.121).
- Eat plenty of fresh vegetables, fruit and salad.
- Cut down on red or processed meat, and fast foods.
- Drink eight glasses of water a day.
- Eat a banana or drink a glass of milk before bed.
- Take a warm bath in the evening.
- Avoid processed soft drinks such as cola and fizzy drinks because they contain phosphorus.
- Stretch before going to bed.
- Avoid standing for long periods of time.
- Don't sit with your legs crossed.
- Rotate your ankles and wiggle your toes when you can.

- When cramp strikes, massage the muscle and then walk it off.

What can my doctor do?

- Recommend a good pregnancy multivitamin and mineral supplement.
- Check for a blood clot, especially if your calf pain persists and the area is red and tender.

Which complementary therapies can I try?

- Aromatherapy
- Homeopathic remedies such as arnica cream

Nausea and vomiting

A feeling of queasiness, sometimes accompanied by vomiting, is the commonest medical condition of early pregnancy. The condition – which can mar the joy of learning you're pregnant – is caused by increased hormone levels together with a heightened sense of smell. Nausea and vomiting is different to severe sickness, in which you can't keep anything down. This is known as hyperemesis gravidarum (see p.230).

What can I do?

- Avoid any foods or smells that make your stomach churn.
- Stay away from rich, spicy, acidic or fried foods.
- Aim for high-protein foods and those rich in Vitamin B.
- Eat little and often, before you get hungry.
- Keep well hydrated.
- Drink ginger, peppermint or spearmint tea.
- Sniff cut lemons.
- Wear acupressure or seasickness wristbands.
- Get as much rest and relaxation as possible.
- Keep some plain crackers by your bed to nibble on in the morning.
- Tell your family and friends how they can help you.

What can my doctor do?

- Recommend a safe pregnancy multivitamin.
- Prescribe medication, if necessary.
- Treatment becomes more difficult the longer you leave it, so make an early appointment.

Which complementary therapies can I try?

- Aromatherapy
- Chiropractic
- Homeopathy
- Hypnotherapy
- Osteopathy
- Reflexology

Nosebleeds

Nosebleeds are a common problem during pregnancy. They are caused by your increased blood supply putting extra pressure on your nose's delicate veins. The membranes inside your nose may also swell and dry out, especially in cold weather and this, too, can lead to nosebleeds.

What can I do?

- When your nose bleeds, remain seated and put pressure on the bleeding nostril for at least four minutes.
- Consult your doctor if you frequently have heavy nosebleeds.

What can my doctor do?

Not a lot. As annoying as nosebleeds can be, it's a temporary problem, likely to disappear after you have your baby.

Piles (haemorrhoids)

Piles are varicose veins of the bottom. They can give you symptoms of itching, pain and sometimes bleeding.

What can I do?

- Don't wait when you get the urge for a bowel movement.
- Clean the affected area after a bowel movement (try baby wipes).
- Eat a high-fibre diet to avoid constipation.

Getting ready for pregnancy

Staying safe and healthy

Your pregnancy diary

Birth and beyond

- Drink fruit juices and at least eight glasses of water a day.
- Take regular, gentle exercise.
- Try deep breathing.
- Do pelvic floor exercises.
- Take a warm bath.
- Use an ice pack.
- Sit on an inflatable ring.
- Don't sit or stand for long stretches of time.
- Don't wear clothes or shoes that are too tight.
- If you smoke, stop.
- Avoid high heels.
- Sleep on your side, not your back.

What can my doctor do?
- Recommend safe topical anaesthetics or medicated suppositories.
- Arrange minor surgery after pregnancy.
- Confirm that any bleeding is coming from the piles and that nothing else is the matter.

Which complementary therapies can I try?
- Acupressure
- Aromatherapy oils in the bath
- Homeopathic remedies, such as pulsatilla, nux vomica or hammamelis
- Osteopathy
- Reflexology
- Witch hazel

Stuffy nose
What is it?
A runny or stuffed-up nose is a common condition during pregnancy. It has a name – allergic rhinitis of pregnancy – but unfortunately there is no cure. There are measures you can take to help yourself, though.

What can I do?
- Fill a bowl with hot water, then cover your head with a towel and lean over the steaming bowl as if you were giving yourself an old-fashioned facial. Inhale and exhale a few times.

- A hot shower may also help.
- You might find a nasal spray provides relief (but only use one on your doctor's or midwife's advice).

What can my doctor do?
- Advise you on nasal sprays and decongestants that are safe to use in pregnancy.

Swollen hands and feet (oedema)
Swollen hands and feet are the result of a chain reaction in your body. First, you acquire extra blood during pregnancy. Second, your growing uterus puts pressure on your blood vessels, which causes your blood to pool. Third, pressure from the trapped blood forces water down into the tissues of your feet and ankles – and that results in the swelling. Some pregnant women also retain excess water, which adds to the swelling. Some oedema is normal, but if you have severe swelling in your hands and face, you should call your doctor or midwife.

What can I do?
- Raise your feet when possible.
- At work, keep a stool or pile of books under your desk; at home, try to lie on your left side when possible.
- Put on waist-high support tights before you get out of bed in the morning.
- Drink plenty of water to keep yourself hydrated.
- Exercise regularly, especially by walking, swimming or riding on an exercise bike.
- Eat well, and avoid sodium and salty foods like olives and salted nuts.

What can my doctor do?
- In the third trimester, test you for pre-eclampsia.

Thrush in pregnancy
This is a thick, white and creamy vaginal discharge, which can cause itching. It is caused by the vagina being

rich in a sugar called glycogen during pregnancy. This promotes the growth of candida, the fungus that causes thrush.

What can I do?
- Reduce your consumption of sugar and sugary foods.
- Avoid getting too warm down below.
- Wear cotton underwear and abandon your tights.
- Wash your clothes in a non-biological soap powder at 60°C (140°F) in order to kill the fungus.
- Don't lie in a hot bath for too long.
- Apply a cloth soaked in witch hazel or diluted tea tree oil to the inflamed outer area of the vagina.
- Press an ice pack to the inflamed, outer area.
- Eat natural live yoghurt.
- Apply natural live yoghurt to the affected area.
- Use garlic in your food.
- After using the toilet, wipe your genital area from front to back.
- Do not use vaginal deodorants.

What can my doctor do?
- Prescribe some suitable pessaries or creams.

Which complementary therapies can I try?
- Acupuncture
- Homeopathy
- Probiotic supplements

Tummy cramps
Carrying a baby puts a lot of pressure on your muscles, ligaments, veins and the rest of your insides, so it isn't surprising if you sometimes feel pains in your stomach. These pains on their own are rarely anything to worry about but if you have other symptoms, they may be a sign of a more serious problem.

What can I do?
- Most tummy cramps can be eased by getting into a new position or finding a way to relax.

- Mild cramps on one or both sides could be stretching ligaments – resting comfortably when the pain occurs usually clears it up.
- Cramps during and after orgasm can be eased by a gentle back rub.
- For cramps and persistent lower back pain in late pregnancy, resting on the sofa may help, or possibly going for a more active walk.

What can my doctor do?

- Examine you if you experience cramping along with spotting, heavy bleeding, fever, chills, vaginal discharge, tenderness and pain, or if the cramps don't subside after several minutes of rest. These additional symptoms can be a sign of underlying problems, such as ectopic pregnancy (see pp.44–5), miscarriage (see pp.42–3) or premature labour (see pp.280-81).

Vaginal discharge

All women have some vaginal discharge that changes according to the stage they're at in their menstrual cycle. During pregnancy, it is quite common for women to experience an increase in their vaginal discharge. It is almost always nothing more than leucorrhoea – a mild-smelling milky fluid discharge that is caused by an increased blood flow to the area around the vagina.

For some women the discharge increases as they approach labour. The discharge can then be quite heavy. If this happens to you, it may be a sign that you are approaching labour.

What can I do?

- Keep your genital area clean.
- Wear cotton underwear.
- Avoid tight or nylon trousers, perfumes and deodorant soaps.
- If you need to absorb the flow, use pantyliners, not tampons.
- Contact your doctor if you notice a brownish discharge.

What can my doctor do?

- Test you for a vaginal infection. A foul-smelling, thick, yellowish-green discharge, or one that causes itching or burning, could be a sign of thrush or other infection. You'll need to treat it before you deliver your baby.

Vaginal spotting or bleeding

Spotting is light bleeding from the vagina that can vary in colour from red to brown. It is similar to, but lighter than, a period. About 15 to 25 per cent of women experience some sort of bleeding in the first trimester. It is usually just "one of those things". However, it can be a sign of a more serious problem such as miscarriage (see pp.42–3). This is why it's always best to get it checked out.

In early pregnancy, severe, persistent abdominal pain with bleeding can be a sign of ectopic pregnancy (see pp.44–5) – go to hospital immediately. In the third trimester, it can signal placenta praevia (see pp.231–2), placental abruption (see p.232), or premature labour (see pp.280–81).

What can I do?

- Call your doctor, midwife or hospital straightaway for advice.

What can my doctor do?

- You may need a vaginal examination or an ultrasound to rule out any complications, such as fibroids or an inflamed cervix.
- In early pregnancy, your doctor will probably also do a urine pregnancy test and a blood test in order to check your hormone levels.
- An examination using "transvaginal" ultrasound is often the best way to check whether or not all is well.
- Your doctor may switch you to consultant-led rather than midwife-led care so that any potential problems are monitored more closely.

Varicose veins

Varicose veins in the legs occur when the blood is unable to travel back up the legs to the heart.

Unfortunately, varicose veins are more likely to develop during pregnancy because the growing uterus increases blood pressure in the veins of your legs. On top of that, an increase in the hormone progesterone causes the walls of the veins to relax so they fail to push the blood through.

If you have varicose veins, you may just see the blue veins under your skin, or the veins may bulge; you may feel some pain, or no discomfort at all.

What can I do?

- Exercise daily – even just a brisk walk around the block can help.
- Raise your feet and legs whenever you get a chance.
- Try to lie down on your left side with your feet raised on a pillow when you are at home.
- Before getting out of bed in the morning, put on special support tights.
- Don't stand on your feet for long periods of time.
- Don't cross your legs when you are sitting down.
- Be aware that excessive weight gain can contribute to the problem.
- If you have a tender, reddened area on the surface of a varicose vein, coupled with fever, leg pain, or a rapid heartbeat, report it to your doctor or midwife without delay. In rare cases, rapid heartbeat and/or shortness of breath could be signs of a pulmonary embolism (when the blood clot has travelled to the lungs). You should go to the nearest accident and emergency department, or call an ambulance.

What can my doctor do?

- If you have a major problem with varicose veins, your doctor can prescribe some support tights for you.

Getting ready for pregnancy

Staying safe and healthy

Your pregnancy diary

Birth and beyond

Birth and beyond
Becoming a parent

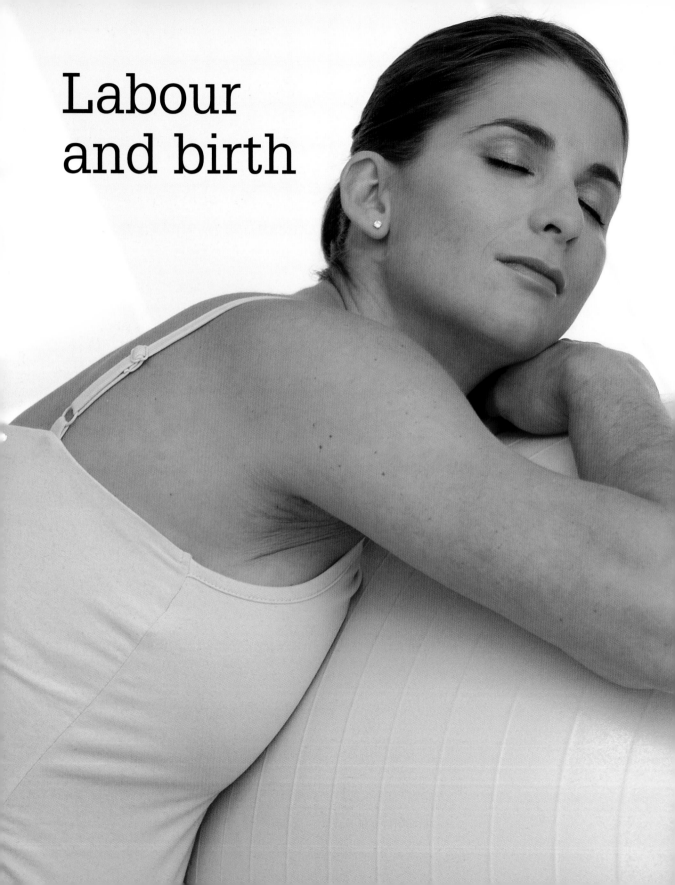

Labour
and birth

You're going to be a parent

Your baby will arrive around 266 days after you conceive. However, most babies arrive before or after, with only about 5 per cent born on their due date. Each labour and birth is different, but knowing what's involved helps you understand and deal with any issues that may arise.

An overview

Labour begins when your body's hormones respond to triggers from the baby's adrenal gland. Your uterus starts to contract and your waters may break. If you are overdue, you may be induced.

During the first stage of labour the contractions, which open the cervix become progressively stronger, longer and more frequent. The cervix begins tightly closed and quite firm, but thins and stretches as labour progresses. So dilation starts slowly but speeds up as labour progresses. Once the cervix has dilated to 10 centimetres, it is fully dilated and the baby can move through it and down the vagina.

Now the second stage of labour begins. You will feel a very strong urge to push downwards, unless you've opted to have an epidural. In this case your midwife will tell you when to push. The second stage can take anything from a few minutes to a couple of hours or more, and it can be hard work! Your midwife will guide you when to push. Usually the baby's head comes out first and, after a few more contractions, the baby is fully born. If you are very tired or the baby is in distress, either forceps (like large sugar tongs) or ventouse (vacuum extractor) may be needed to help the baby to be born. Occasionally, if the baby needs to be delivered very quickly, an emergency caesarean may be necessary.

After the birth

After birth, the umbilical cord is usually clamped and cut then, if all is well, you'll be able to hold your baby. The third and final stage of labour is the delivery of the placenta, which takes five to 30 minutes. You can have a medically managed third stage or, if you have no blood pressure problems and there is no risk of haemorrhage, the uterus can be left to contract naturally.

It's never too early to look into where and how you want to give birth. The majority of women in the UK have their baby in hospital. However, home birth is enjoying a revival, and midwife-led maternity units (birth centres) are becoming increasingly popular.

Labour is hard work but when it's all over and your baby has arrived, you and your partner can start enjoying being parents.

Getting ready for pregnancy

Staying safe and healthy

Staying safe and healthy

Birth and beyond

Preparation and choices

There's a lot to think about when you're planning your baby's birth. Will you give birth in hospital or at home? Who do you want with you? How will you manage the pain of contractions? Thinking your options through before the birth will help to give you confidence on the day.

Where to give birth: home or hospital?

The majority of British women – around 97 per cent of them – give birth in hospital. If you live in a big city, you may have a choice of two or three different hospitals. In rural areas, the possibilities are often limited, although you sometimes can choose between giving birth in a small, local midwife-led unit or in a large consultant unit in your nearest town or city.

Hospitals have set ways of doing things, but it's your right to make it clear how you'd like to be treated when you're there. Talk to your midwife about what the routine procedures are during labour in the maternity unit where you'll give birth. If there's anything you don't like the sound of, say so. Talk through how you'd like things to go, and write a birth plan (see pp.174–5) to keep with your

notes. Make sure your birth partner is aware of your wishes, too.

Home birth, which was frowned on by health professionals for many years, is enjoying a revival. For a woman experiencing a normal pregnancy, research shows that it is just as safe to give birth at home as it is to have your baby in hospital. However, you may find that there are not enough midwives

---

Home birth versus hospital birth

This checklist sums up the pros and cons of home and hospital births. It will help you to choose what suits you.

Home birth pros

- You have your own toilet and bathroom. There is no risk of cross-infection or hospital-acquired infections.
- You'll have one-to-one midwife care.
- You are more likely to have a straightforward, normal vaginal birth.
- Your own home comforts and distractions are always available.
- You are less likely to need pain relief.
- You can have as many people as you like with you at the birth.
- After the birth, you can relax at home in the comfort of your own bed.

Home birth cons

- Some pain-relief options are not available at a home birth, including an epidural. If you want pethidine, you'll need to discuss it with your midwife in advance.
- There is a 40 per cent transfer to hospital rate for first-time mothers.
- Birth can be messy. You will need to protect carpets and furniture.
- You may worry about noise disturbing the neighbours.

Hospital birth pros

- You may prefer knowing that doctors are close at hand in case of emergency.
- There is direct access to an epidural should you want one. Gas and air, pethidine and a birth pool should also be available.

- You may feel more comfortable making a lot of noise in hospital than you would if you were at home.

Hospital birth cons

- You are unlikely to know the midwife who is caring for you in labour and she may be caring for more than one woman at a time.
- You are more likely to have interventions such as forceps and ventouse, and you are twice as likely to have a caesarean.
- You will need to travel to the hospital in active labour.
- The hospital ward may be noisy and you'll have to share a bathroom and toilet with other women.

available to attend a home birth when you go into labour, and you'll also have to be prepared to go into hospital if complications arise. If you'd like to know more about having a home birth, talk to your midwife.

It's your right to have an "active" birth as well as to refuse "routine" interventions, such as having your waters broken, electronic fetal monitoring, and drugs such as Syntometrine.

If you hire a birth pool to use at home, you may like to get one that is large enough for your partner to get into and help you.

Stand-alone birth centres

Birth centres are small maternity units that are staffed and, mostly, run by midwives. They offer a comfortable, low-tech environment where birth is treated as a "normal" process rather than a medical one.

Most birth centres are independent or "stand-alone", but lots of hospitals now have midwife-led centres alongside their conventional or "consultant-led" maternity units.

Birth centres are a kind of halfway house between home and hospital. They provide a homely, relaxed atmosphere, but they are also well-equipped and staffed with highly skilled midwives. Birth centres can offer facilities that may not be available in your local hospital, such as family accommodation, water pools, complementary therapies and comfortable, low-tech birthing rooms. You are more likely to have one-to-one care from a midwife throughout your labour in a birth centre than in a busy consultant-led unit.

Birth centres also have a high standard of postnatal care. You'll probably have a private room with your own bathroom facilities, which will give you the opportunity to relax with your baby in peace. Other family members may be able to stay overnight and women are encouraged to stay until they feel ready to go home.

A birth centre may be able to offer you a low-tech birthing room where you will feel more relaxed during the birth process.

On the other hand, you are unlikely to have the full range of pain relief on offer – you won't be able to have an epidural, for example. There is also no special-care baby unit on hand in the event of an emergency. However, midwives are generally skilled in life-support and resuscitation techniques and in managing emergency situations. You may not be able to have an assisted delivery with forceps or ventouse at a birth centre although some birth centre midwives are now trained so they are able to use ventouse.

If you do happen to get into difficulties during labour, you will be transferred to hospital by ambulance, accompanied by your midwife. Despite the lack of medical facilities, evidence shows that giving birth in a birth centre is just as safe for you and your baby as having your baby in hospital.

Eligibility criteria vary from one birth centre to another, but you will generally only be able to book in if your pregnancy is low-risk and you have a good chance of having a normal birth at full term.

Hospital births

There's no shortage of information out there about the physical process of giving birth. But for those women who've opted for a hospital birth, they're not always sure what awaits them when they finally reach the maternity ward.

Some of your fears can be allayed and your questions answered if you visit the hospital where you are "booked in" to give birth during your pregnancy. From about 34 weeks onwards, you may

care of you will ask you to tell her what has happened so far: have you had a show (a brownish or blood-tinged mucus discharge), for example, or have your waters broken? She'll also need to see your maternity notes, so don't forget to take them with you.

Next she'll check your blood pressure, temperature, pulse and urine. She'll measure and feel your bump to find out which way round your baby is

"Women **are not** always **sure what will** happen **at hospital**."

be offered a chance to visit. As well as having a tour of the delivery suite, your visit gives you the chance to become familiar with the layout and find out how things are done there.

On the day

When you arrive at the hospital, you'll be directed to the maternity ward reception. The midwife who'll be taking

and whether her head is engaged in your pelvis or not. She'll also assess how long, strong and frequent your contractions are and how much pain you are in.

Checking your baby

The midwife will want to check that the baby is OK so she may ask to see your sanitary pad if you've had a show, or if your waters have already broken. She'll be checking for bleeding or meconium (your baby's first bowel movement) in the amniotic fluid. She'll also listen to your baby's heartbeat. Next, she may ask your permission to do an internal (vaginal) examination to see how many centimetres dilated you are. You don't have to have this examination if you don't want to.

Everything your midwife does is written down on your partogram, a special chart that records every detail

The receptionist on the maternity ward will welcome you and hand you over to your midwife to check how your labour's going.

of your labour. It means that if your midwife goes off duty, the next midwife will be able to see at a glance how you're getting on.

What happens next

If the midwife sees that you are in very early labour, you might choose to go home again and wait for the contractions to get stronger. If you decide to stay in hospital, you will probably be sent to the antenatal ward, or perhaps to a special waiting area on the delivery suite.

If you're in active labour – more than 3cm dilated – you'll be taken straight to a delivery room where you'll stay until your baby is born, unless you've booked a water birth (but bear in mind that the birth pool may already be in use, so it may not be available).

In the delivery room

Many hospital delivery rooms are designed to look like a bedroom to help you feel more relaxed. As well as the bed and a chair, there will be pictures on the walls and perhaps a TV. Some even have an en suite bathroom. Normally, gas and air (Entonox; see p.276) and oxygen are available for you to use in the room when you need them.

Throughout your labour, your midwife will regularly check your pulse, temperature, blood pressure, urine, cervix and the baby's position and heart rate. If you find that you do need some form of medical intervention – such as an epidural (see pp.278–9), an assisted birth (see pp.282–3) or an emergency caesarean (see pp.288–91) – all the specialist professionals will be on hand.

You don't have to get into bed. You can move around during labour. In fact, being mobile in active labour can help your labour progress. Once you're in the delivery room, try to make it feel "yours".

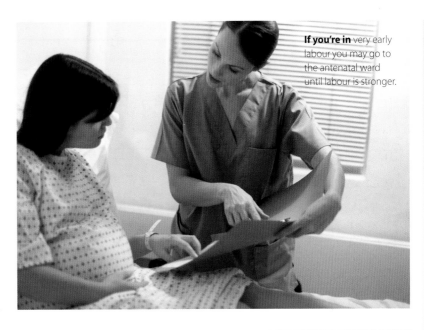

If you're in very early labour you may go to the antenatal ward until labour is stronger.

You may want to move the bed to one side to allow more space to walk around. Perhaps the lighting is too bright. You can turn it off and just have a lamp on. Use the time in early labour to get comfortable and relax. Have a bath or a shower. It often helps with the contractions.

65%
of pregnant women say they plan to give birth in a hospital; 20 per cent say they'd like to give birth at home. A further 14 per cent plan to give birth in a stand-alone birth centre.

ParentsAsk...

Can my partner stay with me during labour?

Yes, in fact it may be invaluable. One study showed that women meet an average of six or more unfamiliar professionals during labour, so a friendly face can make all the difference. A birth partner can also provide practical help. Another study found that a birth partner who offered encouragement in pain control made an epidural less likely and meant that women were less likely to feel panicky and exhausted.

Can I eat and drink in labour?

Yes. Studies have found that there are no harmful effects for either the mother or the baby if you eat and drink while you are in labour. This is provided you don't use a painkiller, such as pethidine, (see p.276) or develop any complications during labour that might mean you need a general anaesthetic later on. Don't worry, though. If you've been snacking and then find later that you need some pain relief, you won't be denied it.

Eating or drinking liquids that have some calories in them during labour will help to prevent ketosis. This is when the body starts to break down its own fatty stores for energy. Ketosis can make you feel nauseous, might make you vomit and can give you a headache. It is best to avoid ketosis during labour because you have a lot of hard physical work ahead of you.

Getting ready for pregnancy

Staying safe and healthy

Your pregnancy diary

Birth and beyond

Perineal massage is worth considering to help prepare your vagina for the work ahead.

"From the time I was around 33 weeks pregnant, I started giving myself a daily perineal massage using vitamin E oil. I would put some on my fingers and thumbs before putting my thumbs a little way into my vagina. Then I'd push downwards and sideways until I could feel a slight tingling. When I went into labour, the very intense stretching sensation when my baby's head crowned was already familiar. I didn't panic but felt positive enough to start pushing. My midwife even used perineal massage in the later stages of my labour to help relax my vaginal muscles. It really boosted my confidence because it made me feel like I had been doing something right all those weeks and that it was going to pay off. "

Preparing yourself

Labour could start at any time now. As this reality hits home, it's very normal to feel apprehensive, even a little scared. Being prepared both mentally and on a practical level is the key to dealing with fear and pain during childbirth.

If you're still a bit hazy on the three stages of labour (see pp.262–5, 268–9, 270–71), now is the time to refresh your memory. When things get underway you

Make sure, too, that you have your birth plan (see pp.174–5) ready and review it one final time. Of course, no one knows in advance what sort of birth experience they will have, but a written plan will at least help explain to the midwife or medical staff what really matters to you.

Having a birth plan also helps you think through some of the options you might have to face, so that you won't

> "If you're a **bit hazy** about the **three stages of labour** now is the time to **refresh your memory**."

will feel much more in control if you recognise the early signs of labour and what to expect as it progresses. With your baby's birth perhaps only hours away, there's nothing like a time limit to focus the mind!

have to make certain decisions when you're in labour. But remember – your birth plan is not a list of demands. You need to acknowledge that things might not go according to plan on the day, so be prepared to be flexible.

Parents**Ask...**

Can I try for a vaginal birth after a caesarean?

Just because you've had one caesarean doesn't mean that you'll have one next time. Guidelines recommend women be supported if they want a vaginal birth after a caesarean (VBAC), provided they are informed about all the pros and cons.

Many of the advantages of VBAC are the same as those of a vaginal birth. After a normal delivery, for example, you're less likely to need a blood transfusion, your baby is less likely to have breathing problems and your hospital stay will be shorter.

Disadvantages of VBAC may include perineal pain or stitches, more chance of stress incontinence in the first three

months after birth and an increased chance of your womb "dropping" (prolapse) in later years. One disadvantage that is specific to VBAC is that, very rarely, your uterus may rupture, which could put you and your baby at risk. Studies show that the rate of rupture in women having a VBAC after one previous caesarean section is one in 200.

Your chances of having a successful VBAC are higher if you have delivered at least one baby vaginally in the past and if your last caesarean was for a breech baby.

About 72 to 76 per cent of women who choose VBAC after a single previous caesarean go on to have a successful vaginal birth. Women who have previously had a vaginal birth, particularly a successful VBAC,

have an even higher rate of success for planned VBAC of 87 to 90 per cent.

What happens to my vagina and pelvic floor after birth?

Directly after a vaginal birth, the opening of your vagina will be bigger and not as neat as it was. But the area will regain its shape over time and with regular pelvic floor exercises.

Your pelvic floor muscles may initially feel "switched off" due to pain and swelling. Start doing your pelvic floor exercises (see p.135) as soon as you can. These will increase the blood flow to the area, aid healing and help tighten and strengthen the pelvic floor.

Mental preparation

Finally, it is useful to have some mental strategies ready to help you cope with the birth. Remember the breathing techniques (see below and p.274) that you learned at antenatal classes. These help you work with your body, reframe the pain and keep you focused.

Some women also find visualisation really effective – for example, repeating the thought "My body is strong and is working well for me". Many mums have used strategies like these to delay or avoid the need for additional pain relief or medical interventions during labour. Remind yourself, too, that you only have to deal with one contraction at a time and each contraction is one closer to your holding your baby.

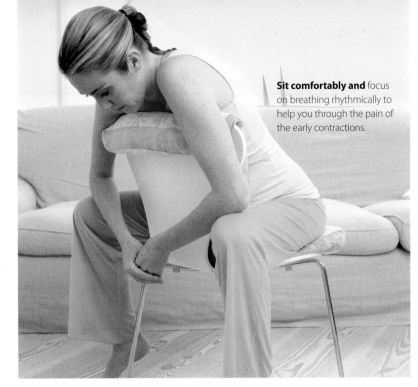

Sit comfortably and focus on breathing rhythmically to help you through the pain of the early contractions.

Breathing techniques

Practising rhythmic breathing while you are in labour maximises the amount of oxygen available to you and your baby. It can also help you cope with the pain of contractions.

It can be very hard to keep your breathing rhythmical and to relax every time you breathe out when you're having painful contractions. You're tired, and labour seems to be endless. This is where the support of your birth partner is essential. He can help you keep your breathing steady by breathing with you.

You need to be in eye contact with him, and he can hold your hands or place his hands on your shoulders. Then you can follow his pattern of breathing as he breathes in through his nose and blows out softly into your face. Practise this during pregnancy.

During the second stage of labour, you will be pushing your baby out into the world. Follow your urges and push

as many times per contraction as feels right for you. You may find that you feel the urge to push briefly three to five times with each contraction, taking several breaths in between.

Sometimes women get the urge to push before their cervix is fully dilated. In this case, depending on how far dilated you are, your midwife may ask you to try not to push to give your cervix more time to open. This can be extremely difficult!

You can help by changing your position, perhaps onto your side or kneeling on all fours with your bottom in the air and your cheek resting on the ground. When a contraction arrives, give four short pants, then a quick in-breath, followed by four more short pants and so on. You can also repeat the phrase "I must not push" in your head as you pant. Try to breathe normally between the contractions.

Overcoming your labour fears

It's natural to have anxieties over giving birth, especially if this is your first baby. But there are strategies to help you overcome your fears:
- Talk to someone who knows you very well about how you have dealt with pain in the past. When you compare labour with other painful experiences, you may realise that you are stronger than you thought.
- If you have your baby in hospital, you will have a range of pain relief options, such as an epidural. Talk to your midwife or doctor about these, and ask them to help you prepare a birth plan, so that your wishes are clear to everybody looking after you.
- If you have a strong fear of childbirth, talk to your doctor or midwife about counselling. This can help you to understand and come to terms with your fear.

Overdue babies

Your due date's arrived but your baby hasn't. What now? Don't worry too much – lots of babies arrive after their due dates. You may want to learn a bit more about induction in the meantime but, more importantly, put your feet up and get some rest.

Coping strategies after 40 weeks

If time has slowed to a crawl as you wait for your baby to arrive, try these coping strategies:

● Have something planned for every day. Don't stay home thinking about what's (not) happening.

● If you haven't already stocked up the freezer, do so now.

● Tell friends and relatives not to ring to find out what's happening. You'll call them when there's news.

● Go out for lots of last-minute treats with your partner – it won't be so easy after your baby's born.

● Rest – if you're finding it difficult to sleep at night, take a nap during the day. Put your feet up. Play some music or watch TV. Don't fret if you can't sleep; dozing is fine. Build up your energy stores for labour.

My baby's late

Lots of women go beyond their expected due date. But only about four per cent have what is called a prolonged pregnancy – a pregnancy that lasts longer than 42 weeks.

The reason obstetricians worry so much about "post maturity" (going over your dates) is that the number of babies who die unexpectedly while still in the womb increases after 42 weeks of pregnancy, and again after 43 weeks. However, the numbers are still very small. In the UK, the risk of stillbirth is about one per 3,000 pregnancies at 39 weeks, four per 3,000 at 42 weeks and eight per 3,000 at 43 weeks.

Research shows that membrane sweeping (see opposite) increases the chances of labour starting naturally within 48 hours. But if membrane sweeping doesn't work and your pregnancy has been straightforward, you should be offered the possibility of an induction (see opposite). Many women prefer to be induced at this stage, as they feel that they have had enough of being pregnant, but some others would rather wait and let nature take its course.

If, after talking to your obstetrician, you're not sure about having an induction, you could ask for a day or two to consider. If you decide not to be induced, it's highly likely that you'll go into labour spontaneously before 42 completed weeks (if your due date is based on a dating scan).

An alternative to induction is to have your pregnancy monitored on a regular basis (every two to three days) to check that your baby's OK. Your midwife may be able to visit you at home to listen to your baby with a Sonicaid (portable ultrasound device), or you may be asked to go into hospital to have a trace on a CTG machine, which records your baby's heartbeat, and a scan to check the levels of amniotic fluid

Ultimately, the decision whether or not to have an induction is yours. You should talk to your midwife or obstetrician if you need more advice.

20% of babies per year is roughly the amount of induced births in the UK. An induction is usually done because the risks of prolonging a pregnancy are more serious than the risks of delivering the baby straight away. Most labours begin naturally, but sometimes the birth process may need a little help.

Natural ways to bring on labour

You're ready to go and nothing's happening? The following might be worth trying to get labour going.

- **Nipple stimulation** It's believed that this releases oxytocin, a hormone that causes contractions.
- **Sex** Orgasm may help to stimulate the uterus into action. Semen also contains prostaglandins to open the cervix.
- **Eating curry** There is no scientific evidence for this one! But it is said to stimulate the bowel, which is next to the uterus.

- **Eating pineapple** Fresh pineapple contains the enzyme bromelain, which is thought to help to soften the cervix.
- **Acupuncture** Limited studies suggest that acupuncture may be effective.
- **Walking** If your baby has not "dropped" or is still high in the pelvis, walking is thought to encourage your baby into a better position.

Induction

Although it's usually best to let nature take its course, sometimes the birth process may need a little help. When labour is started artificially, it is said to be induced. You may be offered an induction if:

- Your pregnancy has gone beyond 41 weeks.
- Your waters have broken but labour hasn't started within 24 hours.
- You suffer from diabetes or another condition, such as pre-eclampsia (see p.233) or kidney disease, that could threaten your wellbeing or the health of your baby.

There are a number of methods your midwife can use to try to get your labour started. You will normally be offered the methods of induction in this order:

Membrane sweep – when the membranes that surround your baby are gently separated from your cervix during an internal examination.

Prostaglandin – a hormone-like substance that helps stimulate uterine contractions. Your midwife or doctor will insert a tablet, pessary or gel containing prostaglandin into your vagina. You may

need a second dose of the tablet or gel after six hours if labour hasn't started.

Syntocinon – this is the synthetic form of the hormone oxytocin. It's given via a drip and you are only offered it if your labour hasn't started following a membrane sweep or prostaglandin. Some women say the contractions brought on by Syntocinon are more painful than natural ones. If that is the case, you may choose to have an epidural for pain relief.

There is some evidence that you are more likely to need instruments such as forceps or ventouse to help deliver your

A Syntocinon drip (synthetic oxytocin) may be used to start your labour.

baby following an induction, whatever method is used. This may be due to complications in the pregnancy that led to the induction and/or it may be due to problems caused by the induction itself.

ParentsAsk...

How will I know if induction will work?

There are various methods of induction. Your midwife or doctor may suggest that one method is better than another, depending on how soft and ready for labour your cervix is.

The ripeness of your cervix is assessed using what's called the Bishop Score, which gives your cervix a mark out of 10 based on its condition. A score of eight or more indicates that your cervix is "ripe" and ready for labour.

About 15 per cent of inductions started with an unripe cervix fail. In these circumstances, your doctor will discuss your options with you to help you decide whether to carry on trying, either with stronger interventions at a later time, or to have a caesarean.

Home birth

Research shows that, for women with normal pregnancies, a home birth is just as safe as a hospital birth. If you're expecting a straightforward birth and decide that a home birth is the right choice for you, you should find that your midwife or doctor is fully supportive.

All you need to know

For women who've had a normal pregnancy and can expect a straightforward labour, a home birth is just as safe as giving birth in a hospital.

If you've decided to go for a home birth and you're healthy and having an uncomplicated pregnancy, talk to your

Fact: In the UK, it is every woman's legal right to give birth at home. The local supervisor of midwives is obliged to provide midwifery care for you within the National Health Service.

doctor or midwife once your pregnancy has been confirmed. If your doctor isn't keen, you can ask to be referred to a community midwife or another doctor who provides full maternity services. Another option is to pay an independent midwife who can carry out your antenatal care, attend the birth of your baby at home, and provide your postnatal care, too.

You can change your mind at any time. Government guidelines say that doctors and midwives should "develop a flexible system of care so that women are able to take time in making their decision regarding the place of birth,

and can alter that decision close to the time of birth if they so wish". Opting early on for a home birth allows you the greatest possible flexibility, as you can decide to transfer to hospital right up to the delivery itself.

You need very little equipment for a home birth. A few weeks before your due date, your midwife will bring round a "birth pack" containing all the bits and pieces she needs.

You're in labour

Once you go into labour, the community midwife may visit you once, twice or more during your labour. Once she

---

Home birth checklist

A few weeks before your due date, the midwife will have left her "birth pack". You may also need:
- An adjustable floor or desk lamp, used to check your perineum.
- A plastic sheet, plastic shower curtain, or some old newspapers for the floor.
- A birthing ball.
- A birth pool if you want to use one.
- Some large, warm towels to put around you and the baby.
- Plenty of hot water if you want a bath.

- Energy-boosting snacks for you to eat, and drinks with bendy straws.
- A hand mirror so you can see your baby's head crowning.
- A fan to keep you cool.
- A portable heater if necessary.

Offer your midwives food and drink and make sure you're stocked up on beverages. Your birth partner can make up sandwiches to leave out for them.

Finally, pack an emergency bag in case you need to be transferred to hospital.

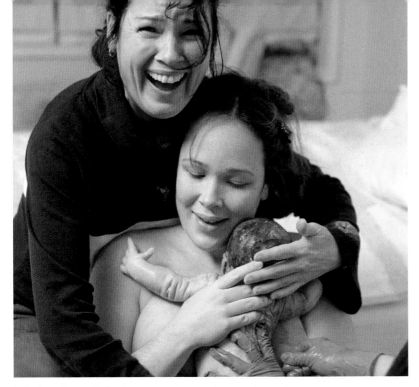

Having a home birth where your mother can be present as well as other family members can be a very moving experience for everyone.

Dad's Diary

A family occasion

"Our first two children were born in a hospital, but Diane was really keen to give birth to our third baby at home. James (seven) and Molly (five) were really excited about the prospect of having a new baby sister. We'd involved them throughout the pregnancy – they went to both scans and they even got the honour of telling Granny and Granddad the good news about their impending grandchild. So, it seemed really natural to have them at home for the birth, too. We explained in the weeks leading up to the birth that Granny would be coming to take care of them while mummy had the baby, but that they'd be able to see her as soon as she was born. They seemed quite happy with that.

When the time arrived, Diane went into labour in the early hours of the morning and gave birth at about 6.30am. The kids were so excited when I woke them up to tell them I had a surprise downstairs. It was lovely to have the whole family together and for them to share in the moment. I can't say how wonderful it was for the three generations to all have breakfast together the next morning."

thinks the birth is imminent, she'll stay with you and will call a colleague to assist her. Who else is present is up to you – it's your home, after all.

If your midwife thinks you need to be transferred to hospital during labour, she will talk to you and your partner about why she believes it would be a good idea. If you agree, she will then call an ambulance. You're far more likely to need to transfer to hospital because your labour has slowed down than because there's a real emergency.

After the birth

Once your baby is born and the placenta (also known as the afterbirth) is safely delivered, the midwives will probably leave you and your partner alone with your baby for a while. They'll then check him over and weigh him, help you with your first breastfeed, clear up any mess, and see you into bed. A midwife will always stay after the placenta has been delivered until she's happy that you are comfortable and well, and when she leaves she'll take away the placenta and any rubbish from the birth.

Your midwife or another community midwife will visit you daily for a few days to check your baby and see how you're progressing. Your doctor will also usually call on the first day and carry out a complete check on your baby.

A home birth is an intimate experience and allows your partner to participate more fully in what is going on.

Your baby's position

Believe it or not, the position your baby is lying in when you go into labour is one of the key indicators of whether or not you'll have a straightforward birth. Find out which positions are likely to allow your baby a smooth birth and how to encourage her into them.

Lie, presentation and position

Most babies get into the best position for birth before labour begins. This is in a head-down position, lying with the back of her head slightly towards the front of your tummy. This is called an "anterior" position (see opposite, centre).

During labour, most babies also curl their back over and tuck their chin into their chest. This is nature's way of helping your labour to progress and making birth easier. During contractions in the first stage of labour, the top of your baby's head puts rounded and even pressure on the cervix and helps it to dilate. Then, in the pushing stage, your baby comes through the birth canal with the part of her skull that has the smallest diameter leading the way.

If your baby has her chin up or her head extended back, then her face or her brow will be coming first (see p.197). This doesn't happen very often, but when your baby's at this angle, the diameter of her head is much bigger, and this makes it more likely that she'll get stuck during the birth. Try putting on a tight polo neck top using different parts of your head to push through and you'll understand why a tucked-in chin works best for birth!

 Laid-back mum

Listening to your body in labour rather than pre-planning each detail is often the way to go.

"I really wanted to go with the flow during my labour, and listen to my body rather than plan everything too closely. And when it came to it, my body was saying 'Help, this really hurts!' It turned out my baby was in the posterior position (see opposite, right) so I had the most excruciating backache, and it slowed my labour down loads. The pain went on for ages, so I finally opted for an epidural. It took the pain away completely, so I could just relax, and push when my midwife told me to. I did end up having an assisted forceps delivery, though – he didn't want to turn and decided to be born with his face looking up at me!"

ParentsTalk...

"My baby had his back next to my spine when I went into labour and it was really uncomfortable in the early stages. The only thing that helped was getting on all fours so he dropped away from my spine. He did eventually turn before making his grand entrance."
Joely, 28, mum to two-month-old Kieran

"My daughter was in a breech position right up until the week before my due date. I was willing her to get into the right position because I really didn't want to have a caesarean with my first baby. I wanted to try to do it without any assistance first. Thankfully, she turned nine days before I went into labour and I delivered her naturally."
Maeve, 30, mum to one-month-old Cath

"My baby wasn't in the right position when I went into labour and I was terrified of having to deliver him with the help of forceps or ventouse. Luckily, though, he decided to do mummy a favour and turn just as I reached 10cm."
Pritty, 31, mum to six-month-old David

About one in 10 babies are head down but lying "back-to-back" at the start of labour. This "posterior" position (see below, right) means that the back of the baby's head is toward the mother's spine. Most babies in this position are born vaginally but your labour may be longer and you may need an assisted birth.

It's rare, but your baby may be lying across your tummy – this is called a "transverse" or "oblique" lie. If your baby stays in this position you'll need a caesarean birth.

Babies lying with their bottom down and their head up are in a breech position. If your baby is breech as you start the third trimester, don't panic. At this stage, about one in five babies is breech but most turn on their own into a head-down position before labour starts. Only one in about 29 babies is still breech at 40 weeks. Although they can sometimes be born vaginally, in the UK most breech babies are born by caesarean section.

Common positions for your baby

As you approach your due date, you may notice that your midwife writes notes about your baby's position. When she does her routine examination, she'll feel for the position of your baby's head and then try to work out where her back is and where her arms and legs are. Here are the most common positions that your baby may be in:

Left occipitolateral (LOL) Your baby is lying on your left side with her back towards your left side.

Left occipitoanterior (LOA) Your baby is lying on your left side with her back towards your bump.

Left occipitoposterior (LOP) Your baby is lying on your left side with her back towards your back.

Right occipitolateral (ROL) Your baby is lying on your right side with her back towards your right side.

Right occipitoranterior (ROA) Your baby is lying on your right side with her back towards your bump.

Right occipitoposterior (ROP) Your baby is lying on your right side with her back towards your back.

Getting ready for pregnancy

Staying safe and healthy

Your pregnancy diary

Birth and beyond

Signs of labour

It's the question that's uppermost in most heavily pregnant women's minds: "How will I know when I'm in labour?" Persistent lower back pain and breaking waters are two possible signs. Read on to discover the other signs that say your baby's finally on his way.

Something's starting

Everyone's labour is different, and pinpointing when it begins is not really possible. It's more of a process than a single event. A number of changes in your body work together to help deliver your baby. Signs of the approach of labour include:

● Lightening (when the baby's head begins to drop into position in your pelvis); you may notice that you can breathe more deeply and eat more, but you'll also need to urinate more often.

● Vaginal discharge becomes heavier and full of mucus.

● More frequent, and noticeably more intense, Braxton Hicks contractions (see box, left).

● Vomiting and diarrhoea.

In early labour, also called the latent phase, you may experience some or all of the following:

● Persistent lower back or abdominal pain, often accompanied by a crampy premenstrual feeling.

● A bloody show (a brownish or blood-tinged mucus discharge). If you pass the mucus plug that blocks the cervix, labour could be imminent or it could be several days away. It's a sign that things are moving along.

● Painful contractions that occur at regular and increasingly shorter intervals and become longer and stronger in intensity.

● Broken waters, but you're in labour only if it's accompanied by contractions that are dilating your cervix.

How you will feel in early labour depends on whether you've had a baby before, how you perceive and respond to pain, and how prepared you are for what labour may be like.

What you do when you are in early labour will depend on what time of day it is, what you like doing and how you're feeling. Keeping calm and relaxed will

True contractions or Braxton Hicks?

Most women who are pregnant for the first time will ask their midwife or friends how to tell the difference between Braxton Hicks contractions (see p.177) and real labour. The answer is usually maddeningly vague: "You'll know real labour when it begins."

Labour contractions are noticeably longer as well as more regular, frequent and painful than Braxton Hicks contractions. Also, labour pains are persistent, and they increase in frequency, duration, and intensity as time goes on, while Braxton Hicks contractions are always unpredictable and non-rhythmic.

If your contractions have become longer, stronger, more regular and more frequent, then your labour may well be starting. Your midwife will probably have talked to you about what to do at this stage, but if you're in any doubt, give her a call.

If you have lower back pain that simply won't go away and a crampy feeling, you could be in the early stages of labour.

help your labour to progress and will also help you to cope with the contractions, so do whatever you like that will help you to stay relaxed.

Try to relax

Relaxing could mean watching a favourite film, reading, or asking a friend or relative over to keep you company for a couple of hours. You could alternate between walking and resting, or try taking a warm bath or shower to ease any aches and pains. If you can, try to get some rest to prepare you for the work ahead. You may feel hungry so eat and drink if you feel like it.

Early labour is a good time to try out different positions and breathing techniques (see pp.249 and 274) to see if they help you cope with the contractions, now that you're having them for real. If you've got a TENS machine (see p.272), early labour is the time to start using it.

Believe it or not, it is possible to have contractions and not be in labour. When you are in labour your cervix becomes progressively thinner (called effacement) and dilated. Some women are sensitive to the pain of contractions before the

The cervix is thick and firmly closed

The cervix starts to thin and open

Before labour starts, the cervix is thick, tough, short and firmly closed. The baby's head is engaged.

When labour starts, the cervix begins to thin out, stretch and open. This is known as "effacement".

"The start of **labour** is a **process** not a **single event.** It's not possible **to pinpoint** it exactly."

cervix has started to dilate. A midwife can confirm whether or not cervical changes have started by doing an internal examination.

If your baby is in a posterior position (with his head down but his back to your back; see p.255) it can take longer for your baby's head to engage and for

labour to get started properly. Your contractions may come erratically and may not be very intense, and you may also have a lot of backache.

Your midwife will advise you on ways to cope at home until labour becomes stronger. You could try a warm bath or massage to relieve the pain.

Parents**Talk...**

"There was no mistaking it when my contractions started. They were very low down like period pains but with an extra strong 'sting' at the peak of them. Just enough to make you go 'Ooooh, something's happening and it hurts!'"
Shona, 24, first-time mum

"I was trying to get to sleep when I felt a weird, rippling sensation down on my left-hand side. I thought maybe the baby had turned his head and scraped against something. Anyway, I turned over to try and get comfy and felt a gush of fluid – I went to the loo and saw that I was leaking fluid. It smelled like honey and had very

small blobs of blood in it. My midwife said it sounded like my waters had broken, so I called a taxi!"
Lesley, 30, mum to one-month-old René

"The night before my due date I kept waking up with what I thought were practice contractions, but I wasn't sure if I was in labour. I hadn't lost my mucus plug and my waters hadn't broken. When the contractions jumped to being every three to six minutes and each one felt stronger than the last. I knew this was it. I never did spot the mucus plug, but I did have a beautiful baby boy on my due date!"
Mei, 27, mum to two-month-old Alex

Getting ready for pregnancy

Staying safe and healthy

Your pregnancy diary

Birth and beyond

Parents**Talk...**

"My waters broke four weeks early while I was in the supermarket. I was so embarrassed that I told my husband to finish the shopping. I went to wait for him in the car."
Rhian, 27, mum to two-month-old Dylan

"A few days before my due date, my waters started trickling out while I was out for dinner with my husband. I dashed to the loo to dry off. It was only when I saw the pink-coloured liquid that I realised it couldn't be wee."
Maria, 30, mum to seven-month-old Angelina

"My waters broke when my husband and I were having a spot of lovemaking – so it kind of ruined the mood!"
Penny, 29, first-time mum

"When my waters broke I was on an underground train on my way home from some last-minute baby shopping – I quickly got off at the next stop, leaving a wet seat behind and hailed a taxi home as fast as I could."
Gemma, 25, mum to year-old Leah

"When I was 9cm dilated and they were encouraging me, I suddenly got the urge to push. I screamed, 'No, my waters haven't broken!'. With that said, my waters gushed out with a huge push, exploding all over my husband. I couldn't help it. I started laughing and kept laughing in between intense contractions. Just the look on his face was enough to set me off."
Fiona, 32, second-time mum

My waters are breaking

During pregnancy your baby is protected and cushioned inside your uterus in a bag of membranes full of amniotic fluid. If a tear forms in the bag then the fluid leaks out via the cervix and vagina. This is known as your "waters breaking". It is written in your notes as SROM (spontaneous rupture of membranes).

Most women's waters break towards the end of the first stage of labour. For about one in 10 women the waters break at the end of pregnancy but before labour starts (prelabour rupture of membranes at term or PROM).

Prelabour rupture

If your waters do break before you go into labour, don't panic. Put on a sanitary pad for protection. This will also make it easier to see the colour of the fluid you are losing. The fluid is almost clear with a yellow tinge, and possibly a little bloodstained to begin with.

The amount of fluid you lose may vary. It may be a slight trickle or a large "gush". If there is a lot of fluid, a sanitary pad will not be enough and you'll be better off using an old hand towel. While undignified, it's more practical, especially if you need to travel by car to hospital or the birth centre.

It's important that, regardless of how many weeks pregnant you are when your waters break, you should be seen fairly quickly for an assessment. Once your waters have broken, there is less protection against getting an infection.

Once you have been examined, provided you are at least 37 weeks pregnant, you can choose to be induced. This will usually be done about 24 hours after your waters have broken. Alternatively, the staff at the hospital might decide on a "wait and see" policy – to see if you go into labour after the 24 hours are up. About nine out of 10 women at full term give birth naturally within 24 to 48 hours of their waters breaking. If your waters break earlier than 37 weeks – between 34 and 37 weeks – you may also have a choice of induction or to wait and see.

If all is well with you and your baby, you can go home if you wish while you wait. A wait-and-see approach carries a slight risk of infection (about 1 per cent of women compared to 0.5 per cent of women whose waters haven't broken). In the meantime, it's safe for you to have a bath or shower but don't have sex once your waters have broken as this increases your risk of infection.

70% of women whose waters have broken will go into labour within 24 hours, almost 90 per cent within 48 hours, and 95 to 96 per cent go into labour within 72 hours.

The "wait and see" approach

While you wait to see if you go into labour naturally, you will need to:

- Have your baby's heart rate and movements checked by a midwife or doctor every 24 hours until you go into labour or are induced.
- Check your temperature every four hours while you're awake to see if you're developing a fever.
- Check for changes in the colour and smell of the amniotic fluid (waters), which could indicate an infection.
- Check that your baby is still moving as usual.

If you have any signs of infection or fever (such as shivering and flushing), or you've noticed a decrease in your baby's movements, contact the hospital immediately. If an infection is diagnosed you'll need intravenous antibiotics and to be induced straight away.

If you have no signs of infection but your waters have been broken for more than 24 hours, you're advised to give birth in hospital. This is because your baby may need immediate access or transfer to neonatal care.

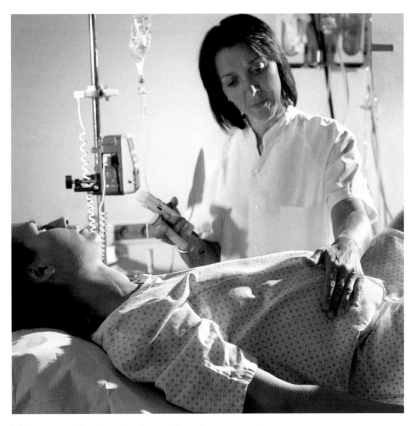

After your waters have broken you'll need an assessment. If everything's OK with you and your baby, you can choose to be induced, or wait to see if you go into labour naturally.

ParentsAsk...

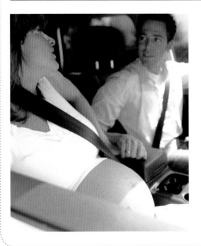

It's unlikely during a first labour that you won't have enough time to get to hospital. The first phase of labour can take a long time.

How will I know if it's too late to get to hospital?

When you are having a first baby, it's very unusual for labour to progress so quickly that you'll leave it too late to get to hospital. First labours can be very long. The so-called "latent phase" (before the cervix has opened to 3cm; see p.262) may last for many hours. Second and subsequent labours, however, tend to be quicker because your pelvis and vagina have already been stretched once and so are more elastic than last time around.

If you are still at home, and you have an uncontrollable urge to push, then it might well be too late to go to hospital. If you find yourself in this situation, call the hospital – or call 999 if you don't happen to have the hospital number to hand. The emergency services will arrange for either a paramedic or a midwife to come out to you at home. They'll also stay on the telephone with you until help arrives.

If you've had a previous labour that was fast and furious, it's important to be especially attuned to the signs of labour. Be prepared to make a mad dash for the hospital, because subsequent labours can go even faster.

False labour

You're having contractions, but they're coming and going. Are you in labour or not? Some women experience "false" labour at full term, in which contractions are sporadic and your cervix fails to open. Try to relax – it's a positive sign that your baby's birth is not far away.

If you think labour may be starting don't feel embarrassed to call your midwife to check what you should do next.

Is this the real thing?

As you approach your due date, the Braxton Hicks contractions (see p.177) that you may have been feeling since mid-pregnancy sometimes become more rhythmic, relatively close together, and even painful, possibly fooling you into thinking you're in labour. But, unlike true labour, this so-called false labour doesn't cause significant, progressive dilation of your cervix, and the contractions don't grow consistently longer, stronger and closer together.

Sometimes it's hard to tell the difference between false labour and the early stages of true labour. Not every woman has bouts of false labour. And in some cases, the strong, regular contractions of true labour come on with little or no warning.

What might be happening

If you're 37 weeks or more, here are some clues to what's going on:

● False labour contractions are unpredictable. They come at irregular intervals and vary in length and intensity. Although true labour contractions may be irregular at first, with time they start coming at more regular and shorter intervals, they become increasingly more intense, and they last longer.

● With false labour, the pain from the contractions is more likely to be centred in your lower abdomen. With true labour, you may feel the pain start in your lower back and wrap around to your abdomen.

● False labour contractions may subside on their own or when you start or stop an activity or change position. True labour contractions will persist and progress no matter what you do.

If you're not yet 37 weeks, don't waste time trying to work out what's going on. If you notice any signs of

---

When to contact your midwife

You and your midwife have probably talked about what to do when you think you're in labour. But if you're not sure whether or not the time has come, don't be embarrassed to call. Midwives are used to getting calls from women who need guidance; it's part of their job.

The truth is that they can tell a lot by the tone of your voice, so talking to her helps. She will want to know how close together your contractions are, whether or not you can talk through a contraction, and any other symptoms you may have.

If you're planning to have your baby in hospital or a birth centre, she may ask you to come in so that she can make an assessment. If she thinks you're still in early labour, depending on how you're coping and whether you've got a birth partner to support you, she may encourage you to go back home until you're in stronger active labour.

You should contact your midwife or doctor if:

● Your waters break, or if you suspect you're leaking amniotic fluid.

● Your baby is moving less than usual.

● You have vaginal bleeding (unless it's just a little blood-tinged mucus).

● You have a fever, severe headaches, any changes in your vision, or any abdominal pain.

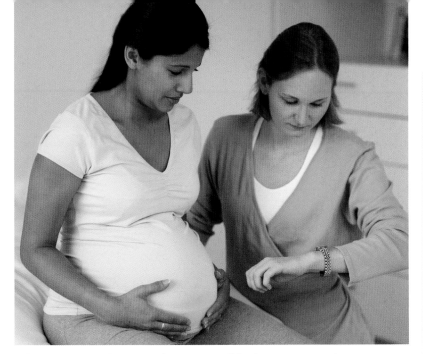

Time your contractions to see what is going on. If they become more regular, closer together, more intense and longer-lasting, then your labour has started.

labour, call your doctor or midwife right away, especially if you have a watery or bloody discharge from your vagina.

After 37 weeks, you can sit out the contractions (whether they are false or from true early labour) at home and see what develops. The exceptions to this are if you think your waters have broken (see pp.258–9), if you have any bleeding or if you think your baby's movements have decreased.

False labour contractions can be a real drag, interfering with your sleep and making you tired and irritable. You might also feel anxious, wondering when true labour will start. If you feel discomfort, it sometimes helps to lie down or, conversely, to get up and take a walk – it's the change in activity that can help ease any pain you feel. A warm bath sometimes helps, too.

Now is a good time to practise staying relaxed during contractions, too. Take a deep breath and, as you breathe out, let your muscles relax so that they feel loose and soft. This way, by the time you eventually go into labour you will automatically be able to identify areas of tension in your body and to relax them.

If you have an older child, you might be constantly wondering whether it's time to call the babysitter. When in doubt, make the call – there's no harm done, even if you don't end up in labour, and you may be able to rest more easily knowing that help is at hand.

Time your contractions until you get a sense of what's going on. And don't hesitate to call your doctor or midwife to check in if you're concerned, confused, or just need a little encouragement or reassurance.

Dad's **Diary**

False alarm story
"**1.00am** Emma wakes up, she has some sharp pains in her sides.
1:45am Emma: 'I'm getting the BH contractions at seven-minute intervals, very regular.'
2:00am Check pregnancy books – should BH contractions be random or what? Neither of us can remember. OK – it seems like they're just BH contractions. Attempt to relax.
2:15am Emma: 'OK… brown mucus discharge. Looks like the "show"'
2:16am Me: 'DON'T PANIC! CALL THE HOSPITAL!'
I then panic and grab the bags for hospital. Emma calls the hospital who advises us to go straight there.
2:45am 'RABBIT!' screams Emma as I swerve across the slip road of the motorway. Those suicidal rabbits are a nightmare! Luckily I avoid hitting him – karma remains balanced.
3:45am After various discussions, samples and examinations, Emma is hooked up to a machine to check her contractions. We're told that the figure needs to read 90 to 100 for it to be 'the real thing' but Em is peaking at 50. The midwife leaves us on monitor for more time to check contractions.
4:15am The midwife checks Emma's cervix. It's confirmed that things aren't really happening but it was wise to check. She reassures us that, although the cervix isn't yet dilating, Em's body is getting ready for labour and that's a good sign. Doctor comes in and says Em can stay in if she chooses but we politely decline and head home.
05:45am Finally get to bed! So it was our first 'false alarm'. It was a good test run, though."

"False **labour contractions** come at **irregular intervals** and vary in length **and intensity**."

First stage of labour

Early labour is an enjoyable, exciting part of your baby's birth. While contractions are still mild it's time to tune in to your body and do whatever feels right. Taking a nap, eating a healthy snack or just watching TV will help you to gather strength for the hard work ahead.

Latent and active phases of labour

The early phase of labour is sometimes called the latent period or pre-labour. The uterus starts to contract or tighten regularly and the contractions gradually become more painful. As the cervix begins to open, its position in your pelvis changes, moving forwards. It softens and effaces, which means that it gets thinner and springier.

At this stage, you'll probably be able to potter around the house, go for a walk, watch a DVD, take a warm bath or have a nap. Relax as much as you can and have lots of snacks to keep your energy levels up. If you want to use a TENS machine (see p.272), put it on during this early phase as it seems to work best when used from the very start of labour.

Midwives and doctors say you are in active labour when your cervix has dilated, or opened, to 3 to 4cm. Your contractions will be getting stronger and more frequent. They will also be getting longer. Eventually they may be coming as frequently as every three to four minutes and lasting as long as 60 to 90 seconds.

The time to go to hospital or the birth centre is when you and your birth companion feel you would be more

The cervix
becomes springy
and thinner

The cervix
has opened
to 3–4cm

During the latent phase of labour, the cervix begins to stretch and thin. This is the start of effacement.

During the active phase of labour, contractions are stronger and the cervix thins to 3 to 4cm.

Coping with backache labour

If you are having a "backache labour", try one or more of these tactics to help relieve the pain:

● Get on all fours. This position may reduce the pressure of your baby's head on your spine.

● Do pelvic tilts (see p.151). These simple exercises may also help to minimise the pressure on your spine.

● Ask your labour coach to rub your lower back between or during contractions, or both – whatever feels best to you.

● Many women find that steady counter pressure on the lower back helps to relieve some of the pain. Ask your labour partner to push on this area with his fists during contractions or massage it with a tennis ball.

● Take a warm bath or shower, or apply warm compresses or a hot-water bottle to your lower back. Heat may ease the achiness and bring you some comfort. On the other hand, some women find cold packs more soothing, or that alternating hot and cold is helpful. You may want to give both a try. Just be sure to use a towel to protect your skin from direct contact with heat or cold.

● If you don't have your heart set on natural childbirth, consider getting an epidural. In most cases, it provides total pain relief.

relaxed there than at home. If you're having a home birth, call your midwife when you need some reassurance. Contractions may start to feel as if they are coming one on top of another. Try to work with your body. What is it telling you to do? Would you be more comfortable in a different position? Would it help if you went to the toilet?

Breathing and relaxation techniques really come into their own now; your partner can remind you how to use them. You could try some gas and air to take the edge off the contractions. Consider taking a warm shower or bath or getting into the birth pool. Many women find the warm water relaxing and it's easier to change position in the pool. You hear stories of women who sink into a bath or pool when they're 5 or 6cm dilated, relax, and are fully dilated an hour later!

During the first stage of labour, try to find a position that's comfortable for you. This will allow you to focus on your breathing.

Using a birth ball can help to keep you upright and leaning forwards, which is a good position for helping your baby descend.

Monitoring your baby in labour

Your midwife will listen to your baby's heartbeat during labour to get an idea of whether she is coping well with labour or is becoming distressed. There are two ways she can listen.

Using an electronic fetal monitor enables your baby's heartbeat to be checked while you are in labour.

Intermittent monitoring

During labour, listening to your baby's heartbeat using a Sonicaid or Pinard is an essential part of your care. You only have to keep still for a minute or so while your midwife listens in and then you can move around again. Your midwife will monitor your baby at least every 15 minutes during the first stage of labour, and once every five minutes during the pushing stage. This is called intermittent auscultation.

Women who are considered to have a high-risk pregnancy should be given continuous electronic fetal monitoring (EFM; see below)

Electronic fetal monitoring (EFM)

This type of monitoring is done using two electronic sensors that are held in place with elastic belts. One is placed on top of your tummy and one over your baby's heart. Each sensor is attached to a wire which, in turn, is attached to a machine. The machine produces two lines on a piece of graph paper. One line records your baby's heartbeat and the other, your contractions. By studying the relationship between the two, your midwife and doctor get an idea of how your baby is doing. Sometimes, a small clip is placed on your baby's head and this monitors her heartbeat instead of the abdominal sensor. The clip is called a fetal scalp electrode and it may provide a more accurate reading.

First stage of labour: transition

For lots of women, transition is the toughest part of labour. As your cervix dilates fully to allow your baby to pass through, your contractions become stronger and you may start to wonder if you can cope. Hang on in there – it won't be long until you can start pushing.

The cervix is now fully dilated so your baby can be pushed out via the birth canal.

The neck of the cervix now measures 10cm

Now what's happening?

Transition is the last stage of the first phase of labour. It is the time when your cervix dilates from about 8 to 10cm. This stage of labour can be a stormy time, physically and emotionally, but the end is in sight.

Your contractions may start to come one on top of another. Instead of peaking and fading away, the contraction may peak, start to fade and then rev up again to a second peak. These contractions may be longer, but

they may also be less frequent, giving you a bit of time to recover in between.

Transition may last for just a few contractions or it may feel like it's never going to end. The muscles of your uterus start to work differently during transition, and you may begin to feel some expulsive, pushing contractions. If you feel like pushing but your cervix isn't fully dilated, your midwife may ask you to not push, but to pant through these contractions instead.

How to cope with the transition phase

If you're labouring without an epidural, this is when you may fear you can't handle the pain. You'll need lots of support from those around you.

● Some women appreciate a light massage (effleurage), some prefer a stronger touch, and others don't want to be touched at all.

● A change of position can bring relief – for example, if you're feeling a lot of pressure in your lower back, getting on all fours may reduce the discomfort.

● A cool cloth on your forehead or a cold pack on your back may feel good, or you may find a warm compress more comforting.

On the other hand, because transition can take all of your concentration, you may want all distractions – music or conversation or even that cool cloth or your partner's loving touch – eliminated.

It may be useful to focus on the fact that those hard contractions are helping your baby make the journey out into the world. Try visualising his movement down with each contraction.

The good news is that, if you've made it this far without medication, you can usually be coached through transition – one contraction at a time – with constant reminders that you're doing a great job and that the end is near.

Ask your birth partner to put a cool cloth on your forehead to help to soothe you during the transition stage.

Dad's **Diary**

Our labour story

"Jenny was surprisingly calm and polite between contractions, but then I'd hear the most blood-curdling howl I'd ever heard in my life. You meet ultra-butch, Alpha-male dads who've fainted at this point, and you can understand why fathers used to be barred from births.

But the worst thing is that there's not a lot you can do. Your instinct is to cuddle your partner and to try to make the pain go away but, of course, it won't. It's horrible. And the last thing she wants is the man who put her through all this telling her, 'Don't worry honey, it'll be all right.' Your main role is as an advocate – to convince overworked midwives that your wife's contractions really do hurt, that she's started dilating, that she still wants to stick to her birth plan and, no, she still doesn't want an epidural.

Like bare-knuckle boxing, labour is an endless barrage of noise, blood and bodily fluids. And yes, chances are that there'll be some tearing involved.

I became an auxiliary midwife as my wife was choreographed through more and more improbable birthing positions (on your knees, on your back, bend double, lean against me, try squatting, don't forget to breathe). Woe betide the man who hasn't done his homework."

ParentsTalk...

"Things weren't great for me during the transition phase – each contraction went on for ages and was so painful. I was just screaming and gripping my husband's hand so tightly that I bruised him. (But despite him yelling from the pain, there's no way it came close to what I was going through!)"
Pippa, 29, mum to month-old Owen

"For me, the transitional phase was the most physically difficult part of the whole of the labour process – I felt shaky and nauseous from the pressure and pain my body was enduring as the contractions were pushing my cervix to its limit before the big push."
Yoko, 31, mum to year-old Ricky

"The transitional stage had no effect on me – I couldn't feel a thing because of the epidural! The only problem came when I had to push. I had to wait for my midwife to give me the cue as I couldn't feel the contractions. That was a really odd sensation."
Frances, 24, first-time mum

"The pain was so intense, I felt like I was having an out-of-body experience during the transitional stage of my labour. I'd been doing my breathing through my contractions the whole time and, as they got stronger and longer, I just had the feeling that I was floating away on a cloud! It felt quite blissful."
Rachel, 30, mum to month-old James

Usually there is some sort of change in your behaviour, which marks the transition phase. You might feel shaky, shivery or sick. You may feel so out of control that you want to shout and scream, and demand pain relief. You may feel that you really can't carry on any more! Or, you may feel sleepy and go within yourself during this stage. Some call this experience the "rest and be thankful" stage.

Partners are often quite worried by this stage of labour. You may feel the need to shout, cry out or even swear as a way of coping, but your partner may see it as a sign that you need help and he may feel alarmed. Make sure he's

Your partner needs to be extra patient while you are in the transition stage, especially if you feel like shouting at him.

"Some **call this** experience the **'rest and be thankful'** stage."

well prepared for this stage. If he is aware of what is happening, he is more likely to be able to get through it himself – and to give you the support you need to help you get through it.

Recognising that you're in transition, in whatever form it takes for you, can give you a boost. It means that you're nearly there! Think of it as a bridge you need to cross to reach your baby.

Getting ready for pregnancy

Staying safe and healthy

Your pregnancy diary

Birth and beyond

Positions for labour

Forget those pictures you've seen on TV of women flopping around in bed during labour. Giving birth is a bit like running a marathon – it requires strength and stamina – and using active, upright positions is one of the things that will help your body to do its important work.

First stage positions

When labour starts, you'll probably feel restless. You'll want to move around but don't get over-tired before your labour is properly underway. Have short rests in a chair or lying down. If labour starts at night, try to stay in bed and relax for as long as possible.

As contractions get stronger, you'll need to concentrate on them and practise your breathing and relaxation exercises. Now is the time to find the positions that best help you cope with your contractions. Your midwife should help you find a comfortable position.

You might think that you'll be most comfortable lying down. However, keeping upright will help your labour to progress and you and your baby to cope better during labour.

Sitting facing the back of a chair with your arms on the back for support gives you the chance to have a back massage.

Sitting on an exercise ball keeps you upright. This position helps you concentrate on your rhythmic breathing.

Lying down helps you conserve your energy during the first stage. Try tucking a pillow under your bent leg for comfort.

Transition stage

As you reach transition, upright positions can help lessen the pain of contractions and make it easier for your birth partner to massage your back or breathe with you. You could put your arms around your partner's neck and lean on him, or lean on a work surface or the back of a chair, Some women prefer to go onto all fours or kneel on one leg with the other bent. Rock your hips backwards and forwards or in a circle to help your baby through your pelvis.

You'll probably find that you don't want to move around a great deal. You'll need all your strength simply to cope with each contraction as it comes along.

Leaning on a pillow with your legs wide apart can help open your pelvis, which makes space for your baby to get through.

Positions for pushing

Finding a comfortable upright position is recommended for the pushing stage of labour. You are less likely to need help with instruments to deliver your baby if you're upright. The combination of the muscular action of your uterus, your pushing efforts, a wider outlet through the pelvis and gravity is a powerful one.

Alternatively, you could try kneeling on the mattress and leaning against a large pile of pillows placed at the top end. Some women find it very helpful to kneel on the bed and put their arms around their partner's neck as he stands at the bedside.

If your midwife is happy for you to give birth on the floor, you could try kneeling. When it's time for your baby's head to be born, kneeling on all fours is an excellent position. Gravity is not so effective in this position, so your baby's head is able to emerge very gently from the vagina.

An all-fours position is very good for giving birth gently as it reduces the effect of gravity.

The knee-chest position helps slow things down while you adjust to stronger contractions.

Getting ready for pregnancy

Staying safe and healthy

Your pregnancy diary

Birth and beyond

Second stage of labour

Once your cervix is fully dilated, the work and excitement of the second stage begin. This is the stage of labour when your uterus pushes your baby down the birth canal and out into the world. The hard work is nearly over and you're about to meet your baby.

Descent and birth

During the second stage, your contractions change to expulsive, pushing contractions. You will feel pressure between your legs as your baby moves down your vagina.

As your baby descends you may get an overwhelming urge to push and hear yourself grunting deep in your throat with each contraction. For many women the urge to bear down and vocalise is instinctive and feels completely natural.

Not everyone feels "pushy", though. If you've had an epidural, the pushing

Seek reassurance and encouragement from your birth partner while you are doing the difficult job of pushing your baby out.

urge may be delayed for a while. Some women don't get the pushing urge at all. Your midwife may suggest you wait a while to see if the urge comes on or she may help you get into a good position for pushing and guide you to bear down with each contraction. She might ask you to push down into your bottom, as if you were having a really big poo!

The walls of your vagina are a bit like the folds of a concertina. Each contraction helps your baby stretch and move down the folds until his head appears at the entrance of your vagina. "Crowning" is when his head stays visible at your perineum and doesn't slip back at the end of a contraction. At this

ParentsAsk...

Will I need an episiotomy?
Your vagina is soft and stretchy and is designed to stretch around your baby's head as he moves down the birth canal. However, around 14 per cent of women need an episiotomy during labour.

An episiotomy is a small cut made in the skin and muscle from the entrance of the vagina towards the back passage. Your midwife will give you a local anaesthetic before the cut is made. An episiotomy will

need to be stitched afterwards using water-soluble stitches. You'll be given some more local anaesthetic.

The most common reason for having an episiotomy is during an assisted birth with forceps or ventouse. An episiotomy may also be used if your baby is in distress and needs to be born quickly or if your baby is very premature (the episiotomy may help to protect his head). Other reasons why you might need an episiotomy include if you are

distressed or very tired, or if it is taking a very long time for the tissues of the vagina to stretch.

You may have feelings about having an episiotomy. It can be useful to discuss these with your midwife during your pregnancy and also during labour. Having a birth plan (see pp.174–5) will help to get the conversation started and ensure that your wishes are heard and noted by the staff who are caring for you.

Getting ready for pregnancy

Staying safe and healthy

Your pregnancy diary

Birth and beyond

The head crowns, which means that it appears at the vaginal opening. When this happens, your midwife will tell you to pant instead of pushing to give the perineum time to stretch a bit more and to allow the head to emerge gradually.

The head emerges fully so it is free of the perineum. Your baby will extend his neck and automatically turn to face left or right to the inside of one of your thighs. His shoulders will now be in the best position for a smooth delivery.

The first shoulder slips under the pubic bone, quickly followed by the other shoulder. Now the rest of his body is free to slip out and he can be put on your tummy.

point, you may want to reach down and touch the top of his head.

Listen to your body during this second stage and push when you get a strong urge. You'll probably want to push down several times during the course of a contraction, taking breaths in between, particularly when you start to push your baby's head out. Try not to hold your breath to push, as bearing down for long periods is more likely to result in you tearing. It's best not to hurry this stage.

Pant, don't push

You'll probably get a hot, stinging sensation as the tissues of your perineum and the entrance of your vagina stretch. Rather than pressing on through this "ring of fire", try to pant instead of pushing. Give the tissues of your perineum time to stretch a little more with each contraction.

When your baby's head is born you'll feel a sudden release. With the next contraction your baby's shoulders and body will be born. First-time babies usually take longer than second or later

babies, just because your body has done it all before.

Once your baby has emerged, he'll be dried and, if there aren't any complications, he'll be put on your tummy so you can touch and marvel at him. The skin-to-skin contact will keep him nice and toasty, and he'll be covered with a warm blanket – and perhaps given his first hat – to prevent heat loss. Your midwife will clamp the umbilical cord in two places and then cut between the two clamps – or your partner might like to do the honours.

The second stage can take from a few minutes to two or three hours. You'll feel proud, but relieved it's all over.

Fact: With each contraction and every push, your baby will move down through your pelvis a little, but at the end of the contraction, he'll slip back up again! Don't despair. As long as the baby keeps on moving on a little further each time, you're doing fine.

Working mum

Work and being promoted are important, but giving birth is a unique experience.

"Ever since my first job, my work has always been really important to me. I've never resented doing overtime or putting the hours in at home if I needed to meet a deadline. Every promotion has meant the world to me because I know it's something I've earned on my own merits. My family have been really pleased with how far I've come, too.

However, that has all paled into insignificance now. When I gave birth to my son, after more than 20 hours of labour, I felt like I was going to burst with pride. Looking into his eyes, and at his perfect fingers and toes, I knew instantly that he was my greatest achievement. Nothing would ever top this feeling of pure satisfaction that I had made him. I've never felt happier or more content."

Third stage of labour

In the third stage, you deliver the placenta – the life-support system that has supplied your growing baby with nutrients and taken waste products away. Be prepared for a few more contractions and then, at last, the chance to relax and admire your beautiful new baby.

It's not quite over yet!

After your baby is born, contractions resume a few minutes later, but at much less intensity. These contractions cause the placenta to peel away from the wall of the uterus and drop down into the bottom of your uterus. You will probably feel as if you want to push. The placenta, with the membranes of the empty bag of waters attached, will pass down and out of your vagina. Once this has happened, your midwife will carefully examine the placenta and membranes to make sure that nothing has been left behind. She will also feel your tummy to check that your uterus is contracting, as this is nature's way of stopping the bleeding from the place on the uterus where the placenta was attached.

Delivering the placenta usually takes from five to 15 minutes, but it can take up to an hour. You may hardly be aware of the third stage, as your focus has probably shifted to your baby. Seeing and handling your baby, and offering her the breast will stimulate hormones that help the placenta to separate.

You may hardly notice the third stage of labour as you lie there with your newborn baby on your tummy.

How you will feel

Now that the birth is over, you may feel shaky due to adrenaline and the adjustments your body immediately starts to make. Or you may simply be on a high, ready to pick up your baby and dance around the room.

Some women find it hard to pay attention to the baby if they've had a long labour, or if they've had pethidine or a similar drug. There's nothing wrong with their maternal instincts; they're simply exhausted. If this happens to you, take your time. After a rest, you'll be much more interested in getting to know your baby. A lot of women are hungry and ready for tea and toast, while others want to telephone all their friends and family and tell them the wonderful news.

A natural or managed third stage?

You have the choice between a managed or a physiological (natural) third stage.

● A managed third stage involves an injection in your thigh as your baby is being born. The cord is clamped and cut immediately and the injection makes the uterus contract strongly so the placenta comes away and is delivered quickly.

This is all over quickly, usually in five to 10 minutes. There is little blood loss and less risk of you having heavy bleeding.

● A physiological, or natural, third stage means waiting for the placenta to be delivered naturally. This can take from 20 minutes up to an hour. You will need to actively help the delivery of the placenta by pushing. Cord clamping is delayed until the cord has stopped pulsating. This ensures that your baby gets the maximum amount of oxygenated blood from the placenta. There is a higher risk of blood loss if you opt for a natural third stage.

The placenta is attached to your baby's umbilical cord (yellowish-white). After the placenta has been delivered, the midwife will check to make sure it is all present.

ParentsAsk...

What is postpartum haemorrhage?

A primary postpartum haemorrhage (PPH) is heavy bleeding in the first 24 hours after the birth. It happens in about 5 per cent of births with a managed third stage and in 13 per cent of births with a natural or physiological third stage.

Most cases of primary PPH are due to the uterus not contracting down properly after the birth to shut off all the blood vessels where the placenta was attached. You may feel the blood trickling out or sometimes it builds up inside your uterus, so you may not be aware of the haemorrhage until signs of shock appear: a drop in blood pressure and a rise in your pulse rate, and you may feel faint and dizzy.

Your midwife regularly checks your uterus after birth to make sure it is firm and contracted. If it is soft she will massage the top of the uterus to encourage it to contract. She may give you another oxytocin injection and an intravenous drip to help your blood to clot. If the bleeding is severe, you may need a blood transfusion.

Complications in the third stage

Retained placenta means that all or part of the placenta or membranes are left behind in the uterus during the third stage of labour. You'll be treated for a retained placenta if the third stage takes longer than usual or if there are signs that a small piece of placenta that was connected to the main part of the placenta by a blood vessel is still attached to the uterus.

The midwife will examine the placenta and membranes very carefully after delivery to ensure that they are complete. If she notices a blood vessel leading to nowhere, this should alert her to the possibility that part of the placenta has been left behind in the uterus.

Sometimes a part of the placenta may adhere to a fibroid or to a scar from a previous caesarean. Sometimes a full bladder will prevent the placenta from being delivered, so your midwife may insert a catheter to drain your bladder.

Normally after the placenta is delivered, your uterus contracts down to close off all the blood vessels inside it.

If the placenta only partially separates, the uterus cannot contract properly, so the blood vessels inside will continue to bleed. If small fragments of placenta or membrane are retained and are not detected immediately, this may cause heavy bleeding (see Parents Ask, above) and infection later on.

If the third stage is taking a while, you could try breastfeeding your baby or rubbing your nipples. This can make the uterus contract and may help to expel the placenta. If you're sitting or lying, try changing to a more upright position so that gravity can help.

If the placenta still can't be removed, it may need to be removed manually. You'll be given a regional anaesthetic, although you can ask for a general anaesthetic if you prefer.

Dad's **Diary**

My big thrill

"The midwives had me holding up one of my wife's legs at a bizarre angle while I tried not to look at what was going on between her legs. Jenny told me afterwards that I proved to be a big, safe, chunky cushion to lean against.

After the most protracted scream I'd ever heard in my life, out it popped. I picked up our wonky-headed, blood-covered, prune-faced little baby, with a furry back and alarmingly hairy ears. The fruit of my loins. 'It's a girl!' I shouted excitedly. (This was a relief. Our boys' names were all rubbish, but we both liked the same girl's name – Lilah.)

Then I was given the honour of cutting the umbilical cord. I hadn't really planned to do this. I thought I'd be too squeamish but, after everything I'd seen Jenny go through during the last few hours, this was a breeze. It was the first thing I did to care for my new baby daughter and it made me feel like a daddy for the first time."

Getting ready for pregnancy

Staying safe and healthy

Your pregnancy diary

Birth and beyond

Natural pain relief

We're lucky to live in an age when we can have effective pain relief during labour if we want to. Some forms of medical pain relief, though, can have side effects for you and your baby, so it pays to be clued up on natural pain-relief methods, too.

Your choices

Gone are the days when pain relief in labour meant using a magic charm. You now have a range of natural options to choose from.

TENS

TENS stands for Transcutaneous Electrical Nerve Stimulation. A TENS machine is a small box with a clip that you can attach to your clothing. Leading out of the box are four wires connected to sticky pads. These give out pulses of electrical energy which are thought to help block pain messages to the brain.

Your birth partner can place the pads on your back for you. Two are placed on either side of your spine at about bra-strap level. The other two go lower down, at about the level of the dimples in your bottom.

The TENS machine has dials that you can adjust to control the frequency and strength of the pulses. There's also a boost button for you to hold in your hand and press when you want maximum output from the machine. This can help you with a particularly difficult contraction.

TENS seems to work best and give you the most effective pain relief if you start using it at the very beginning of your labour. Start with the controls at their lowest settings and turn them up gradually as your contractions get stronger. Use the boost button at the peak of contractions.

Acupuncture and acupressure

Acupuncture, which uses fine needles inserted into specific energy points of the body, may help to induce labour and reduce labour pains. You'll need to have a private acupuncturist with you in labour if you wish to use it. Acupressure involves finger-tip pressure on these same energy points.

If your contractions are painful, ask your partner to massage very firmly into the small of your back. He can also use his thumbs to press firmly into the dimples on either side of your lower spine, starting at your coccyx (tailbone)

Music can help you relax during any stage of your labour.

Sitting in a bath or birth pool can be so relaxing that your labour sometimes slows down.

and moving up to your waist. Ask him to apply pressure to each pair of dimples for two seconds, then move up to the next pair, and so on. When he reaches your waist area, he needs to start again at your coccyx. He can do this about four times during each contraction.

Reflexology

Reflexology is based on the idea that your feet represent a map of your body. Reflexologists believe that pressure on particular points of the feet will alleviate symptoms in the corresponding part of the body.

If you are finding contractions hard to cope with, ask your birth partner to squeeze your heels several times during a contraction. Your heels are supposed to represent the reflexology zone for the pelvis. Squeezing your heels is a way of "hugging" the part of your body that is doing all the work during labour.

If your contractions slow down, your partner could massage the back of your big toes. There's a reflexology point here which is believed to relate to the pituitary gland in your brain, from which labour hormones are produced.

Hypnotherapy

Hypnotherapy can help to reduce pain by preparing you mentally for labour and birth, and by using the power of suggestion to help you relax. It may also help to alter your perception of pain.

You can learn self-hypnosis techniques from specialist CDs, or do a special hypnotherapy course while you're pregnant. Some women find their own registered hypnotherapist. She may use traditional hypnosis techniques both before and during your labour.

Hypnosis may shorten the first stage of labour but it can lengthen the second stage slightly. If you choose to have medical pain relief in addition to hypnotherapy, you might find that you can cope with much lower doses.

Water and water births

It's quite common for women to get into a shower, bath or special birth pool to help cope with labour, and many midwives are experienced and skilled in supporting this.

If you are using a birth pool in hospital, you may not be able to get into the pool until your labour is well

Natural pain relief methods

This handy summary of natural pain relief shows what you – and your partner – can easily do to help ease those labour pains.

- ask for information: the more you know, the more relaxed you'll feel
- breathe rhythmically
- cuddle your partner
- drink sips of isotonic drinks or water in between contractions
- eat carbohydrate-rich foods little and often if you feel hungry
- fan yourself with a small electric fan
- groan and moan – making a noise is a great coping strategy!
- hold your partner's hand
- imagine your baby moving down through your pelvis with every contraction
- joke with your partner and your midwife
- kisses (from your partner, mum, sister, friend)
- listen to music
- move around
- nestle down in a large pile of pillows
- open your pelvis as wide as possible, for example, by kneeling on one leg with the other out to the side
- positive thinking is a must
- question what you don't understand
- rock your pelvis
- sigh out gently with every breath
- trust your body
- understand the treatment offered
- visit the toilet regularly – a full bladder will slow your labour
- walk around to ease aches and pains
- more kisses!
- yell, loud and long
- zzzzzzz: doze off in between contractions

established. This is because getting into the pool may cause labour to slow down. Once you get in, you might find either that your contractions are less intense for a while, or that they suddenly become more frequent and stronger. Either way, you will benefit.

Remember that the pool is there for you to use as it suits you. This may mean getting in and out several times, or staying in all the time, or getting out completely if it doesn't seem to help.

As the end of the first stage of labour approaches and contractions are coming thick and fast, you might want to get out of the pool, even if you had originally intended to give birth in it. Or, alternatively, you might feel that you simply cannot get out, although your

plan had been to give birth on dry land. Unless your hospital has a strict policy about women not giving birth in the pool, you are free to choose what you want to do when the time comes.

Breathing techniques

In labour, you need to conserve your energy as much as possible and give your baby plenty of oxygen to help him cope with the birth process. Rhythmic breathing can help you do this and focusing on your breathing is a great way of getting through each contraction.

Take a deep breath at the beginning of the contraction and, as you breathe out, re-lax. Then breathe in through your nose and breathe out through your mouth, keeping your mouth and cheeks very, very soft. Don't worry too much about how deeply you're breathing, just keep a good rhythm going. Breathe in through your nose, and out through a

soft mouth. And again. And again. Concentrate as hard as you can on your breathing as the contraction builds up, and as it fades away. When the contraction's over, re-lax.

Or you can try counted breathing. As you breathe in, count slowly up to three or four (or whatever number seems comfortable for you) and, as you breathe out, count to three or four again. You might find that it's more comfortable to breathe in to a count of three and out to a count of four.

Massage

Massage stimulates the body to release endorphins, which are natural pain-killing and mood-lifting substances. Childbirth experts recommend it because it has been shown to ease pain and reduce anxiety in the first stage of labour. The use of massage is also linked with shorter labours and a lower risk of postnatal depression.

Massage can also bring you closer to the person who is caring for you: your midwife or your birth partner. Tell them where you'd like to be massaged. You might like massage at the very base of your back during contractions. Or you might like your shoulders massaged in between contractions to help you relax. Give feedback when you can, so that you get the best out of it.

A massage that starts slowly is best – frantic rubbing will simply make you feel panicky rather than relaxed! And it's firm pressure that's needed. This will help to stimulate your body to release endorphins, which is what makes massage such a positive experience.

Aromatherapy

Aromatherapists believe that essential oils – extracts of certain plants and flowers – can stimulate and balance hormone levels and soothe stress.

Ask your birth partner (above) to massage your temples or shoulders to help you relax between your contractions.

Focusing on your breath (left) when in labour helps you through contractions and gives your baby plenty of oxygen.

Drinking sips of water or an isotonic drink can help you to relax between contractions, and also keep you well hydrated.

Massage with essential oils during labour can help to reduce anxiety and increase our levels of "feel good" hormones such as oxytocin, which help labour to progress normally. If you don't like the idea of massage, you can just inhale the odours of the oil by putting one or two drops on a tissue.

Grapefruit, bergamot, ylang ylang, mandarin and lavender essential oils can all help to relieve tension in labour. Frankincense is particularly recommended: it is especially useful for easing any feelings of panic you may experience when contractions are getting difficult to cope with.

Warmth

Using warmth is a traditional way of relaxing tense muscles. It can also be used to provide relief from labour pain.

You can warm your back, tummy or groin using a wheat bag or a hot-water bottle. A wheat bag is filled with wheat husks. You heat the bag up for a few minutes in the microwave, then apply it. The wheat bag will drape and shape itself to your body and will stay warm for an hour or more. You can buy them online or in pharmacies. Some hospitals sell them at antenatal clinics.

If you are planning to use a hot-water bottle, you should fill it with hot (but not boiling) water, and carefully wrap it in a towel or soft cover before using it. Do this to make sure you don't get burned by the hot rubber.

Don't forget that massage provides warmth as well. Having someone rub your back will warm your skin as well as stimulate your body to release natural pain-killing endorphins. Using a birth pool is yet another way to envelop yourself in all-encompassing warmth.

When your baby's head is being born, a soft warm flannel or compress placed over your perineum (the tissue between the back of the vagina and the back passage) may make you feel more comfortable as the perineal tissue stretches. However, the warmth won't necessarily prevent any tears.

Homeopathy

Homeopathy uses minute, highly diluted doses of substances which, if they were taken as a full dose, would actually cause the same symptoms that the diluted dose attempts to treat. We don't fully understand the way in which homeopathy works, but homeopathic remedies are very gentle and they do not interfere with any prescribed medicines.

Homeopathic remedies, like other complementary therapies, are best administered by an experienced homeopath or a midwife who is trained in homeopathy. Some homeopaths will prescribe a "birthing set" of remedies which are specially designed to suit you for your labour.

Homeopaths recommend taking arnica for treating any shock, trauma or bruising you may experience during and after giving birth. Start taking the arnica within an hour of your baby's birth, and take it three to four times a day for up to five days. If you needed an assisted birth or a caesarean section, it is recommended that you take the tablets more frequently.

Medical pain relief

Nobody knows exactly how labour will feel for them until it starts. Some of us find that labour is bearable with little or no pain relief, although many of us are likely to want help at some point. Either way, it's useful to read up about your choices early on.

ParentsAsk...

I'm really scared of labour. What if the pain relief I'm offered doesn't help?

There are many strategies you can adopt. All labour involves some pain, which can be frightening, but thinking about it beforehand, and accepting it, can help you to cope with it better.

Talk to someone who knows you well about how you have dealt with pain in the past – you may have coped better than you thought.

Having good one-to-one support can help you, too. Think about who would be the best person to help you in labour: it may be your partner, a friend or relative, or you may be able to employ a birth supporter or a doula.

Remember that there are very effective methods of pain relief available to you in hospital, such as an epidural. Talk to your midwife or doctor about these and other options, and ask them to help you prepare a birth plan, so that your wishes are clear to everybody looking after you.

Make sure you understand what happens during labour. Knowing how your body works can help with the fear. Try to work out which aspects of labour are worrying you. Is it the fear of losing control? Do you worry that something might go wrong? Once you have put your finger on the key worry you can talk it through with your doctor, midwife or antenatal teacher.

Your choices

We've moved on since the days when Queen Victoria and Mrs Charles Darwin opted for chloroform to ease their pain in childbirth. Women today have more – and safer – options.

Entonox (gas and air)

Entonox, or gas and air, is a colourless, odourless gas that is made up of half oxygen and half nitrous oxide, or laughing gas, as it is commonly known. It has a calming effect and takes the edge off labour pain, rather than blocking it out completely. Gas and air should be available wherever you choose to give birth, whether that's in a birth centre or at home.

You can have gas and air whenever you want in labour. You breathe it in through a mask or mouthpiece:
● Simply bring the mask up to your face or put the mouthpiece between your lips or teeth.
● Keep it there as you breathe deeply and evenly.
● Continue to breathe deeply until you start to feel a little light-headed, then take the mask or mouthpiece away from your face.

You'll need a bit of practice to get the timing right. It takes at least 30 seconds of breathing for the gas to build up in your bloodstream to give you some benefit. Start breathing the gas and air the very second you feel a contraction beginning. If you wait until the contraction really hurts, and then start breathing it in, it will take effect between contractions.

You'll probably be given gas and air through a mouthpiece. However, if you're offered a rubber facemask, and the rubber makes you feel queasy, you can ask to swap to a mouthpiece. It's quick and easy to do. Have lots of sips of water in between contractions to keep your mouth moist.

When you're pushing your baby out in the second stage of labour, you may find it easier to concentrate on what you're doing if you don't use gas and air. Or you could have a little gas and air to help you at the beginning of each contraction, then put the mouthpiece to one side, and PUSH!

Pethidine

The pain-killing drug Pethidine is rather similar to morphine. It also works as an antispasmodic, which means that it helps you to relax. Pethidine should be available wherever you give birth, including in labour wards, birth centres and at a home birth.

Your midwife can both prescribe and give injections of Pethidine for pain relief. She doesn't have to consult a doctor first. It is often combined with another drug to control sickness (an anti-emetic) because Pethidine often causes sickness.

It can also be given through a vein in your arm (intravenously). A fine tube is inserted into the vein and the other end of the tube is attached to a pump. You can operate the pump to give yourself small amounts of Pethidine. This is called Patient-Controlled Analgesia or PCA. It's not available everywhere.

The time to have Pethidine is during the first stage of labour, when your cervix is opening. You shouldn't have Pethidine if your midwife thinks you're close to giving birth because it could have an adverse effect on your baby.

Pethidine works quickly and it won't slow your labour down if you're already in established labour. It may help you to postpone or avoid having an epidural if you're struggling with contractions. On the down side, some people find opiate drugs such as Pethidine unpleasant, and may feel drowsy and "out of it" or nauseous. Some women find that they can't remember the baby being born, especially if drugs are given in late labour. Some mums fall asleep and wake at the peak of contractions, in pain but unable to help themselves by breathing through contractions.

Pethidine also crosses the placenta. It may affect your baby's breathing and make her drowsy for several days after she is born, particularly if she is born within two hours of the drug being given to you.

Meptid

Meptid, or meptazinol, is an opiate pain-relieving drug. It shares many of the advantages and disadvantages of Pethidine, which is more commonly used, and is usually given by injection.

You're most likely to be offered Meptid during the first stage of labour when you might need some extra help to cope with the strong contractions. Meptid may make you feel less drowsy than Pethidine and is less likely to affect your baby's breathing. One disadvantage, though, is that Meptid is more likely to make you feel and be sick than Pethidine.

Meptid is less commonly used than Pethidine, so do check that Meptid is available at your hospital before deciding that this is what you want to have in labour. If you have a vaginal examination and find that you are further on in labour than you thought, you might decide that you don't need Meptid after all. It takes approximately 15 minutes for the drug to start working, so use your breathing techniques to help you until it takes effect.

Diamorphine

Diamorphine, otherwise known as heroin, is a powerful opiate pain reliever that is derived from the opium or poppy plant. It seems to work better at relieving labour pain and to have fewer side-effects than other similar drugs such as Pethidine and Meptid. When diamorphine is used to relieve pain in labour, it doesn't result in dependence on the drug – so don't worry; you're not going to end up as a heroin addict if you have it during your labour.

Drugs like diamorphine, or more commonly, Pethidine, should be available wherever you choose to give birth. The usual dose is between 5 milligrams (mg) and 10mg, depending on your body size. It is given by injection but can also be given intravenously. A fine tube is inserted into a vein in your arm and the other end of the tube is

Your doctor or midwife will be able to give you information about the various methods of pain relief, so discuss them beforehand to help you decide.

attached to a pump, which you can operate yourself.

You're most likely to be offered diamorphine during the first stage of labour if you need some extra help to cope with strong contractions. It is probably more effective at relieving labour pain than either Pethidine or Meptid, and is less likely to make you feel sick or drowsy.

Like Pethidine and Meptid, diamorphine provides only limited relief from the pain of labour and can make you feel drowsy, feel sick or be sick. It also crosses the placenta, which means that it may affect your baby's breathing for several days after her birth and may interfere with breastfeeding.

If you think you would like diamorphine for pain relief during your labour, you should check whether or not it is available at your hospital before writing it into your birth plan, as it's not available everywhere.

Getting ready for pregnancy

Staying safe and healthy

Your pregnancy diary

Birth and beyond

Epidural

An epidural is where pain-killing drugs are passed into the small of your back via a fine tube. The drugs are injected around the nerves that carry signals from the part of your body that feels pain when you're in labour. The result is very effective pain relief.

When you have an epidural, your anaesthetist will first give you an injection of local anaesthetic in your lower back. She then guides a hollow needle between the bones of your spine into the space between the layers of tissue in your spinal column (the epidural space). A fine tube is then passed through the needle. Once the tube is in place, the anaesthetist removes the needle. The tube is taped up your back and over your shoulder. Once your epidural is in place, it should stay in until after your baby is born and your placenta is delivered.

In the UK, most hospitals use low-dose epidurals. These contain a mixture of pain-killing drugs, usually a local anaesthetic, bupivacaine, and an opioid – fentanyl. Having a low-dose epidural means that you may still have some sensation in your legs and feet.

You can have an epidural at any point during your labour, but most women choose it when their contractions are getting pretty strong, which is often when their cervix has dilated by about 5 or 6cm. You'll also be offered an epidural if your labour has to be speeded up with a Syntocinon drip, because this can make your contractions difficult to cope with.

An epidural usually provides excellent pain relief during labour. Top-ups can be given by an experienced midwife, so you don't usually need to wait for an anaesthetist once the epidural is in place. Another advantage is that your mind remains clear. You may still be aware of your contractions, but feel no pain.

One disadvantage is that the epidural may not work properly at first. You may find that you are numb in only parts of your tummy. If you are not free of pain within half an hour of being given the epidural, ask for the anaesthetist to come back to adjust it or to try again.

Epidurals have other disadvantages, too. Once you have had one you will have to stay in bed. With a low-dose epidural you may be able to shuffle around on the bed but you won't be able to walk around. You may also need to have a catheter inserted to empty your bladder, and your baby's heartbeat will be monitored continuously for at least 30 minutes when you're first given the epidural, as well as after each top-up.

There's also more chance of your baby needing to be born with the aid of forceps or ventouse (see pp.282–3). This may be because an epidural can make it difficult for your baby to move into the best position to be born. An assisted delivery means you will have more bruising, stitching and postnatal pain, as well as an increased risk of long-term incontinence.

There is a small risk of you having a severe headache. This can happen if the epidural needle punctures the bag of fluid that surrounds the spinal cord, causing a leak of fluid. There is about a one in 100 chance of this happening.

Even maternity units equipped to give epidurals may not offer a 24-hour service, so be prepared for the possibility that you may not be able to have one.

Walking epidural

A walking, or ambulatory, epidural is similar to a standard low-dose epidural; it gives excellent pain relief, but also allows you to retain some sensation in your legs so you should be able to move about and even to walk around to some extent, but you will need help to do so. The main aim of this kind of epidural is to relieve pain; keeping you mobile is only a secondary concern. Some women find that they're not really mobile at all.

A walking epidural uses the same lower-dose combination of drugs as the low-dose epidurals that most hospitals in the UK offer as standard. It is a regional anaesthetic, which means the drug is injected around the nerves

Systemised mum

Knowing that pain relief is on hand can help you through the worst of labour.

"I felt that it was much better to be prepared and make a definite decision beforehand about pain relief, instead of deciding at the last minute and then feeling flustered and panicked. I knew I wanted my birth to go as smoothly as possible, and to be controlled but relaxed.

I did as much research as I could about all the methods of pain relief and what would be best for me. My final birth plan was to have Pethidine during the first stage of labour, as the contractions started. Then, as they grew stronger and more painful, I intended to have an epidural. When I actually went into labour, I found that knowing that pain relief was definitely on the way stopped me from panicking. And I knew exactly how the Pethidine and an epidural would be administered, and was prepared for how I would feel when the pain relief took effect. In the end, I was so pleased I'd made this decision – I don't think I'd have coped with the pain easily, as my labour ended up being a long one!"

Epidural space
Vertebra
Syringe attachment
Plastic tube
Spinal cord

In an epidural, anaesthetic is injected via a fine tube inside a hollow needle that has been positioned in your back.

When you have an epidural, a sterile cover is put over your back and you are given a local anaesthetic. The hollow needle is then guided between the bones of your spine.

that carry signals from the part of your body that feels pain when you're in labour.

The few hospitals that offer walking epidurals have procedures in place to ensure that it is safe for you to move about with an epidural in place, and that they have enough staff to support you while you're doing so. If the medical

Spinal block

A spinal block is a single pain-killing injection that gets to work faster than an epidural. An anaesthetist will give you a local anaesthetic in the small of your back, into the fluid surrounding the spinal nerves, using a very fine needle. The local anaesthetic numbs the nerves

Sometimes, doctors will use a spinal during a forceps or ventouse birth (see pp.282–3). They may also use one if they think that your baby won't be able to be born vaginally and may need to be born quickly by caesarean.

Otherwise, you will be given a spinal if you are having a caesarean, if you

"A spinal block provides **rapid pain relief** as it **works within** five or **10 minutes**."

staff agree that you are safe to walk, you must always be accompanied and monitored while you are moving around.

You may find that you only have a very limited amount of movement. Some women can manage to move from the bed to a chair, and a few can walk with help. You may also find the extra monitoring you'll need intrusive.

Check in advance whether or not your hospital offers walking epidurals. Very few UK maternity units offer them, because of the extra resources that are needed for them.

supplying your uterus and cervix so that you can no longer feel your contractions, or so that you can have a caesarean section if it is needed.

You can have a spinal during the first stage of labour, as part of a combined spinal epidural (CSE). The spinals used in CSEs are called mini-spinals and use a low dose of pain-killing drugs. Full-dose spinals are only given in an anaesthetic room or operating theatre. They can be used if you haven't already got an epidural in place, or if your epidural needs boosting.

want pain relief for stitches after your baby is born or if you need a manual removal of the placenta if you have retained placenta.

A spinal block provides rapid pain relief, working within five or 10 minutes. Unlike an epidural, it can be given in a single injection, so there is no tube left in your back. However, spinals are short-acting. Mini-spinals last between 60 and 90 minutes, and full-dose spinals last about two hours. They can't be given more than once and, unlike an epidural, a spinal can't be topped up.

Getting ready for pregnancy

Staying safe and healthy

Your pregnancy diary

Birth and beyond

Premature labour

About 10 per cent of babies are born prematurely (at less than 37 weeks), and about one per cent arrive very prematurely (at less than 32 weeks). Here's how to spot the signs of premature labour and what to expect if you deliver your baby early.

What is premature labour?

A premature birth is when a baby arrives before 37 completed weeks of pregnancy. Seven per cent of babies in the UK are born prematurely each year. A baby who arrives at 34 weeks is unlikely to have any problems, although he may be a bit small and may have breathing difficulties.

However, babies who are born earlier than this still have a lot of growing to do and their internal organs need to mature (see opposite). They may be quite weak and find sucking and breathing difficult. It is still very difficult for doctors to predict whether a healthy woman will

go into labour prematurely. There is evidence to show that the presence of certain bacteria in the urine makes premature labour more likely. Because of this, it is now recommended that all women have their urine tested for bacteria early in pregnancy.

There are a number of other risk factors for premature labour:
- Infections of the vagina and of the urinary tract.
- Expecting twins or more.
- Smoking.
- Using recreational drugs, such as cannabis, ecstasy or cocaine.
- Some abnormalities of the uterus.
- Previous premature birth.

If your waters break, or you start having contractions before 37 weeks of pregnancy, contact your midwife, doctor or hospital immediately, even if it's the middle of the night. You will almost certainly be asked to go to hospital. Don't drive yourself. If you have nobody to give you a lift, the hospital will send an ambulance for you.

At the hospital, you will be given a vaginal examination to see if your cervix

A baby born before 34 weeks will have to go straight into intensive care. You'll be able to visit and sometimes touch him.

is shortening and opening. A number of tests may be carried out to check for infection, including a urine test and vaginal swab. You may be offered a vaginal ultrasound scan to see how long your cervix is. A short cervix may indicate that labour has started. Another test is for a substance called "fetal fibronectin" in the fluid in your vagina. Finding this substance often indicates that the baby will be born soon.

If labour's underway

Unfortunately, doctors can't stop labour if it's really underway and resting won't help either. However, if you are less than 34 weeks pregnant, your doctor can offer you a drug to delay the birth for a while so there's time to transfer you to a hospital with an intensive baby care unit. You'll also be offered steroid drugs to help your baby's lungs mature. If you are more than 34 weeks pregnant, your doctors will probably allow labour to continue at its own pace.

It's probably hard to describe the shock of finding that you are going to give birth several months earlier than you had anticipated. You will naturally feel very worried, and perhaps out of control because of all the medical attention you are receiving. Do ask your midwives and doctors to explain everything that's happening to you.

Your baby's heartbeat will be monitored throughout labour. Although labour is premature, you won't necessarily need a caesarean. However, you might if you've gone into labour following a haemorrhage or if your baby is severely distressed.

If your baby is born before 34 weeks, he may need to go immediately to the Special Care or Intensive Care Baby Unit (see p.297). This is very frightening and you'll need the support of your midwife. She'll understand how you are feeling.

A baby born between 34 and 37 weeks may not need any medical treatment and may be able to go to the postnatal ward with you. Or you may both be admitted to a special ward with a high ratio of staff to mothers. You may be encouraged to carry him close to your breasts. This seems to provide the right physical and emotional conditions for your baby to grow quickly.

Future risk

If you have already had one premature birth you are at an increased risk of having another premature baby. There is about a 15 per cent chance that your next baby will also be premature. At the moment, doctors don't know how to prevent a woman giving birth prematurely. However, if you smoke or use recreational drugs, giving these up will certainly reduce the risk. At least, if you have had one premature birth then, next time around, you will be able to make preparations for the possibility that your baby may arrive early. During a subsequent pregnancy, your midwife will monitor the pregnancy closely and she will help you to cope with the anxiety you are bound to feel.

If your baby is born prematurely

Number of weeks	Possible problems	Treatment
Pre 28 weeks	Most of these babies weigh less than 1kg (35oz). They can't suck, swallow and breathe at the same time. They have little muscle tone, and most move very little.	All need oxygen and mechanical assistance to help them breathe. They must be fed through a vein (intravenously) until they're able to suck and swallow. They have a high risk of one or more medical complications and may face an extended stay in the neonatal intensive care unit.
28 to 31 weeks	These babies usually weigh 900 to 1800g (2 to 4lb). About 90 to 95 per cent survive. If they weigh less than 1.5kg (3lb 4oz) they are at risk of serious disabilities.	Most require oxygen and mechanical assistance to help them breathe. Some can be fed breastmilk or formula through a tube placed through their nose or mouth into the stomach, although others will need to be fed intravenously.
32 to 33 weeks	More than 95 per cent of babies born at this time survive. Most weigh 1.4 to 2.3kg (3 to 5lb). Some can breathe on their own, and many just need supplemental oxygen to help them.	Some can be breast- or bottle-fed, but those who have breathing difficulties will probably need tube feeding. These babies are less likely than babies born earlier to develop serious disabilities, although they remain at a slightly increased risk of having learning and behavioural problems.
34 to 36 weeks	Babies born at this time are almost as likely as full-term babies to survive. They have a higher risk than full-term babies for health problems, including breathing and feeding problems, difficulties regulating body temperature and jaundice. These problems are usually mild, and most babies make a quick recovery.	Most of these babies can be breast- or bottle-fed, although some (especially those that have mild breathing problems) may need tube feeding for a brief time. It's estimated that, at 35 weeks' gestation, the weight of the brain is only around 60 per cent that of full-term babies. Late preterm babies, which is what babies born at 34 to 36 weeks' gestation are called, are unlikely to develop serious disabilities resulting from premature birth, but they may be at a very slightly increased risk for subtle learning and behavioural problems.

Getting ready for pregnancy

Staying safe and healthy

Your pregnancy diary

Birth and beyond

Assisted birth

Chances are you'll push your baby out into the world with nothing but a bit of encouragement from those around you. Now and again, though, babies need a helping hand to be delivered – what's known as an assisted delivery. The two main methods are forceps and ventouse.

The whys and hows

In about one in eight births in the UK, a baby needs help to be born. An assisted birth uses instruments – either forceps or ventouse – that are attached to your baby's head so that she can be pulled out.

Forceps look like and have sometimes been described as "stainless steel salad servers" or "large sugar tongs". They have two intersecting parts and a pair of curved ends to cradle your baby's head. There are many different types and makes of forceps.

The ventouse, or vacuum extractor, has a cup attached to a small vacuum pump, and a handle for pulling on. The cup fits on top and towards the back of your baby's head.

baby's body is born and then there is difficulty delivering your baby's head.

Avoiding an assisted birth
It's not always possible to avoid an assisted birth, but the following factors can help reduce your risk. These include:
● Having continuous support during labour from a birth partner or doula.
● Using upright positions during labour.
● Avoiding an epidural (see pp.278–9).
● If you've had an epidural, waiting for

"Some factors **can reduce** your **risk of** having an **assisted birth**."

Your midwife and doctor might recommend an assisted birth if:
● Your baby has become distressed during the pushing stage of labour.
● You are very tired and simply can't push any more.
● Your baby isn't making any progress through your pelvis.
● There's a medical reason why you shouldn't push for too long (for example, if you have heart disease).

Forceps may also be used during a vaginal birth of a breech baby (see pp.286–7). This might happen if your

at least an hour after you are fully dilated or until you feel the urge to push, before trying to push your baby out.

For an assisted birth you will need to put your legs into stirrups or supports at either side of the bed. The end of the bed will be removed, and your legs will be draped in sterile green sheets. You will be given pain relief, which may be a local injection (a pudendal block) inside the vagina, an epidural or spinal anaesthetic. A thin tube called a catheter, attached to a bag, may be put into your bladder to empty it as you

Dad's **Diary**

My ventouse baby's head
"I'd seen the pictures in books. I knew that newborn babies came out looking a bit blue or grey, and covered in greasy white stuff. But I wasn't prepared for how ours looked after his ventouse birth. A ventouse is basically a suction device. His head was bruised and a bit swollen, and his scalp was grazed. It was very worrying at first, but our midwife was quick to reassure us that this was entirely normal and that the marks would clear up within a week or so. The next day, we noticed that he had a blood blister on his head where the ventouse had been attached. He was jaundiced, too, which they said may have been related to the blister. He was a little tender for a couple of weeks, so we were careful to be especially gentle with him. The blister took a few weeks to go away, but there were no lasting problems. Now, at 12 weeks, his head looks perfectly normal."

need to have an empty bladder for an assisted birth. A paediatrician (a doctor specialising in the care of babies and children) may be present. This is quite usual, so try not to worry.

Ventouse birth

Many doctors prefer to use a ventouse for an assisted birth because it's often less painful. You're less likely to need an episiotomy, and there's less risk of perineal tearing. The doctor or specially trained midwife will place the ventouse cup on your baby's head inside the vagina, and then suck the air out of the cup using a foot-controlled vacuum pump or a hand-held pump.

Once the cup is securely fixed on your baby's head, the doctor will ask you to push when your next contraction comes along, and she will pull on the cup to help your baby out.

Forceps birth

Your doctor will need to make a cut (episiotomy) through the back of your vagina to enlarge the opening so that the forceps can be placed around the sides of your baby's head.

Once the forceps are in place, the doctor will gently pull while you push during a contraction to help your baby move down through the birth canal and be born. If your baby is not moving down with each pull or is not born after three contractions/pulls then normal practice is for the forceps to be abandoned and for your baby to be born by caesarean section (see pp.288–91).

Ventouse and forceps

In a ventouse birth, a cup is attached to the baby's head and the air is pumped out of the cup. This creates a vacuum that holds the cup in place. Pulling gently on the cup helps the baby through the vagina.

The cup is attached to the baby's head

The curved blades of the forceps cradle the baby's head

In a forceps birth, the baby's head is cradled by the forceps, which are inserted into the mother's vagina. Pulling on the forceps in time with the contractions helps the baby out.

ParentsAsk...

How will I feel after an assisted birth?

After an assisted birth, you may have:

● Soreness and bruising from a tear or episiotomy.

● Pain or numbness in your perineum when you go to the toilet.

● Problems with leaking urine when you're not on the toilet.

Your midwife should give you pain relief and check to ensure that you're able to urinate properly after the birth.

How will my baby feel after an assisted birth?

Your baby may have some bruising or marks after an assisted birth.

● Forceps babies tend to have marks or bruising on the face or side of the head.

● Ventouse babies may have a bruised swelling or slight grazing to the scalp, or a blood blister.

● Very occasionally the facial nerve is damaged, causing a palsy, so that your baby's mouth droops at one corner; this is usually temporary.

These marks usually clear up within a week or so, although a blood blister may take several weeks to disappear. Bruises and trauma may cause your baby some discomfort, so handle her gently.

Getting ready for pregnancy

Staying safe and healthy

Your pregnancy diary

Birth and beyond

Twin/multiple birth

As you probably already know by now, there are some additional risks linked with giving birth to twins or more. The best option is to discuss your babies' birth fully with your doctors and midwives so that, together, you can make sure it is as safe and positive as possible.

ParentsAsk...

What are the chances my twins will be born prematurely?

Twins and higher multiples do tend to arrive ahead of schedule. Although some twin pregnancies go to 40 weeks or even longer, 37 weeks is considered to be full term in a twin pregnancy. Anything earlier than this is considered premature. Around 30 per cent of twin pregnancies go into premature labour, and around half of all women expecting twins give birth before 37 weeks.

Premature labour is more common in identical (monozygotic) twins, especially if the babies are sharing the same placenta, membranes or amniotic sac.

Premature babies born between 34 and 37 weeks generally do very well. Extremely premature babies born before 28 weeks may survive, but they'll need intensive medical care and a little luck. However, advances in neonatal care mean the outlook for premature babies is improving all the time.

The factors behind whether you will go into labour prematurely have little to do with your behaviour or lifestyle. While you shouldn't get too anxious about whether this may happen, it's important to familiarise yourself with the signs of pre-eclampsia and premature labour.

Eating healthily during your twin pregnancy is also important, as it gives your babies the best chance of being born healthy and at a good weight.

Delivering more than one

If you are expecting more than one baby, it's very likely that you'll give birth in hospital, because of the potential risks associated with giving birth to twins or more. It may be possible for you to have your babies in a birth centre or at home, although this happens very rarely.

Some doctors argue that it is safer to plan for your twins' birth at about 37 to 38 weeks of pregnancy, either by induction or by planned caesarean. This limits your place of birth to hospital, as neither induction nor caesarean can be carried out at home or in a midwife-led birth centre. Ultimately the choice is yours, and if you do want to consider either a home birth or having your babies in a birth centre, you should discuss your options with your midwife or ask to have an appointment to discuss it with the consultant midwife at your hospital.

The chances of a caesarean

You don't automatically have to have a caesarean, although your chances of having one are higher than if you were pregnant with just one baby. Whether you have a caesarean or not will most likely depend on the position of your first twin. If she's in a head-down position and the placenta isn't in the way of the cervix, a vaginal birth is generally possible. Many doctors and midwives will also do their best to deliver your second baby vaginally rather than by caesarean, even if he is in a breech position (see pp.286–7).

Of course, you may need to have a caesarean for the same reasons any other pregnant woman would – for example, if:

- There is a complication with your labour.
- The babies don't fit through your birth canal.
- One or both babies' heartbeats drop drastically.
- You have severe pre-eclampsia (see p.233).
- There is placental abruption (see p.232).
- There are other signs that your babies could be in danger – for example, if they are small for their gestational age.

50%
is the approximate percentage

of twins born before 37 weeks' gestation. Some twin pregnancies go to 40 weeks or more, but 37 weeks is considered full term.

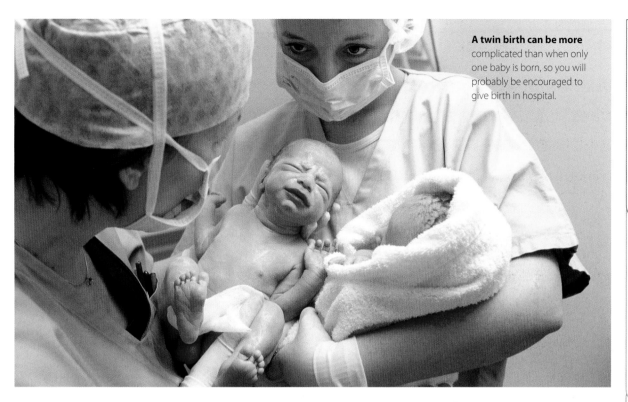

A twin birth can be more complicated than when only one baby is born, so you will probably be encouraged to give birth in hospital.

Unfortunately, all of these potential complications are rather more common in the case of multiple births.

It may help you make a decision about the sort of birth that you want if you can choose a doctor who has experience of delivering twins. If you don't want an unnecessary caesarean, discuss your birth options with her. Ask if she's comfortable delivering twins if one is in the breech position, and what she'll do in order to avoid a caesarean.

Although some things are beyond your control, such as your babies' positions in the uterus and any complications you may have developed, you can take steps to stay as healthy as possible during pregnancy by eating well (see pp.48–51, 120–21, 148–9 and 182–3). You should also try to remain active during labour. This may, in turn, improve your chances of avoiding a caesarean. When you're in labour, also try to use positions that will help your babies to turn if necessary.

Most twins are born early, often by induction or planned caesarean. However yours are born, you'll be thrilled to hold your two new little ones in your arms.

ParentsAsk...

What will my recovery be like?

That depends on whether you've had a vaginal birth or a caesarean and whether or not you've had other complications. If everything goes well, you can be discharged from hospital within two days after a vaginal birth and within four days after a caesarean. Some babies can't go home right away.

Because twins tend to have more complications, particularly those related to being born earlier and smaller, it's not uncommon for them to be admitted to the special care unit. All mothers can use lots of help taking care of a new baby, but you'll be even more exhausted if you're taking care of multiples. Arrange to get as much help as you can. Many dads of twins save up some annual leave and combine it with their paternity leave, so they have more time at home.

Getting ready for pregnancy

Staying safe and healthy

Your pregnancy diary

Birth and beyond

Breech babies

As labour approaches, most babies settle into a head-down position. However, a few end up bottom down – a breech position – which can make birth more difficult. That's why a doctor or midwife should offer to turn your breech baby before she is born.

Planning for a breech birth

If your baby is breech, it means that she is in a bottom-down position. When labour begins, 96 per cent of babies are lying head down in the uterus, but a few settle into a breech position.

If your baby is breech at 36 weeks, your doctor or midwife should offer you the chance to have your baby turned manually into a head-down position. This is called external cephalic version (ECV; see Parents Ask, opposite). ECV is more likely to work if you've given birth before. Sometimes, however, a baby just refuses to budge or she will rotate back after ECV.

Most, but not all, breech babies in the UK are currently born by caesarean. A review of the research on breech births in 2004 suggested that it is safer for breech babies to be born by caesarean section. But some midwives and doctors challenge this. They feel that a normal birth is just as safe, provided that the midwife or doctor has the special skills needed to help a woman give birth to a breech baby vaginally.

A vaginal birth

If you want a vaginal birth with a breech baby, your doctor may be more likely to be supportive if:

- You've given birth vaginally before.
- A midwife or doctor who is trained

Breech-baby positions

There are several types of breech presentation. Your midwife will be able to tell your baby's position when she examines you towards the end of your pregnancy. You may also be able to tell by your baby's movements. If you feel strong kicks on your bladder and you can feel something hard and uncomfortable under your ribs, your baby may be breech.

Complete breech   **Frank breech**   **Footling breech**

Complete breech This is one of the most common of the breech presentations. Your baby has her feet tucked beside her bottom, and her knees and arms are close to her body. A vaginal birth is sometimes possible.
Frank breech This is another of the most common of the breech presentations. Your baby sits bottom down with her legs fully extended, straight up towards her head. This is the best position for achieving a vaginal breech birth.
Footling breech This is the rarest breech presentation. Your baby is bottom down with one or both feet extended below her bottom. A vaginal birth is unlikely.

If your baby is in a breech position, once you've reached 36 weeks of pregnancy, you should be given the chance to have your baby turned by hand.

and experienced at breech birth will be present at the birth.
- Facilities for a caesarean (in case one is needed) will be available nearby.
- There are no other features of your

situation and discuss the risks and benefits of both a caesarean section and a vaginal birth so that the two of you can choose what's likely to be best for you and your baby.

"Sometimes a **breech baby** refuses **to budge** or rotates **back**."

pregnancy that would make having your breech baby vaginally more risky for you or your baby.

Before making a final decision, you and your doctor should evaluate your

As the number of breech vaginal births continues to fall, it may be more difficult for you to find an obstetrician with the skills and knowledge needed to deliver your breech baby vaginally. If your local hospital doesn't have an obstetrician with this experience, you should ask to be referred to a hospital where this option is available if you wish.

If you still want to give birth to your breech baby vaginally and your doctor isn't happy, you could consider going to an independent midwife, although you'll have to pay for this.

Fact: A breech labour is usually slower than a normal one because a baby's bottom doesn't exert as much pressure on the cervix as a baby's head. Some breech labours are quick and straightforward, though.

ParentsAsk...

Are there any safe and proven methods available for turning a breech baby?

Many breech babies spontaneously turn around before, or even during, labour without any assistance. Some babies who remain in the breech position can be turned by hand, using a technique called external cephalic version (ECV).

This technique has been practised by doctors for thousands of years and a great deal of research has been carried out to test its safety. The Royal College of Obstetricians and Gynaecologists recommends that: "All women with an uncomplicated singleton breech pregnancy at 36 weeks should be offered external cephalic version."

ECV can be carried out at any point from 36 weeks of pregnancy; there is no upper limit. Sometimes, it is even carried out at the beginning of labour, if the waters haven't already broken.

The procedure will be carried out in hospital, where there is equipment to monitor your baby's heartbeat and ultrasound to check your baby's position. You will be given a drug to make the muscles of your uterus relax. If you are rhesus negative, you will have an injection of anti-D (see p.233). It is not painful, so you will not need to have a general anaesthetic.

Why are some babies breech?

A lot of babies are breech before 30 weeks, so if your baby is premature she may be in the breech position. Sometimes a baby cannot turn because something is in the way – a fibroid perhaps. Sometimes there is a problem with the cord – it may be too short for the baby to turn. If you have a small or unusual-shaped pelvis, and your baby can't fit her head through it, she may turn around and put her softer and smaller bottom there instead. In most of these cases, the baby would need to be born by caesarean.

Getting ready for pregnancy

Staying safe and healthy

Your pregnancy diary

Birth and beyond

Caesarean section

Caesareans, or C-sections, are carried out for a wide variety of reasons and roughly a quarter of women have them in the UK. While caesareans are very safe, it is a major operation, and you will take longer to recover after the birth than if you give birth naturally.

The lowdown on C-sections

Some women know that they will need a caesarean before they go into labour. This is called an elective or planned caesarean. In other cases the decision to opt for a caesarean is made during labour. This is called an emergency caesarean. The risk of you needing a planned caesarean is greater if:

- Your baby is in a breech (bottom first; see pp.286–7) or transverse (sideways; see p.197) position.
- You are having three or more babies.
- Your baby has a fetal illness or abnormality.
- You have an infection such as herpes (see p.226) or HIV (see p.227).
- You have placenta praevia (see pp.231–2) and the placenta is so low in the uterus that it's blocking the baby's exit.
- You have pre-eclampsia (see p.233) and it is rapidly worsening, making it dangerous to delay delivery.

- You have a history of invasive uterine surgery or multiple caesarean sections.

You may also need an unplanned caesarean during labour if:
- Your baby's heart rate has become irregular.
- The umbilical cord prolapses, or slips, through the cervix.
- Your baby is not moving down the birth canal.

What happens in a caesarean?
During a caesarean, the doctor will make a cut in your abdomen and uterus and will remove your baby through it. In most cases, your partner will be allowed to be with you for the birth. He will only be asked to leave in a true emergency, or if you need a general anaesthetic.

Most caesareans are carried out using an epidural or spinal block so you can be awake and see your baby straight after the birth. As well as having the epidural in your back, you will have a catheter inserted to drain your bladder, and a drip in your arm or hand to give extra fluids or pain relief if needed. You will also have to wear a heart monitor.

A screen will be put up while the caesarean is taking place. Once you are completely numb the doctor makes a straight cut in your skin above your

Systemised mum

Choosing an elective caesarean may suit you as it can bring certainty and peace of mind.

"When I reached 36 weeks, my baby was showing no signs of moving from the breech position. My midwife offered to try to turn the baby manually but, as this was my first, it had less chance of working than if I'd given birth before. We did try and my baby refused to budge!

I could have gone ahead and had a vaginal birth anyway, but I felt that the best thing for me was a caesarean, seeing as this was my first baby and I was worried about the risk of complications. I admit I was slightly disappointed at not having a vaginal birth, but I also felt relieved knowing that my baby would arrive safely – and I had the date written on the calendar so I could prepare for his arrival!"

For a bikini incision the doctor makes a horizontal cut just above the public hair line. After healing, the scar is hardly noticeable.

Parents**Ask...**

I'm having a planned caesarean as my baby is breech. Will I be able to hold him straight after he is born?

As soon as your baby has been lifted out, he will be checked over, then shown to you. Your partner will probably hold him while the placenta is delivered and you are being stitched up. After this, you may be able to hold him or you may be moved to a side ward, where you will be able to breastfeed him if you want to. The only circumstances in which you won't be able to hold him are if he is very small or very unwell and needs to go straight to the special-care baby unit (see p.297).

After your baby is born you should be able to hold him once the placenta has been delivered and he's been checked over.

pubic bone (this is called a bikini cut; see opposite), and then makes a second cut in the lower section of your uterus. Your baby is then lifted out. It takes only a few minutes.

Your baby will be quickly checked by the paediatrician and then you or your partner can hold him while the placenta is being delivered and you are stitched up using a double layer of stitches. The external wound will be closed with stitches or staples.

Reducing the risk

Caesareans can be life-saving for both mothers and babies, so not all should be avoided. But there are some ways you can reduce your chances of having one. These include:

● Staying healthy during pregnancy, eating well (see pp.48–51, 120–21, 148–9, 182–3), exercising (see pp.56–7, 134, 184) and getting plenty of rest (see pp.162–3, 198–9). Then, when labour starts, you'll be in optimal condition.

● If you have a choice of hospitals, check out the caesarean rates at each

and compare them. You may want to avoid a hospital that appears to have a high rate of caesareans. You can check out the caesarean rates at your local hospital at www.birthchoiceuk.com.

● Having a female birth partner, as well as your midwife, to support you during your labour can reduce your chances of having a caesarean. You'll need good, solid support from the moment your labour starts. You could ask a female friend or relative, or a doula, to be there to help you.

● If your baby is in a bottom-down, or breech, position as you near the end of your pregnancy, you could talk to your doctor or midwife about trying to move your baby into a head-down position (see p.286).

● If your pregnancy is considered to be low risk, your baby should be monitored now and again during labour rather than continuously. Continuous electronic fetal monitoring (EFM; see p.263), which stops you from moving around during labour, is linked with an increase in caesarean section rates.

 ### Single mum

Choose a birth partner who can truly sympathise with you when you're giving birth

"When I found out that I'd have to have an elective caesarean, it confirmed to me that my sister really was the best choice to be my birth partner. Her second baby was delivered by emergency c-section, and knowing that she'd been through the same experience gave me confidence that she'd be the most supportive and sympathetic person to have at my side during the birth. Also, knowing that she'd made a great recovery afterwards was a great help.

She knew exactly what to do and say to me: she kept telling me I was doing great and that it was all going well. I couldn't have done it without her. She knew just what to say and when because she'd been there herself. We're closer than ever now."

Getting ready for pregnancy

Staying safe and healthy

Your pregnancy diary

Birth and beyond

ParentsAsk...

How many caesareans can I safely have?

Although vaginal delivery after a previous caesarean is now common and safe (VBAC; see pp.221 and 248), sometimes another caesarean section is your only option. Your consultant will give you individual advice on the health of your uterus and any risks to you of another operation. There are many things that need to be considered, including your weight, age, medical history, fertility history, childbirth history, as well as personal choice. The choices you make will also depend on why you needed to have a caesarean with your first baby, so you should be sure you understand what happened last time.

If you have a caesarean birth, you should always seek advice from your consultant about the best way for you to have your next baby.

As a precaution after a caesarean you shouldn't lift anything heavy for six weeks – not even your toddler.

After a caesarean

Everyone knows a caesarean is major surgery, but you may still be surprised by how much it hurts afterwards. You may feel you can't do anything on your own – to even move up the bed a little you'll probably need something or someone to hold on to. Trapped wind is another problem, especially by about day three – tightening the abdominal muscles on an outward breath helps expel the gas. Peppermint water also helps and will be available.

It will hurt when you cough or laugh, but less if you support your wound (with your hands or by holding a pillow over your stomach) as you do so. Wearing knickers that are a size bigger than you really need (boxer shorts or disposable maternity knickers are good alternatives) may make the wound feel more comfortable, and you'll need to use sanitary pads because the lochia, or bleeding from the uterus, is the same as after a vaginal birth.

If you had an epidural, you'll probably have the catheter left in place for a few hours afterwards so that top-ups of painkiller can be given when you need them. If you had a general anaesthetic, you'll be offered pain-killing injections in the hours and days after the birth. Doses of painkiller you can control yourself, or patient-controlled analgesia (PCA; see p.277), are often used soon after a caesarean. This gives you pain-relieving drugs through a fine tube into a vein in your arm. You can control the dose by pressing a button.

Getting out of bed

At first you'll probably feel as though you'll never walk again but, as soon as six hours after the birth, your midwife will probably cajole you out of bed. However hard it seems, do try to move – the earlier you can, the better for your circulation and general recovery. Also, you'll have to try it sometime – and when you've got out of bed once, next time will be easier. As well as moving around out of bed, you'll be encouraged to do ankle exercises while you're in bed, to improve blood circulation to your legs and help prevent clots.

You'll probably have to stay in hospital for about three days. You'll be encouraged to start gentle postnatal exercises the day after your operation to help speed your physical recovery. A physiotherapist will show you what to do. You should not start a more strenuous exercise programme until six to eight weeks after delivery.

There's no reason why you shouldn't breastfeed after a caesarean. But the pain from your scar may make it a bit difficult in the early days (see below).

ParentsTalk...

"I had an emergency caesarean and I hate it when people say I gave birth the easy way. Believe me, the pain afterwards is not easy! I needed help on hand to do everything for the first couple of days afterwards. Just moving in my bed was excruciating."
Sara, 23, mum to six-month-old Jo

"I had a lot of leftover adrenaline after my caesarean. There was such a huge build-up of excitement for nine months, and then – within a few hours – the baby was here. Being confined to bed with stitches in my tummy really didn't help!"
Emily, 31, first-time mum

"My midwife persuaded me to get out of bed for a walk a few hours after my caesarean. Despite the pain, it was nice to spend quiet time holding and feeding my baby."
Lizzy, 32, mum to one-month-old Aaron

In some ways life will be easier once you're home – your bed, for example, will almost certainly be lower than the hospital bed and easier to get in and out of – but you can't expect to be back to normal straight away and there are some precautions you should take (see opposite). In fact, it may take your body maybe your partner, need to ask the midwife who was at your baby's birth, and maybe the obstetrician involved, to talk to you about it.

Some maternity units offer a debriefing service. You can also request a copy of your labour notes by writing to the medical records department there.

"It may **take your body** up to **six** months **to recover** after a section."

up to six months to recover and many women say they don't feel completely themselves for up to a year.

Following a caesarean, most of us are just glad it's over and grateful we – and the baby – have survived. You may feel elated and delighted – or you may be weepy, and disappointed that you didn't give birth to your baby vaginally.

If things changed quickly during your labour, you may still feel traumatised by what you have been through. It may help your emotional recovery to go over again, and perhaps again and again, the reasons why a caesarean section became necessary. To do this you, and

Talk to your partner about how you feel as well. If your relationship with your partner or your baby is affected, you may need to seek professional help. Your partner may also be affected after witnessing what happened to you and may be in need of as much help as you.

Speak to your local health visitor and find out if there are any support groups local to you or women who have had similar experiences that she can put you in touch with. If you are really struggling to come to terms with the caesarean, speak to your doctor. It may be that you need some counselling or that you are suffering from postnatal depression.

Dad's Diary

Coming to terms with a caesarean

"After our baby was born by caesarean section, Sally felt really disappointed that she hadn't been able to give birth naturally. She had high hopes for an active labour, with no medical pain relief, but after 18 hours, we were told that the baby was in a very awkward position and that a vaginal birth would be extremely difficult. Sally eventually agreed that a caesarean would be the best option. As I walked down to the operating theatre with her, she kept saying that she felt like a failure – which, of course, she absolutely wasn't. I was proud of her for going through so much for so long. I'm sure I couldn't have done it. James was born 20 minutes later.

Sally recovered well physically, but it took longer for her to get over her disappointment. I found it hard to understand why – I was just relieved that it was all over and they were both safe and healthy. A week or so after the birth, we were able to meet up with the midwife to talk about it. It helped Sally to come to terms with the decision once she knew exactly why she'd had to have a caesarean. She quickly saw that it really was the only option."

Emergency deliveries, fast labour

If you've planned to have your baby in hospital, chances are she will arrive safe and sound once you're there. Sometimes, though, babies have other ideas and arrive on the way to hospital or even before you've got out the door! Here's how to cope if it happens to you…

No time to get to hospital

National statistics describe any birth that happens at home as a "home birth" whether or not it was planned. So it's difficult to know how many home births were actually intended to take place in hospital. However, the number is probably quite small and, if you're expecting your first baby, it's really very unlikely that she'll arrive unexpectedly on the hearthrug! Still, it's always wise to be prepared, so here is your quick guide to emergency home birth.

If you think your baby is coming too quickly for you to get to the hospital:

● Don't panic! Women are made to have babies. Babies are meant to be born. If your baby has been nine months in the womb, and she's coming quickly, it's probably because she's finding it very easy to get out. Your pelvis is clearly a nice spacious one with lots of room to help babies be born easily!

● Ring the emergency number that's given on your maternity notes. Then, if you're on your own, ring someone who can come over quickly – perhaps your mum, friend or neighbour.

● Make sure the front door is unlocked so that all the people coming to help you can get in. Then find a large clean towel ready to wrap the baby in.

● If you've got an overpowering urge to push, you may simply have to go with it. However, if you can, try panting instead. Give three quick pants and a long blow. Three quick pants and a long blow, and so on. This might just delay your baby's arrival for a few minutes.

If your baby insists on putting in an immediate appearance, don't worry. When her head is delivered, if there's a loop of cord around her neck, if you can do so gently, ease it over her head. Then leave the cord alone. You don't need to do anything else with it. Don't pull on it! Wait for your baby's body to be born with the next contraction.

Your baby may well be screaming lustily. If not, breathe on her face and stroke down the sides of her nose to press out any mucus or fluid that's trapped inside.

Pick her up, dry her and cuddle her. She's probably just as amazed as you at this sudden transition from being inside you to being outside.

Above all, keep her warm. Place her against your skin and drape a towel or blanket over her. Being warm and held close to you will help her to calm down.

If you are planning to breastfeed – or even if you're not – place your baby against your breast so that she can

Emergency home birth and the law

In the UK, it is legal to give birth at home without any professional or medical help, whether deliberately or accidentally. However, it is illegal for an unqualified, unregistered person to perform the role of a doctor or midwife during the birth.

If your baby's birth occurs accidentally, and only your partner (or a friend or relative) is with you, neither of you will be in any trouble. However, it is always best to have someone with you who knows what they're doing, for your own and your baby's sake.

If you've already had a baby that arrived quickly, be attuned to the first signs of labour as subsequent labours can go even faster.

1% or fewer women who have had no symptoms of labour or who have only had intermittent contractions, suddenly feel an overwhelming urge to push. This may signal the imminent arrival of the baby.

Parents**Talk...**

"My midwife arrived 10 minutes after Mia was born! I thought I'd be in labour for hours, but after an hour, I realised I was ready to push. That's when I phoned her. Luckily David had been to my antenatal classes."
Lynda, 29, mum to two-month-old Mia

"They say second babies are often quick, but it took less than an hour from start to finish for me. I wouldn't have made it to the hospital, so luckily I'd planned a home birth – although it did end up taking place in my parents' home

rather than my own. They weren't too pleased about the mess I'd made of their spare room!"
Emma, 36, mum to Joely and Laura

"I gave birth in the ambulance on the way to the hospital. When I started pushing I demanded that the driver stop by the side of the road, as I was being bumped around in the back. My husband told me later that our son was officially born outside a Chinese takeaway – classy!"
Christine, 27, mum to three-month-old Andrew

---

nuzzle. If she manages to suck just a little, this will stimulate the release of the hormone oxytocin, which helps the placenta to be delivered.

After the birth

Probably quite soon after your baby is delivered, you will feel the urge to push again. This is your uterus contracting to expel the placenta. The placenta will feel quite soft and slithery as it slips through the vagina. You might be

Keeping your baby warm after the birth is most important. Put her against your skin and lay a blanket or towel over her.

surprised by how large it is (about the size of a dinner plate). If you don't want to look at it, get whoever's with you to pop it into a plastic bag or bucket. So now you have your baby in your arms with the cord still attached to her, which is still attached to the placenta, which is in a plastic bag or bucket. Relax. The midwife and/or ambulance crew will deal with the cord and placenta when they arrive.

Congratulations! You've managed to do it all on your own. And as your baby grows up, she will be able to tell her friends the amazing story of her unexpected arrival.

If you feel upset by this unexpectedly quick birth, do talk to your midwife. Contact the Birth Trauma Association or NCT and ask to be put in touch with someone who's been through the same experience. With your next baby, you may decide to have a home birth again (planned this time!) or, if you choose a hospital birth, you'll know to go in at the first sign of labour. Planned home births are great, but unplanned ones are best avoided, if possible.

Don'ts in an emergency

You probably know the "do's" about an emergency home birth – but what about the "don'ts"?

● Don't panic – stay calm, get comfortable, phone the midwife and the hospital and, if you're alone, phone a friend or family member who can come over immediately to help.

● Don't try not push if the urge is overpowering. Your baby wants to get out!

● Don't cut or pull on the cord when your baby has been born. The midwife or ambulance crew can deal with it when they arrive.

● Don't hold back if you need to push again after your baby has arrived – this is your uterus contracting to expel the placenta. Stay where you are until you've delivered it. Ask whoever is with you to pop it in a plastic bag or bucket when it comes out.

● Don't give birth standing up – without professional help, your baby could fall and be seriously injured.

● Don't lift your baby up high. Lay her on your tummy or thigh and cover her with a blanket.

Getting ready for pregnancy

Staying safe and healthy

Your pregnancy diary

Birth and beyond

Life with your new baby

A life's begun

You're exhausted, emotional and feel a wreck. But you've also never felt so happy. Welcome to the confusing but wonderful world of parenthood. Most of your hours are now spent caring for the new little person in your life, but don't forget to look after yourself, too.

New parents sign on here

Depending on how the birth has gone, you may be feeling alert and happy, even exhilarated, or you may feel bruised and exhausted. Either extreme – or anything in between – is perfectly normal. Remember – you're recovering from a huge physical upheaval (and major abdominal surgery, if you had a caesarean). So be kind to yourself and allow yourself time to rest and recover.

If you're both fine, you may be discharged from hospital the same day or within a day or two. Whether at home or in hospital, sooner or later you'll want

Breastfeeding will help your uterus shrink back more quickly – you may feel a few contraction-like "afterpains" as it happens. Any minor grazes and tears to the neck of the womb, vagina and perineum usually heal within days but, if you've had stitches, these may take a little longer.

As you hold your newborn, the realisation that you are responsible for this precious new life can feel daunting, but don't forget that every mum and dad was a new parent once. Relax – no one expects you to be perfect.

"**Responsibity** for this **precious new life** can feel **daunting**."

to freshen up. Make sure someone is near as you shower or wash, in case you feel a bit wobbly. Take a plastic bottle into the loo with you and pour some warm water over your vagina as you wee, to stop any sore bits stinging. You'll also need to put on a sanitary towel to absorb the lochia (postnatal bleeding).

Holding your newborn may feel strange but you have a whole lifetime to get to know each other better.

 Green mum

Now you're a mum, thinking about the future of the planet is even more important.

"There are so many things us mums can do to help the environment. For a start, I'm breastfeeding, which is completely natural. And I'm also using reusable cotton nappies as well as specially designed reusable wet wipes. All these can be washed carefully and dried on the line. Recycling's even more important to me, too, and it's not just baby jars and toy packaging – I've been buying as many things as I can second hand, like clothes, toys and nursery furniture.

When my baby starts solids, I plan on making everything myself from scratch using fresh ingredients and, if I've got time, I'll even have a go at growing some of my own vegetables. My husband's been talking about getting a couple of chickens so we have an unlimited supply of eggs! And I've been walking as much as I can with the buggy. It not only saves on using the car, but also gives me some much-needed exercise."

Getting ready for pregnancy

Staying safe and healthy

Your pregnancy diary

Birth and beyond

After the birth: your baby and you

As you'll soon discover, newborns don't need much. All your baby needs to thrive is regular feeds, cuddles and nappy changes. For now, try to sleep when he sleeps and ask for help whenever you need it. Your midwife will be around for at least 10 days to support you.

ParentsAsk...

Will it be love at first sight?
Bonding is a very individual experience. Some parents feel an intense love for their baby within minutes of the birth. For others, it may take days, weeks or even longer. However, parents who are separated from their newborns for medical reasons or who adopt their children when they're several months old can still develop enormously close, loving relationships.

Your stay in hospital

Make the most of your time in hospital to recover from the birth and bond with your baby. If there haven't been any problems, you and your baby may be able to go home on the same day. If not, you may stay in hospital for a day or two. If you had a caesarean you'll probably have to stay three to five days.

You'll be feeling very tired after giving birth. Postnatal wards can be noisy with other babies and mothers, so remember to bring earplugs with you to hospital. Try to sleep when your baby sleeps – it's harder to bond when you're physically exhausted.

If you need to stay in hospital for a while, remember that the midwives and nurses are there to help you. If you need help with breastfeeding, don't struggle on alone, your hospital may have a breastfeeding specialist, or one of the midwives can come to see you.

Newborn tests and checks

After the birth, your baby will have examinations to check that he is healthy. The first is the Apgar (see right; the name is an acronym for Appearance, Pulse, Grimace, Activity and Respiration). It is done at one minute, then again at five minutes, after birth. Shortly afterwards, your baby will be weighed and the circumference of his head measured.

A full examination is done between four and 48 hours from birth. Among other things, your baby's ears, eyes, spine, mouth, genitals and feet will be checked.

Before your baby is one week old, a heel-prick blood test is also carried out to check for conditions such as sickle cell disorders and cystic fibrosis.

Apgar scoring system	Score of 0	Score of 1	Score of 2	Component of acronym
Skin colour	blue all over	white at extremities; body pink	pink all over	Appearance
Heart rate	absent	slow	fast	Pulse
Reflex response	no response to stimulation	grimacing when stimulated	crying and coughing	Grimace
Muscle tone	limp	some bending or stretching of limbs	active movement	Activity
Breathing	absent	weak or irregular	good and your baby is crying	Respiration

A doctor or specially trained midwife will carry out standard checks on your baby, both straight after birth and before you take him home.

ParentsAsk...

My newborn's got jaundice. Should I worry?

About half of all normal, healthy babies develop a yellowish tinge to their skin, or jaundice, in their first few days of life. If your baby does, it's probably nothing to worry about, but mention it to your midwife or health visitor. In rare cases it can be a sign of something more serious, such as a liver problem. Breastfeeding should help to clear up the jaundice, but some babies may need treatment in hospital with ultraviolet light.

During your time in hospital you'll learn how to keep your baby clean and how to care for his umbilical cord stump. Don't worry if you don't bond with your baby straight away – everyone is different.

Before you leave hospital a doctor or specially trained midwife will do some checks on your baby (see opposite). He'll have a physical examination and his weight will be noted. He may also have a hearing check.

Your baby in special care

A neonatal unit is specially designed to provide expert, around-the-clock care for newborn babies who are ill or are born prematurely. Between 6 and 10 per cent of all newborns spend some time here, so it is not all that unusual. However, most parents do not expect

that their baby might have to go to the neonatal unit, and it usually comes as a real shock to them.

Every hospital has a neonatal unit, but some may not be equipped to provide the care your baby needs. Your baby might therefore have to be transferred to a unit far from your home. This could also happen if your local hospital does not have enough room.

On the neonatal unit, a skilled team from different professions will care for your baby. Some of the people you may meet include specialist neonatal nurses, a consultant paediatrician or neonataologist, and other specialist doctors, such as surgeons.

Last but not least, there's you, the parents. Your special-care baby needs all the things that other babies need

from their parents. Your touch, voice and presence all help a great deal. The professionals will recognise this and treat you as part of the team.

If you're keen to breastfeed, let the nurses know and they should make every effort to help you. They will help you to express your milk if your baby is not well enough to breastfeed. The expressed milk may be given to him via a feeding tube or will be stored and used to feed him when he is ready.

Most hospitals allow parents to visit their neonatal unit 24 hours a day. Others have more restricted visiting hours. Don't forget that, if you're not at the hospital, you can call the neonatal unit anytime, day or night. Always ask questions or talk to the staff about any worries you may have.

Getting ready for pregnancy

Staying safe and healthy

Your pregnancy diary

Birth and beyond

Breastfeeding while lying down can give you some much-needed rest, especially at night. It's also comfortable after a caesarean.

For breastfeeding while seated, make sure your back and arms are well supported and you are relaxed. It will make you more comfortable if you use a pillow on your lap to bring your baby up to the right height.

Avoiding sore nipples

Sore nipples are common in newly breastfeeding mothers. You well may feel some tenderness at the beginning of a feed during the first few days. But if the pain is intense or lasts longer than a few days, it is a sign that you may need to make some changes.

The most likely cause is that your baby isn't latching on well or that she's incorrectly positioned at the breast. She needs to take a large mouthful of breast – not just the nipple – into her mouth before she begins to suck. If she is just sucking on the nipple, it will probably hurt. It is important for you to get expert help from a breastfeeding counsellor or infant feeding specialist to sort out your baby's latching-on technique.

Feeding your baby

Whether you decide to breast- or bottle feed your baby, giving that first feed can be an emotional experience. If you've never given birth before, the maternity support staff or your midwife will give you the practical advice you need on how to go about it.

Breastfeeding

Offer your baby the breast soon after she's born – babies are sometimes very alert at this time and they feed well. But it doesn't matter if all your baby wants to do is to lick a little and enjoy the loving, close cuddle she gets when you hold her in your arms this way.

The midwife should help you find a comfortable position and will talk to you about how you can help your baby to get "latched on" (see left) so she feeds effectively and doesn't make your nipples sore.

Your baby needs a wide open mouth to take in your breast. Remember to bring your baby onto the breast. Don't try to "slot" your nipple in. You and your baby will get better and better at this, and you shouldn't be downhearted if you don't get it right at first.

Feed your baby as often as she seems to want it. Keep her close to you – next to you in bed, snuggled up against your skin. That way you will both get plenty of "feeding practice" and you can rest a little in between. It's not helpful to wait until your baby is yelling loudly before you feed her. No one learns well when they're upset, and your baby will find it hard to get a good mouthful of breast if she is crying, because her tongue will be in the wrong position. Her tongue needs to be forwards and, when she's crying, it's too far back in her mouth.

Bottle feeding

As with breastfeeding, most experts agree that you shouldn't follow a rigid schedule in the early weeks. Instead, you should offer the bottle every two to three hours, or when your baby seems hungry. Until she reaches about 4.5 kilograms (10 pounds), she will probably take 30 to 90 millilitres (1 to 3 fluid ounces) per feed. Your health visitor will advise you.

Before you first use new bottles and teats, and each time that you use them, they must be washed and sterilised carefully. To do this, you will need a steam steriliser, or a microwave steriliser, or you can use sterilising

solution. You can also boil the bottles and teats for at least 10 minutes to sterilise them. You will need to continue this sterilising routine for the first year of your baby's life.

To make up formula milk, follow the instructions on the packet carefully. Use boiled cooled water (but it should not have been left for longer than half an hour to cool). Fill the bottle to the marked level and measure the milk powder with the scoop provided. Use a knife to level off the scoop, but avoid packing the powder down. Add this to the water in the bottle. Put the teat and cover on and then shake well. Don't be tempted to add extra scoops of formula powder as this can make your baby ill.

If you need to prepare a feed for later, put freshly boiled water in a sealed flask and mix it with formula powder when required. You should never re-warm bottles of milk.

How to bottle feed your baby

Stroking your baby's cheek before a feed helps to stimulate the sucking reflex and encourages her to open her mouth ready for the bottle.

Hold the bottle at an angle to keep the teat full of milk and free of air. If you hold the bottle firmly, she can pull against it slightly to get a good sucking action.

Near the end of the feed, tilt the bottle so the last drops fill the teat. To stop your baby sucking on an empty bottle, slide your finger into her mouth to release the suction.

Getting ready for pregnancy

Staying safe and healthy

Your pregnancy diary

Birth and beyond

Going home with your newborn

After nine months of growing your baby and several hours of giving birth, you're finally at home with your newborn. Feeling overwhelmed, confused and ever so slightly terrified of looking after a baby? We can help. Our survival guide will lead you through these first few hectic days.

The first few days at home

Some women feel completely at ease and can't wait to get home with their new baby; others are overwhelmed by the responsibility – especially when they're still recovering physically and emotionally from labour. Either way, as a new mum you'll need lots of support and help. You will get some of it automatically, but sometimes you may need to ask. You shouldn't think that asking for help is a sign of weakness;

it's simply acknowledging the fact that you need to get enough rest so you are able to care for your new baby.

Now is the time to forget the housework and anything else – just focus on recovering from the labour and bonding with your baby. Get your partner, family and friends to look after the day-to-day chores, and make sure that any visitors are the type that will look after you, rather than expect to be entertained. In the early days a midwife will visit regularly, to check that you are healing OK, continue your baby's medical care, help establish feeding and provide other advice and support.

After three or four days your milk will arrive, making your breasts feel hot, swollen and tender. At first your nipples may feel very sensitive, and the first 10 to 20 seconds of each feed may be uncomfortable. This usually begins to ease off after about the fifth day.

It's common for women to feel weepy around this time – a combination of raging hormones and exhaustion – so don't feel guilty if you're not feeling elated every minute of the day.

Hand your baby over to your partner as often as you can. You need plenty of rest if you are to care for your baby properly.

ParentsAsk...

Is it OK to have my baby in bed with me?

The nurturing and closeness that co-sleeping brings can help create a stronger relationship between you and your child.

Studies have shown that sleep-sharing babies breastfeed more, yet disrupt their mothers' sleep less, than babies who sleep alone. Mothers who co-sleep also tend to breastfeed their babies for longer.

Co-sleeping babies also stay awake for shorter periods of time during the night than solitary sleepers, and they may cry significantly less, too. Sleeping close to your baby allows you to respond quickly if he coughs or cries in the night.

However, it is not safe to take a premature baby into bed with you. Also, to reduce the risk of SIDS, you should never share a bed with your baby if you or your partner have been drinking alcohol, have taken drugs or medication, or if either of you are a smoker. Never sleep with your baby on a sofa or armchair, nor in a water-bed. And you shouldn't ever share a bed with more than one child.

An alternative to sharing a bed with your baby is to use a co-sleeper cot that attaches to your bed. Its mattress is the same level as your mattress, so it creates a level surface. Many mothers find the cost well worth it.

Bathing your baby

You don't need to wait for your baby's umbilical cord stump to fall off, or for the area to heal completely, before you give him a bath. For the first week or so, you may find it easier to stick to sponge baths, often called "top and tailing" (see below). The most important thing when bathing your baby is to keep him warm.

Newborns don't need a daily bath. Until he is crawling and getting into messes, a bath isn't really necessary more than once or twice a week.

While he is tiny, you can bath him in a small baby bath. Fill it with about 5cm (2in) of water, at a temperature that is warm but not hot – about 38°C (100.4°F.)

Always test the water with your forearm, as the skin is more sensitive there than on your hands. Never put your baby in the bath while the water is still running in case the temperature changes. Also, you should avoid using strong cleansers, as they may damage your newborn's skin.

How to top and tail your baby

Clean his face and neck with a piece of damp cotton wool. Don't forget the neck creases. Wipe the eyes from the inner to outer corners. Pat dry with a soft towel.

Gently uncurl his fingers and use a fresh piece of damp cotton wool to wipe the fronts and backs of his hands and in between his fingers. Pat dry with a soft towel.

Take off his nappy and use a fresh piece of damp cotton wool to wipe around his genital area. Clean in between the skin creases, then pat dry with a soft towel.

How to give your baby a bath

Undress your baby and wrap him in a towel. Tuck him under your arm, support his head with your hand, and gently wet his hair. Dry his hair with a soft towel.

Unwrap the towel and lower him into the water, supporting his shoulders with one hand. Always hold him securely. Slowly splash water over him with your free hand.

Lift him out with your free hand under his bottom, then wrap him gently in a towel. Pat him dry thoroughly, making sure you have dried in between the skin creases.

Getting ready for pregnancy

Staying safe and healthy

Your pregnancy diary

Birth and beyond

The first two weeks

You'll probably spend the first two weeks of your baby's life in an exhausted but happy haze. In between feeds and nappy changes, you'll be welcoming visitors keen to see your little bundle and the house will be filled with cards and flowers. Lie back and enjoy the fuss!

Tiredness

While you can't change your baby's around-the-clock schedule, some strategies help you survive the bleary-eyed days and get more sleep at night.

- Simplify your daily routine – keep household chores to a minimum and don't take on anything overambitious, such as trips with your baby to packed shopping malls.

- Say no to caffeine in the late afternoon and evening.
- Nap or rest during the day when your baby sleeps. This isn't a good idea in the long run, but for now it's an important way to keep your energy up.
- Get some gentle exercise and fresh air – a stroll in the park with the pram is perfect.

- If you're falling asleep on the sofa or in the chair in your baby's nursery, make yourself get into bed. Getting into the habit of sleeping anywhere but the bed can lead to sleep problems.
- Avoid heavy meals near bedtime. But if you need an evening snack, choose a high-carbohydrate food, such as a bowl of cereal. It can actually help you sleep.

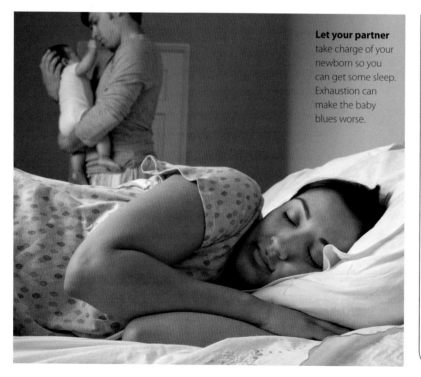

Let your partner take charge of your newborn so you can get some sleep. Exhaustion can make the baby blues worse.

 Active mum

Take every opportunity you can to have a nap while your newborn is sleeping.

"A couple of days after having my baby, the natural high started to wear off and I was hit by a brain-numbing exhaustion! I just felt so physically tired from giving birth and my daughter was waking up several times a night to feed. I started to feel like I'd never catch up on my own sleep. That's when I decided that if she was sleeping, then I needed to be, too. Even though this meant I was napping in the day and still suffering from broken sleep at night, I started to feel so much more human again. Finally she was sleeping through. Bliss!"

Your baby will enjoy it *(above)* if you play with her and talk to her while you are getting her dressed.

Support your baby's head *(left)* as you pick her up, then bring her close to your chest and hold her gently but firmly.

Handling your newborn

Until about four weeks, your baby won't have any head control. Be sure to support her head firmly at all times, but especially when picking her up and putting her down. Use your other hand and arm to cradle her bottom and back, and draw her near you in a fluid motion.

Then you can embrace her gently against your chest. Or hold her up, with her head resting on your shoulder, her bottom in the crook of your arm and your forearm supporting her back. Reverse these steps to put her down.

When your baby is next to your chest, be sure her head is slightly higher than her body. You can also use a sling, as long as her neck and head are well supported and she fits securely in it.

Getting your baby dressed can feel daunting at first. Newborns seem very fragile, and often cry when they are undressed. You can make the process much simpler by choosing clothes for your baby that are quick and easy to put on and take off, and having everything to hand before you start.

Your baby's vest goes on first, over her nappy. Your newborn baby's neck muscles aren't properly developed yet, so support her neck gently as you carefully place her vest over her head. Pull the vest down over her body and do up the poppers at the crotch. Then lay your baby carefully on top of her sleepsuit, ease her arms and legs in gently, and do up the poppers all the way down the front.

As you get your baby dressed enjoy talking to her – tell her what you're doing – or singing to her. Don't worry about sounding silly – your baby will love to hear your voice.

Dad's **Diary**

Where does dad come in?

"Fathers often feel that there's nothing useful they can do when there's a newborn in the house. This is hogwash. Starting with the basics, we can:

- Change nappies.
- Burp the baby.
- Rock baby to sleep (important because, unlike your breastfeeding partner, you won't smell of milk and so won't have your fully fed baby demanding more).
- Read stories (baby won't understand a thing, but it's important to introduce the concept early).
- Keep baby occupied through play (we're the fun parents, remember).
- Talk to baby (she can't talk back yet but it gets her familiar with grammar and vocabulary).

Even helping around the house is useful – and earns us dads extra brownie points. The following easy tasks might provide light relief:

- Doing the washing up.
- Cooking for your partner.
- Loading the washing machine and hanging the clean clothes out.
- Tidying the house now and then.
- Doing the shopping.
- Waiting on your partner unquestioningly, hand and foot."

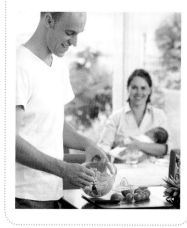

The signs of PND

It is generally thought that about 10 per cent of new mothers suffer from postnatal depression (PND). If you have a lot of the symptoms listed below and you are suffering from them constantly, you should talk to your health visitor or doctor just in case you are one of that 10 per cent. You may be feeling:

● Miserable most of the time and especially bad in the mornings and/or evenings.

● That life is not worth living and you have nothing to look forward to.

● Guilty and very ready to blame yourself.

● Irritable and snapping at your partner or other children.

● Tearful.

● Constantly exhausted, yet not able to sleep.

● Unable to enjoy yourself.

● That you have lost your sense of humour.

● That you can't cope.

● Terribly anxious about the baby, so that you are constantly seeking reassurance about your anxieties from health professionals.

● Worried about your own health, perhaps frightened that you have some dreadful illness.

● Unable to concentrate on anything.

● That your baby is a stranger and not really yours.

You may also be suffering from:

● Loss of sex drive.

● Low energy levels.

● Memory problems.

● Difficulty making decisions.

● No appetite *or* comfort eating.

● Anxiety.

● Disturbed sleep, including early-morning wakefulness.

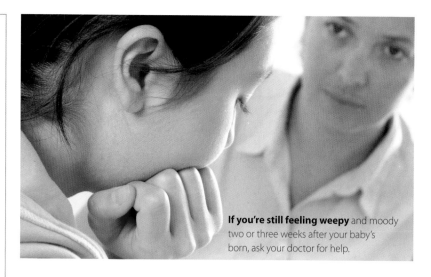

If you're still feeling weepy and moody two or three weeks after your baby's born, ask your doctor for help.

Still feeling blue?

Soon after giving birth, many women have what's commonly called the "baby blues" – weepiness and moodiness. These are often linked to hormonal changes three or four days after delivery, when pregnancy hormones dissipate and milk production starts. They're also linked to the physical and emotional anticlimax after the birth. Returning home from hospital can also increase a new mother's sense of uncertainty.

Baby blues affect 60 to 80 per cent of women shortly after labour, and many find themselves exhausted, unable to sleep, or feeling trapped or anxious. Your appetite can change, or you can feel irritable, nervous, worried about being a mother, or afraid that being a mother will never feel better than this.

All these feelings are normal, and they usually last only a few days. Few women find that their sadness persists for longer. Remember – the responsibility that comes with a baby can be overwhelming, and the reality of what parenthood involves doesn't really hit many women until these first few days at home.

Baby blues are often confused with postnatal depression (PND) because they share common symptoms. But in the first few days after delivery, some emotional upheaval is to be expected. If you continue to feel this way beyond two to three weeks after the birth, you should seek professional support.

 ## Systemised mum

Many mums experience the baby blues in the first few days after their baby is born.

"I had a week of baby blues when my son arrived. I was overwhelmed with the love I felt for him, and spent hours gazing at him. But I felt weepy and emotional at the same time. Being so tired didn't help, either. He's three weeks old now and I feel much more back to my old self and we're starting to form a little routine. My partner and my family were so supportive – they really helped me in those early days."

Colic

About 20 per cent of all babies develop colic. This is a catch-all phrase for uncontrollable crying in an otherwise healthy baby. A baby who has real colic will be crying for more than three hours a day, and for more than three days in one week.

Generally, a baby becomes colicky around two to four weeks and is over it by about three months. In addition to persistent crying, a colicky baby looks truly uncomfortable. He may alternately extend or pull up his legs and pass wind, as well as turn red in the face. Colic usually occurs between 6pm and midnight, although it can occur around the clock, generally becoming worse in the evening.

Colic is often blamed on a baby's immature digestive system or, according to some people, it's the baby's still-developing nervous system simply tensing up. Others subscribe to the theory that the baby is tired or overstimulated, and that colic is his way of blocking everything out so he can sleep. Yet another theory is that babies who are exposed to cigarette smoke are more likely to develop colic.

One theory is that breastfed babies become colicky because of something in their mother's diet, although there's no evidence to support this. Some mums find that if they stop drinking cow's milk and other dairy products, the situation improves. Some breastfed babies seem to be bothered if mum indulges in a lot of spicy food, wheat products, or cruciferous vegetables such as cabbage and cauliflower. To test if these foods are making your baby uncomfortable, try avoding them for a few days and see if it makes a difference.

If your baby is bottle fed, you might try a faster flow teat to see if that improves things. Make sure that you're burping him during and after feeds – it helps to relieve the pressure that builds up when he swallows air. If colic doesn't improve, see your doctor.

Laid-back mum

You'll get lots of advice about caring for your new baby. But it's OK to go with your own instincts.

"My daughter's eight months now and a couple of my friends have babies of a similar age. Francesca wakes up several times a night. I always go to her to see if she's hungry or needs her nappy changed, but I have a feeling that it's just a case of her wanting to hear my voice and know that I'm still there for her.

I don't mind losing sleep to comfort her, but my friends think I'm mad! They both opted for the crying-it-out method and said that, after a few difficult nights, their babies realised that they wouldn't be getting mummy's attention just for the sake of it. They now both sleep through. I just can't bear to hear my daughter cry, though, and despite my friends nagging me for spoiling her, I'm going to keep doing what I'm doing.

We're all different as parents and, as long as we're confident that we're doing our best and the right thing, then I think that's all that matters."

Parents**Talk...**

"Sara had colic from week five to week eight. She'd cry from 6pm to 10pm every night and nothing would soothe her. As I was breastfeeding, my midwife advised me to stop eating spicy foods and to give up dairy products for a while, but that didn't work. I eventually tried gripe water and that seemed to help."
Vanessa, 34, mum to Sara and Ashley

"My health visitor showed me how to do baby massage when Damian had colic. She thought he might be a bit constipated and massage, especially on the tummy, can get things moving. A warm flannel on his tummy at bathtime soothed him, too."
Kate, 31, mum to Damian

"I was really upset when George had colic. He'd scream between midnight and 3am most nights. My midwife suggested using a faster flow teat in his bottle, and it worked immediately. He was obviously swallowing too much air with the old teat."
Nadia, 29, mum to George

Getting ready for pregnancy

Staying safe and healthy

Your pregnancy diary

Birth and beyond

Diet during breastfeeding

Your body is highly efficient at producing milk, so you shouldn't need to take in lots of extra calories while you're breastfeeding. It's best to be guided by your appetite and to eat when you are hungry. There's no right answer about how many calories a day you should have. The amount you need to eat depends on your weight and how active you are.

It's important to get your vitamins, though. Focus on eating whole grains and cereals, fresh fruit and vegetables, as well as foods that provide plenty of protein, calcium and iron. Opt for nutritious snacks such as yoghurt, sandwiches made with wholemeal bread and filled with leafy greens and canned salmon, tuna or cheese, a jacket potato with baked beans, or fruit. The occasional "naughty" treat is fine.

What to drink

You only need to drink enough to satisfy your thirst while you're breastfeeding. Drinking lots of water, or indeed going a bit thirsty, won't affect the amount of milk you make. It's a good idea to have a drink nearby when you are breastfeeding, though. While you are feeding, your body releases the hormone oxytocin, and it makes you feel thirsty.

If you want to drink alcohol, don't have more than one or two units once or twice a week. The Department of Health (DH) says if you're breastfeeding, it's best to follow the same rules that apply to drinking in pregnancy. Alcohol enters your bloodstream – and then your breastmilk – at different speeds, depending on how much you weigh and whether you drink alcohol with food or on an empty stomach. The amount of alcohol in your blood usually peaks 30 to 45 minutes after you have drunk it. You'll need to allow a couple of hours for your body to be clear of one unit of alcohol.

Weight loss

You may have put on a bit of weight while you were pregnant, and it's fine to shed some while you're breastfeeding. Losing about 1kg (2lb) a week shouldn't affect the amount of milk you make. It's not a good idea to go on a strict diet when you're breastfeeding, but eating healthily and doing gentle exercise will help you get in shape.

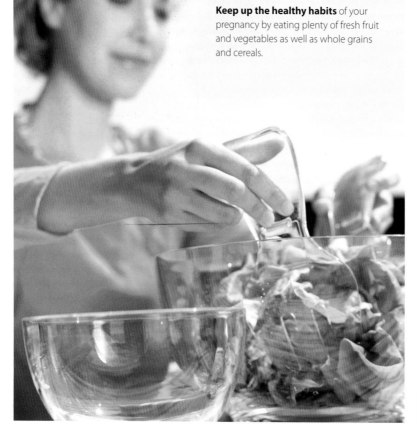

Keep up the healthy habits of your pregnancy by eating plenty of fresh fruit and vegetables as well as whole grains and cereals.

Drinking lots of fluids *(above)* – especially water – will help you to quench your thirst while you're breastfeeding.

Changing a nappy

Your baby will be wearing nappies day and night for the next two to three years. And, believe it or not, she will need eight to 10 nappy changes a day to begin with. Changing her nappy regularly is important, as urine combined with the bacteria in poo can make her skin sore and lead to nappy rash. Wetness doesn't bother most babies so don't expect her to cry every time she needs changing.

Before you change her, be sure you have everything you need nearby. Lay her on a safe changing area with a hygienic, washable surface and use a baby wipe or wet cotton wool to clean her. For a girl, always wipe from front to back. This will help to reduce the possibility of any bacteria getting into her vagina and giving her an infection.

The clean nappy's top half (the one with the tabs) should go under your baby's rear, and the bottom half should come up between her legs. Try not to bunch the nappy up between her legs – this can cause chafing and discomfort. If you are changing a newborn's nappy, you should avoid covering the umbilical cord. For boys, tuck the penis down; that way moisture will be less likely to escape. Fasten the nappy at both sides with the sticky tabs, making sure it's snug, and voilà!

How to change a nappy

Clean your baby's bottom with a baby wipe or some wet cotton wool. Dry her carefully and apply barrier cream (see right).

Lay the nappy flat with the tabs at the back, then gently lift your baby's feet and slide the nappy underneath her bottom.

Bring the front of the nappy up between your baby's legs. The top of the nappy should align with her waist.

Unpeel the nappy's sticky tabs, one at a time, then pull each side firmly over the front of the nappy and press to fasten.

Nappy rash

If your baby has nappy rash, you'll know it. Some of the skin covered by the nappy – probably the genital area, the folds of the thighs and the buttocks – will appear red and inflamed. The affected areas can either be dry or moist and they sometimes look pimply.

The best remedy is to keep your baby clean and dry by changing her nappy frequently. When you're changing your baby's nappy, use just water and cotton wool to clean the nappy area – this will probably clear up the problem if the nappy rash is allergy-based. Leave her nappy off for a while to allow the air to speed up the healing process. You can prevent nappy rash by coating your baby's bottom with a thin layer of barrier cream after each nappy change.

A normal nappy rash should clear up after three or four days of at-home treatment. If your baby's rash persists, spreads, or otherwise worsens, talk to your doctor – he may prescribe a hydrocortisone or anticandial cream to help clear up the rash.

Getting ready for pregnancy

Staying safe and healthy

Your pregnancy diary

Birth and beyond

Life as new parents

The state of your home brings new meaning to the word "disarray", and you're both totally shattered. You've become an exhausted, downtrodden, overburdened mummy, while he may be feeling sidelined and deprived of attention. Welcome to parenthood!

Now's the time for you both to reach deep into your reserves of patience and understanding. Dads who return to work outside the home can start to see their partner and baby as a single unit that excludes them. After all, the parent who is out all day doesn't experience the intense bonding that comes with all those tedious-but-necessary tasks, as well as with the cuddles.

When you're both around, try to divvy up the babycare between you (including the less enjoyable bits). Perhaps bathtime could be dad's job before mum does the bedtime feed. And be considerate if one of you has had more than their share of bum-wiping or rush-hour traffic stress.

Not many things can soothe the tension of a hard day better than a meaningful and encouraging kind word. Don't underestimate the power of occasional reminders that you're both doing a great job. Being a parent really is the toughest, but most rewarding, thing you'll ever do. Try not to forget to remind each other how much you appreciate the effort you're both putting in.

Above all, keep communicating. Pay attention to each other, and make time to talk through things that are bothering you. You got together for a reason, so try not to lose sight of that.

80%

of new mums say that the most surprising thing they've learned about themselves since becoming a mum is that they didn't know they could be so selfless. Now they've got a baby, they always put his needs first.

Systemised mum

Take things one step at a time when it comes to getting your body back to normal.

"Chloe is two weeks old now, and I've already started some gentle exercise. I try to take her out for a walk once a day – even if it's just a stroll to the local shops in her pram. I always feel more energised when I get home, and it helps to have some fresh air and a change of scenery.

Every day, usually when she's asleep, I spend 15 minutes doing some gentle post-pregnancy exercises, which essentially involve me squeezing and lifting my abdominal muscles. I also do my pelvic floor exercises – which are absolutely essential.

I can't wait until my stitches have healed so that I can go swimming again and, after I've had my six-week check, I'd really like to join an exercise class – hopefully I'll be able to find a mother-and-baby one."

It's daunting when you're new parents but staying close and making sure you spend time together helps you both to cope.

ParentsAsk...

When can we have sex again?
You can have sex again when you and your partner both feel that it's right for you. It's assumed that you should wait for your doctor to give you the go-ahead at your six-week postnatal check. But some people think it's a good idea to try making love before your check-up so you can discuss any problems you encounter.

New mothers can feel reluctant or uninterested in sex for a variety of reasons. The most obvious reason is soreness from an episiotomy and stitches. Tiredness is another overwhelming factor and, on top of that, your body image might also hold you back – many women say that they just don't feel "sexy".

If your partner wants sex and you don't, it is important for you to talk about your feelings. Your partner may feel rejected, so it is up to you to explain the physical discomfort or anxieties that are holding you back. Words and cuddles can do much to convey affection and emotion, and you will both benefit from this closeness.

If sex is painful when you do get around to it, despite going carefully and gently, it is worth talking to your doctor about it.

How to cope

Daily life with a newborn can be chaos. Despite little or no previous experience, you are now responsible for the wellbeing, care, nourishment and protection of a tiny new baby, 24 hours a day, seven days a week. No wonder you feel overwhelmed.

The good news is that things will become easier as you get to know your baby and discover what he likes and dislikes, and how he needs to be cared for. Until things settle into more of a routine, here are some ideas to help you get through:

● **Go for a walk** Planning a short walk every day, whatever the weather, may stop you feeling like the walls are closing in on you.

● **Don't try to do too much** If you've always had high standards for housework, accepting that they may need to slip in the early weeks can take the pressure off. Just remember: your newborn doesn't mind if there are crumbs under the toaster. Alternatively, if you can afford one, hire a cleaner.

● **Find some company** Ask your health visitor about mother-and-baby groups that meet in your area and make the effort to go along.

● **Take up any offers of help** If you have visitors, don't make them tea – ask them to make you tea!

● **Set some time aside for yourself** Take a shower, put your feet up and read a magazine, or call a friend for a chat.

Dad's **Diary**

The first week of baby's life
"The first week of Alfie's life was a blur. The three of us settled into something resembling a daily schedule. I would wake during the night with him to change his nappy and hand him to Karen to be breastfed. Then, my alarm would get me out of bed around seven o'clock. I would potter around the house, feeding the dog and making breakfast. Then, I'd wake Alfie and Karen. After another feed, Karen and I would spend time together with Alfie. This was his early-morning full-of-milk cute phase of the day. It was prime-time baby as far as we were concerned. He'd lie on our bed and coo while Karen and I talked to him, sang songs and just enjoyed ourselves as a new family."

"Things will **become easier** as you **get to know** your baby and **his likes** and **dislikes**."

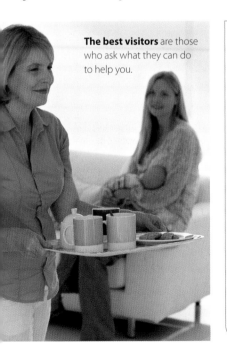

The best visitors are those who ask what they can do to help you.

Knowing when to call the doctor

Life as a new parent means you're on a steep leaning curve. You may worry that you need to call the doctor. Watch out for these warning signs:

● **Change in temperament** A baby who has a runny nose and a big smile is probably not as sick as a baby who has a runny nose and is lethargic.

● **Unusual crying** If your baby is crying more than usual and you can't comfort him, or if his cry is weak or unusually high pitched, he may be seriously ill.

● **Appetite** A baby who tires easily from sucking or loses interest in feeding is probably sick.

● **Abnormal bowel movements** Young babies, especially if breastfed, may have very soft bowel movements. However, if he has watery stools, his tummy may be upset. If he is sleepy and has small, hard, or dry bowel movements, or if his stool is streaked with blood or mucus, or has the consistency of jelly, you should call your doctor.

● **Difficulty breathing** If your baby's breathing is laboured or he's having trouble breathing, get help immediately.

● **Fever** If a baby under three months has a fever higher than 38ºC (100.4ºF), he should be examined by a doctor.

● **Vomiting for 12 hours or more** If this occurs or if your baby has other symptoms with it, such as fever or a rash, call your doctor.

Getting ready for pregnancy

Staying safe and healthy

Your pregnancy diary

Birth and beyond

Glossary

afterbirth The placenta is commonly called the afterbirth once it has been delivered.

alpha-fetoprotein This is a protein which is produced by the baby's liver. It can be detected in the mother's blood most accurately between 15 and 17 weeks of pregnancy. High levels of AFP may be associated with a neural-tube birth defect called spina bifida; low levels may be associated with Down's syndrome.

amniocentesis An amniocentesis is a diagnostic test used to determine possible genetic abnormalities. It is usually performed from 15 weeks of pregnancy. Amniotic fluid is withdrawn from the amniotic sac by inserting a hollow needle through the abdominal wall.

amniotic fluid This is the clear straw-coloured liquid in the amniotic sac in which the baby grows. It cushions the baby against pressure and knocks, allows the baby to move around and grow without restriction, helps the lungs develop, keeps the baby at a constant temperature, and provides a barrier against infection.

Apgar score The Apgar scale is routinely used one and five minutes (and sometimes ten minutes) after birth to assess a newborn baby's health. It assesses five basic indicators of health: activity level, pulse, grimace (response to stimulation), appearance and respiration.

bilirubin Bilirubin is a by-product of the normal breakdown of old red blood cells. Some newborn babies are unable to metabolise it quickly enough, so it builds up under the skin and causes jaundice. If levels become too high, bilirubin is stored in the brain where it can sometimes cause brain damage, which is why some newborns are treated under phototherapy lamps to break down the bilirubin.

bloody show A "show" or "bloody show" is a discharge of mucus tinged with blood that results from the mucus plug dislodging from the cervix as labour approaches.

Braxton Hicks contractions The irregular "practice" contractions of the uterus that occur throughout pregnancy, but can be felt especially towards the end of pregnancy. They can sometimes be uncomfortable and intense, but are not usually painful.

breech presentation A baby is said to be breech presentation, or in a breech position, when it is "bottom down" rather than "head down" in the uterus just before birth. Either the baby's bottom or feet would be born first.

caesarean section A caesarean or c-section is when the baby is born through an incision in the mother's abdomen and uterus. It is used when a woman cannot give birth vaginally or if the baby is in distress or danger.

cephalopelvic disproportion This is when a baby's head is too large to pass through the mother's pelvic opening. It is a common cause of obstructed labour and can result in delivery by caesarean section.

cervical stitch A cervical stitch is used to close a weak cervix to prevent miscarriage and premature labour. It is usually carried out between 14 and 16 weeks of pregnancy.

cervical weakness The condition in which the cervix painlessly opens before a pregnancy has reached full term. It can cause miscarriage in the second trimester or premature labour in the third, but can sometimes be treated with a cervical stitch (see left).

cervix The lower end or neck of the uterus which leads into the vagina, and which gradually opens during labour.

chorionic villus sampling (CVS) Chorionic villus sampling (CVS) is a diagnostic test carried out in early pregnancy, usually between 11 and 13 weeks of pregnancy. Some of the cells which line the placenta, the chorionic villi, are removed through the cervix or abdomen using a needle or catheter. The cells are tested to see whether the developing fetus has Down's syndrome or other genetic abnormalities.

colostrum Colostrum is the first "milk" the breasts produce as a precursor to breast milk. It is rich in fats, protein, and antibodies, which protect the baby against infection and kick-start the immune system. It is gradually replaced by breast milk.

conception Conception or fertilisation is the moment when sperm and egg meet, join and form a single cell. It usually takes place in the fallopian tubes.

congenital problem Any problem with a baby that is present from birth or has developed during pregnancy and is not inherited.

contraction The tightening of a muscle. In labour, the strong, rhythmic contractions of the muscles of the uterus open up the cervix and help push the baby out.

crowning During labour, when the baby's head can be seen at the opening of the vagina, it is said to "crown".

cyanosis A bluish coloration of the skin caused by lack of oxygen in the blood.

cytomegalovirus infection Cytomegalovirus (CMV) is a viral infection transmitted by saliva, breast milk or urine. Relatively rare and relatively mild, the infection does occasionally cause deafness, visual impairment and neurological problems in a developing fetus.

diabetes Diabetes is a disorder in which the body does not produce enough insulin (the hormone which converts sugars into energy), resulting in too much sugar in the bloodstream. It can usually be controlled with appropriate treatment, diet, and exercise.

dilation Dilation, or dilatation, is the gradual opening (dilating) of the cervix during labour. At around 10cm the cervix is fully dilated.

Doppler ultrasound Pocket-sized handheld device which can be used to listen to the baby's heartbeat during pregnancy.

doula A doula is a person who is specially trained to help during labour and after the birth of a baby. A doula might also help a new mother to breastfeed, or cook, clean, and care for older children.

dystocia This term means "difficult childbirth", usually when labour is not progressing. Uterine dystocia is when the contractions are not strong enough to deliver the baby. Shoulder dystocia is when a baby's shoulders get stuck after the head has already been delivered.

eclampsia Eclampsia is a rare but serious condition which can affect women in late pregnancy. If pre-eclampsia (see opposite) is not treated, it can develop into eclampsia, which can cause convulsions and coma. It may require emergency birth of the baby.

ectopic pregnancy An ectopic pregnancy occurs when a fertilised egg implants outside the uterus, usually in a fallopian tube, but it can be anywhere in the abdominal cavity. There is not enough room for a baby to grow, so it must be surgically removed to prevent rupture and damage.

EDD The due date or estimated date of delivery (EDD) is the date when a baby's birth is expected. It is set by a doctor or midwife and is usually based on the first day of a woman's last menstrual period. An ultrasound dating scan may be used to give a more accurate estimate of the due date based on measurements of the baby's size.

effacement This is the thinning and shortening (sometimes called "ripening") of the cervix during early labour. During effacement, the cervix goes from more than an inch thick to paper thin.

electronic fetal monitor An electronic fetal monitor (EFM) is a device that's used to monitor the progress and vital signs of a baby during labour. It records both the baby's heartbeat and the mother's contractions.

embryo The term used to describe a developing baby during the first eight weeks of pregnancy; after that, it is called a fetus.

engagement Engagement, also called lightening or dropping, is when the baby descends into the pelvic cavity. In first-time mothers, this usually happens two to four weeks before birth; babies of other women usually don't engage until labour begins.

episiotomy A surgical cut in the perineum (the area between the vagina and the anus), made to enlarge the vaginal opening to help deliver the baby more quickly, or to avoid a tear.

external cephalic version (ECV) This is a procedure in which a doctor, using ultrasound images as a guide, attempts to massage a breech baby into the more favourable "head-down" position ready for birth.

fallopian tube There are two fallopian tubes, one each side of the uterus, that lead from the area of the ovaries into the uterine cavity. When an ovary releases an egg, the nearest fallopian tube draws it in and transports it down to the uterus.

fetal monitoring Tracking the heartbeat of a fetus and a woman's uterine contractions during labour.

fetus The name given to a growing baby after eight weeks of development; before eight weeks, the developing baby is called an embryo.

folic acid A B-complex vitamin that is essential for creating new blood cells, folic acid has been shown to reduce the incidence of neural tube defects such as spina bifida (incomplete closure of the spine) and anencephaly (partially or completely missing brain). It is recommended that all women trying to conceive should take a supplement of folic acid.

fontanelle Fontanelles are soft spots on a baby's head which, during birth, enable the soft bony plates of the skull to flex, allowing the head to pass through the birth canal. Fontanelles are usually completely hardened by a child's second birthday.

forceps birth A birth in which hinged, tong-like instruments (called forceps) are used to ease the baby's head through the birth canal.

fundal height The distance between the top of a pregnant woman's uterus (called the fundus) to her pubic bone. It is measured to determine fetal age.

gestation The period of time a baby is carried in the uterus; full-term gestation is between 38 and 42 weeks (counted from the first day of the last menstrual period).

gestational diabetes mellitus Gestational diabetes is a type of diabetes (when blood sugar levels become too high) which develops during pregnancy. It can be treated, and usually disappears after pregnancy.

gravida The medical term for a pregnant woman.

haemorrhoids Haemorrhoids, or piles, are swollen blood vessels in the anus. They are caused by increased blood volume and pressure from the uterus on the veins in the legs and pelvis, and are common during pregnancy. Constipation can also cause (or compound) the problem.

health visitor A health visitor is a registered nurse or midwife who has extra training and looks after mothers and young children at home and at a clinic.

hormone A chemical messenger from one cell (or group of cells) to another. Hormones are produced to stimulate or slow down various body functions. The levels of some hormones increase ten-fold during pregnancy.

human chorionic gonadotrophin This hormone is produced by the placenta and triggers the release of oestrogen and progesterone. As it is excreted in urine, hCG is used in testing to detect pregnancy.

intrauterine growth restriction (IUGR) The slow growth of a fetus in the uterus, possibly resulting in a low-birthweight baby.

jaundice Jaundice can bring a yellow tinge to a newborn's skin; it is caused by too much bilirubin in the blood. Newborn jaundice usually begins on the second or third day of life. It may clear up on its own after a few days, or may be treated with special light treatment.

lanugo Down-like, fine hair on a developing baby. Lanugo can appear as early as 15 weeks, and typically begins to disappear sometime before birth.

lightening This occurs when the baby descends lower in the pelvic cavity in the last few weeks of pregnancy.

linea nigra A dark line which may develop during pregnancy, running from below the breasts, over the abdomen and the navel. It often fades after birth but doesn't always disappear entirely.

lochia This is the term used to refer to the vaginal discharge of mucus, blood, and tissue, which may continue for up to six weeks after birth.

meconium The dark, sticky substance released from a newborn's intestines into his first bowel movements. If visible in amniotic fluid prior to birth, it can be a sign that the baby is in distress.

membranes The sac or "bag of waters" filled with amniotic fluid in which the developing baby grows.

midwife A person who cares for women during pregnancy, labour and birth and for a few days after birth.

miscarriage The loss of a baby before 24 weeks. After 24 weeks, the loss is called a stillbirth.

mucus plug The plug which blocks the cervix during pregnancy. It is often released with the onset of labour.

neonatal To do with the first four weeks after birth.

neonatal intensive care unit (NICU) An intensive care unit that specialises in the care of premature, low-weight babies and seriously ill babies.

obstetrician A doctor or surgeon who specialises in pregnancy, childbirth and the immediate postnatal period.

oedema Oedema means swelling. It is caused by fluid retention in the body's tissues, and is very common during pregnancy.

oestrogen A hormone produced by the ovaries which plays many roles throughout the body, but is particularly influential, along with the hormone progesterone, in regulating the reproductive cycle.

ovaries A pair of gonads (sex glands) which produce key female hormones and eggs, and are found on either side of the uterus.

ovulation The moment at which a mature egg is released from the ovaries into the fallopian tubes – the time around when a woman is most likely to conceive.

oxytocin A hormone secreted by the pituitary gland which controls the contractions of the uterus and stimulates the flow of breast milk. Synthetic oxytocin may be used to induce labour.

paediatrician A doctor who specialises in treating babies and children.

palpitation An abnormal heartbeat, often strong and rapid, and often caused by stress.

pelvic floor The group of muscles at the base of the pelvis which help to support the bladder, uterus, urethra, vagina, and rectum.

perinatal Perinatal refers to the period just before, during, and immediately after birth.

perineum The perineum is the area between the vagina and anus. The perineal area often tears slightly during childbirth.

placenta An organ that develops in the uterus during pregnancy, providing nutrients for the fetus and eliminating its waste products. It is also referred to as the afterbirth because it's delivered after the baby.

placenta praevia A pregnancy-related condition where the placenta is placed abnormally low in the uterus, possibly covering the cervix, sometimes resulting in a caesarean section.

postmature A postmature baby is a baby born at 42 weeks or more.

pre-eclampsia A condition a mother may develop in the second half of pregnancy, marked by sudden oedema, high blood pressure and protein in the urine. It can lead to complications such as eclampsia (see opposite), so antenatal care staff monitor women carefully for the warning signs.

pregnancy-induced hypertension A condition where a woman's blood pressure is temporarily elevated during pregnancy. It usually occurs during the last trimester.

premature baby A premature baby is one who is born before 37 weeks of gestation.

premature labour Labour that begins before 37 weeks.

progesterone A female hormone produced in the ovaries. It works with oestrogen to regulate the reproductive cycle.

pudendal block Pain relief induced by anaesthetising the area around the vulva.

Rhesus incompatibility A condition in which a baby inherits a blood type from his father which is different from and incompatible with his mother's. It is usually not a problem in a first pregnancy but may cause problems with subsequent ones. Blood tests will usually determine if there is a problem before delivery.

sciatica Pain in the leg, lower back, and buttocks can be caused by pressure of the uterus on the sciatic nerve. Applied heat and rest may relieve the condition.

show A "show" or "bloody show" describes the discharge of mucus tinged with blood that results from the mucus plug dislodging from the cervix as labour approaches.

special care baby unit (SCBU) A unit in a hospital which provides specialised care to premature babies and babies with serious illnesses.

stillbirth If a baby dies in the uterus before birth at or from 24 weeks, it is called a stillbirth. The loss of a pregnancy before 24 weeks is called a miscarriage.

toxoplasmosis This is a parasitic infection carried by cats' faeces and uncooked meat. It may cause stillbirth or miscarriage if a woman contracts it for the first time during pregnancy. To reduce the risk, pregnant women should avoid touching a cat's litter tray and always wash their hands thoroughly after handling meat.

trimester A trimester is a period of three months. Pregnancy consists of three trimesters.

ultrasound In ultrasound procedures, high-frequency sound waves are used to create a moving image, or sonogram, on a television screen. Often carried out at various stages of pregnancy, ultrasound scans can help to identify multiple fetuses and detect anomalies.

umbilical cord The umbilical cord is the spongy, cord-like structure which connects a fetus to the placenta. It carries nourishment and removes waste via two arteries and a vein. The cord is cut after birth, and when the cord stump falls off, the baby's belly button is revealed.

uterus The uterus is the pear-shaped muscular organ, also called the womb, in a woman's abdomen where an embryo will implant and develop throughout pregnancy.

vagina The canal that leads from the outside world to the cervix (also called the birth canal).

vaginal birth after caesarean (VBAC) This term is used when a woman who has previously had a baby by caesarean section has a vaginal birth for a subsequent baby.

ventouse A suction cup attached to a machine placed on the baby's head to help the baby through the vagina.

vernix caseosa The vernix is a greasy, white substance that covers a baby in the uterus. It protects the baby's skin.

viable The term "viable" describes a baby who is considered capable of living.

zygote This is a medical term for a newly fertilised egg before it implants into the uterus.

Useful contacts and organisations

Fertility

Donor Conception Network
www.dcnetwork.org
020 8245 4369

National Endometriosis Society
www.endometriosis-uk.org
0808 808 2227

Family Planning Service
www.fertilityuk.org

Advice on Preconceptual Health
www.foresight-preconception.org.uk
01243 868 001

Family Planning Association
www.fpa.org.uk
020 7608 5240

Human Fertilisation and Embryology Authority
www.hfea.gov.uk
020 7291 8200

Infertility Network UK
www.infertilitynetworkuk.com
0800 008 7464

Childlessness Overcome Through Surrogacy
www.surrogacy.org.uk
0844 414 0181

Pregnancy

Action on Pre-eclampsia
www.apec.org.uk
020 8427 4217

Antenatal Results and Choices
www.arc-uk.org
020 7631 0285

Eating for Pregnancy
www.eatingforpregnancy.co.uk

Ectopic Pregnancy Trust
www.ectopic.org.uk
020 7733 2653

NHS Pregnancy Smoking helpline
www.quit.org.uk
0800 002 200

Royal College of Obstetricians and Gynaecologists
www.rcog.org.uk
020 7772 6200

Tommy's, the baby charity
Research on miscarriage, premature birth and stillbirth
www.tommys.org
020 7398 3483

Labour and birth

Active Birth Centre
www.activebirthcentre.com
020 7281 6760

Association for Improvements in the Maternity Services
www.aims.org.uk
0300 365 0663

BirthChoiceUK
Information on choosing where to have your baby and whom you choose to look after you in labour
www.birthchoiceuk.com

Doula UK
www.doula.org.uk

Home Birth
www.homebirth.org.uk

Independent Midwives UK
www.independentmidwives.org.uk
0845 4600 105

Association of Radical Midwives
www.midwifery.org.uk

National Childbirth Trust
www.nct.org.uk
0300 330 0772

Royal College of Midwives
www.rcm.org.uk

Breastfeeding

Association of Breastfeeding Mothers
www.abm.me.uk
08444 122 949

Breastfeeding Network
www.breastfeedingnetwork.org.uk
0300 100 0210

National Breastfeeding helpline
www.breastfeeding.nhs.uk
0300 100 0212

La Leche League
www.laleche.org.uk
0845 120 2918

Ask a Midwife
www.midwivesonline.com
01274 427 132

National Childbirth Trust
www.nct.org.uk
0300 330 0771

Rights and benefits

Advisory, Conciliation and Arbitration Service
www.acas.org.uk
08457 474 747

Citizens Advice
www.citizensadvice.org.uk

Directgov Tax Credits help
www.direct.gov.uk
0845 300 3900

Department for Work and Pensions
www.dwp.gov.uk

Equal Opportunities Commission
www.eoc.org.uk
0845 604 6610

Family Rights Group
www.frg.org.uk
0808 801 0366

Child Benefit help
www.hmrc.gov.uk
0845 302 1444

Inland Revenue Tax Credit help
www.taxcredits.inlandrevenue.gov.uk
0845 300 3900

Maternity Action
www.maternityaction.org.uk

Working Families
www.workingfamilies.org.uk
0800 013 0313

Support groups

Action on Pre-eclampsia
www.apec.org.uk
020 8427 4217

Association for Postnatal Illness
www.apni.org
020 7386 0868

Bliss
Support for families of premature and special-care babies
www.bliss.org.uk
0500 618 140

Cleft Lip and Palate Association
www.clapa.com
020 7833 4883

Down's Syndrome Association
www.downs-syndrome.org.uk
0845 230 0372

The National Endometriosis Society
www.endo.org.uk
0808 808 2227

Hyperemesis Foundation
www.hyperemesis.org

Miscarriage Association
www.miscarriageassociation.org.uk
01924 200 799

Obstetric Cholestasis Support
www.ocsupport.org.uk

Postnatal Illness
www.pni.org.uk

Scope
Information and advice on cerebral palsy
www.scope.org.uk
0808 800 3333

Steps
Information and advice on talipes (club foot)
www.steps-charity.org.uk
01925 750 271

Stillbirth and Neonatal Death Society
www.uk-sands.org
020 7436 5881

General

British Association for Counselling and Psychotherapy
www.bacp.co.uk

Citizens Advice
www.citizensadvice.org.uk

Disabled Parents Network
www.disabledparentsnetwork.org.uk
0300 3300 639

Fatherhood Institute
www.fatherhoodinstitute.org
0845 634 1328

Family Planning Association
www.fpa.org.uk
0845 122 8690

Family Action
Charity for disadvantaged families
www.fwa.org.uk
020 7254 6251

Gingerbread
Advice and information for one-parent families
www.gingerbread.org.uk
0800 018 5026

Home Start
Support for families in local communities
www.home-start.org.uk
0800 0686 368

National Childbirth Trust
www.nct.org.uk
0300 330 0772

National Society for the Prevention of Cruelty to Children
www.nspcc.org.uk
0808 800 5000

Parentline Plus
www.parentlineplus.org.uk
0808 800 2222

Twins and Multiple Birth Association
www.tamba.org.uk
0800 138 0509

Tommy's, the baby charity
(See entry under Pregnancy)

Twinsclub
www.twinsclub.co.uk

Index

Page numbers in *italic* refer to the illustrations

Acknowledgments

BabyCentre Acknowledgments:

BabyCentre would like to thank contributing editor Martine Gallie for her work in adapting content from our web pages to make it work on the printed page. Also Victoria Farrimond for her tireless work in managing this project.

Thank you to the BabyCentre team – Daphne Metland, Sasha Miller, Emma Woolfenden, Chess Thomas, Catherine Mendham, Rhianydd Thomas, Bernie Sheehan, Sam Wright, Jenny Leach, and Lynda Hale – for their expertise and contributions. All of our health articles are checked and approved by the team of health professionals on our medical advisory board, but we'd like especially to thank consultant paediatrician and neonatologist Dr Dwight Lindo and GP Dr Philippa Kaye for their advice and assistance during this project.

And, finally, we'd like to thank Penny Warren, Glenda Fisher, Hilary Mandleberg, Emma Maule, Hannah Moore, Kevin Smith, Isabel de Cordova and Saskia Janssen for their hard work in driving this project and for understanding and championing the BabyCentre ethos.

Publisher's Acknowledgments:

DK would like to thank Salima Hirani for proofreading; Hilary Bird for the index; Karen Sullivan for editorial consultancy; Carly Churchill and Sue Prescott for photographic assistance; Joanna Dingley for editorial assistance; Vicky Barnes, Roisin Donaghy, Nadine Wilkie and Alli Williams for hair and make-up; Kate Simunek for designing the icons; Caron Bosler for Pilates advice; and all of our models: Adrian Bewsey; Heidi Carr; Rachel Chan and Niamh Chung; Carmen Ingrid Dillon; Katie, James and Isabella Dockray; Francesca Elliott; Ava Freeman; Kavita Harrison; Carla and Alexa Haslock; Saskia Janssen; Sharmina Karim and Joshua Allen; Sian Lattimer Keller; Dorinda Kemp; Barbara Madley; Lesley Manalo; Zia Mattocks; Emma Maule; Susan Prescott; Nicola Richardson; Nicola Riley; Laura Roberts-Jensen and Quinn Jensen; Andrea Samayoa; Alberta Starr; Phillipa Strub and Molly Statham; Zai Swan.

Picture credits

The publisher would like to thank the following for their kind permission to reproduce their photographs:
(Key: a-above; b-below/bottom; c-centre; f-far; l-left; r-right; t-top)

Alamy Images: Asia Images Group Pte Ltd 18; David J. Green – Lifestyle 219tl; Medical-on-Line 215tl; Paul Mogford 121tr; Picture Partners 275tl; Andres Rodriguez 17; Gary Roebuck 105; Chris Rout 264br; Trevor Smith 221bl; Alena Sudová 297cra; Liba Taylor 270; Andrew Twort 53; **Corbis:** Lisa B. 46–47; Rick Chapman 294; ER Productions 41; Michael A. Keller 123t; Daniel Kroells/Westend61 130; Johannes Mann 14; Marie-Reine Mattera 306bl; RK Studio/Blend Images 21; Andersen Ross/Brand X 253t; Norbert Schaefer 83; Alessandra Schellnegger 216; TH-Foto 183fbr; Bernd Vogel 42; Studio Wartenberg 92; Olix Wirtinger 96; **Getty Images:** altrendo images 15; Anthony-Masterson 306br; J.A. Bracchi 199; Roderick Chen 115; Sarah Cuttle 148; Peter Dazeley 188br; Marc Debnam 95tl; Digital Vision 155t; George Doyle 19, 87bc; Tracy Frankel 57; Eric Glenn 76; Robert Glenn 152; Jamie Grill 89; Dennis Hallinan 52; Noel Hendrickson 80tl; Frank Herholdt 99; Image Source 120bl; Jonathan Kantor 95tr, 125cr; Gavin Kingcome Photography 87br; David A Land 308; Bill Ling 38; Barbara Lutterbeck 183bl; LWA 12–13, 122br; Ericka McConnell 82; Paul Bradbury 117br; Hans Neleman 259t; Bernd Opitz 259bl; Lori Adamski Peek 129; Plush Studios/Bill Reitzel 112; Rayes 119; Andersen Ross 77, 169bl; Richard Ross 183bc (tomatoes); Sam Royds 175; rubberball 143; Stockbyte 25; Jerome Tisne 86; Betsie Van der Meer 20; VCL/Alistair Berg 156; Veer/Mark Adams 65; Visuals Unlimited 251t; Michael Wildsmith 103; Mel Yates 297tl; Yellow Dog Productions 302; David Young-Wolff 231; **iStockphoto.com:** Adrian Albritton 208; Ruth Black 155br; Matjaz Boncina 209; ranplett 144; Vivid Pixels 240–241; **Prof. J.E. Jirasek MD, DSc.:** 125br; **Mother & Baby Picture Library:** Dave J. Anthony 180, 184; Moose Azim 177; Ian Hooton 80tr, 84, 87bl, 90, 127b, 127t, 128, 171cl, 187cl, 223, 232, 243, 247, 274bl, 277; Ruth Jenkinson 181, 210, 245, 251b; Eddie Lawrence 273, 289; Paul Mitchell 101t; James Thomson 85; **Photolibrary:** FoodCollection 55cra; Vladimir Pcholkin 48; zoomphotographics 162; **Science Photo Library:** 137tr, 141br; AJ Photo 224, 304; Samuel Ashfield 280; Biophoto Associate 32; Neil Borden 157cb, 157clb; Neil Bromhall 33; BSIP, Astier 285t; BSIP, Laurent 263bl; CNRI 271; John Cole 171br; Christian Darkin 35cr; Adam Gault 222; Ian Hooton 22, 211, 212, 221t; La La 214; Eddie Lawrence 253b; Dr Najeeb Layyous 179; Living Art Enterprises, LLC 157bc, 157bl; Dr P. Marazzi 215tc; Dr Yorgos Nikas 35bc, 35bl, 35br; Lea Paterson 23; D. Phillips 27tc, 27tl; Antonia Reeve 279; P. Saada / Eurelios 137tl; Saturn Stills 101br; Mark Thomas 285bl; Anatomical Travelogue 117tr; **SuperStock:** age fotostock 183br

All other images © Dorling Kindersley
For further information see: www.dkimages.com

Answers to Dad's Diary Quiz, p. 145

Q1 – a; Q2 – c; Q3 – b; Q4 – d; Q5 – a; Q6 – c